Emergency Pathophysiology:
Clinical Applications for Prehospital Care

Emergency Pathophysiology:
Clinical Applications for Prehospital Care

Samuel M Galvagno, Jr., D.O.
Flight Surgeon
Luke Air Force Base, Arizona

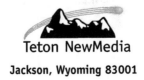
Teton NewMedia

Jackson, Wyoming 83001

Executive Editor: Carroll Cann
Development Editor: Susan L. Hunsberger
Editor: Carroll Cann
Art Director & Production Manager: Anita Sykes
Illustrations: Anne Rains
Design and Layout: 5640 Design, www.fiftysixforty.com
Printer: McNaughton and Gunn, Inc., Saline, MI

Teton NewMedia
P.O.Box 4833
4125 South Hwy 89
Jackson, WY 83001
1-888-770-3165

The views expressed in this text are those of the author, and do not reflect the official policy or position of the United States Air Force, Department of Defense, or the U.S. Government. This work was independently funded by the author and the publisher.

Neither the publisher nor the author are responsible for any injury resulting from any material contained herein. This publication contains information relating to general principles of medical care, which should not be construed as specific instructions for individual patients. Medicine is a dynamic art and science; hence, current protocols should always be followed as required by local jurisdictions. Manufacturers' product information and package inserts should be reviewed for current information, including contraindications, dosages, and precautions.

ISBN # 1-59161007-9

Print number 5 4 3 2 1

    Library of Congress Cataloging-in-Publication Data
Galvagno, Samuel M.
    Emergency pathophysiology: clinical applications for prehospital care / Samuel M. Galvagno Jr.
        p. ; cm.
Includes bibliographical references and index.
ISBN 1-59161-007-9
    1. Physiology, Pathological. 2. Medical emergencies. 3. Emergency medical technicians.
I. Title.
    [DNLM: 1.Emergency Medical Services. 2. Emergencies. 3. Emergency Treatment. WX 215 G183e 2003]
RB113.G35 2003
616.02'5--dc21
                                                                    2002042997

Dedication

For Carmen S. Galvagno.

About the Author

Sam Galvagno, D.O. is presently a United States Air Force flight surgeon for the 63rd F-16 fighter squadron at Luke Air Force Base, Arizona. He graduated from Mount Saint Mary's College in Emmitsburg, MD with a B.S. in biopsychology in 1996. During this time, he attained certification as a Nationally Registered Emergency Medical Technician-Paramedic, and worked for various advanced life support agencies in Maryland, Pennsylvania, and New York. He earned his medical degree in 2000 from the New York College of Osteopathic Medicine in Old Westbury, NY. At the time this text was completed, he was serving as an emergency medicine physician and general medical officer at Osan Air Force Base, Korea.

Acknowledgements

I WOULD LIKE TO THANK THE FOLLOWING:

- Paramedics Danny Hughes, Eric Smothers, Andy Marsh, Dave Chisholm, Ron Crouse, Jim Hepler and Rick Himes—for providing memorable examples of dedication and professionalism, and for teaching me to "think physiologically."

- Robert Sklar and Eric Korneffel—for sharing their years of experience with me, and for carefully reviewing sections of the early manuscript.

- Cindy Roantree, Susan Hunsberger, Carroll Cann, and the staff at Teton NewMedia—for their encouragement and guidance throughout the preparation of the manuscript.

- Anne Rains at Teton NewMedia—for her help with the illustrations in this text.

- Greg Ridenour and the rest of the crew from Staunton—for putting up with my pager(s) during college and paramedic school.

- Mom, Dad, Nanette, Danny, Marc, Kelley, Theresa, and the rest of my family—for their perpetual support over the years.

- Dr. Paul Marino—for being the best teacher and mentor any physician could ever ask for. Without his assistance, this text would not have been made possible.

Preface

For many paramedics and providers involved with prehospital care and emergency medicine, the most engaging, yet challenging, subject areas entail the study of basic sciences. Unfortunately, due to the volume of information conferred over a year's time, adequate attention to these topics is seldom provided. In a quest to further my own understanding of prehospital medications and pathophysiology, I was surprised to find few resources to assist me with this endeavor. With new curricula and college-based EMS training programs, this appears to be changing.

In 1998, the United States Department of Transportation and the National Highway Traffic Safety Administration extensively revised the U.S. DOT curriculum for paramedic education.[1] In addition to a required prerequisite course in anatomy and physiology, the educational model includes preparatory didactic segments on pharmacology and pathophysiology. In the final version of the U.S. DOT Paramedic National Standard Curriculum, the unit terminal objective for the General Principles of Pathophysiology section states:

> At the completion of this unit, the paramedic will be able to apply the general concepts of pathophysiology for the assessment and management of emergency patients.[1]

With the advent of the 1998 U.S. DOT EMT-Paramedic National Standard Curriculum, paramedics are now responsible for a much more detailed understanding of medical emergencies than previously required.[2]

Most paramedic programs in the United States and Canada now require completion of a two-year training program that awards an associate degree in applied science.[3] Once certified, paramedics are required to recertify annually or biannually. Continuing medical education is required on a yearly basis.[3]

The increased scope of practice and new training requirements have drastically changed the approach to paramedic education. For example, prior to 1998, the standard text by Bledsoe *et al.* was limited to one volume with 1,058 pages of text.[4] Under the new curriculum, the text has been expanded to five volumes.[2]

According to the U.S. Department of Labor, there are already 150,000 jobs held by EMTs and paramedics in the United States.[3] In addition, many more paramedics are unaccounted for, working as volunteers in rural areas and small towns. A recent report by the Bureau of Labor Statistics indicated that employment of EMTs and paramedics is expected to increase by 21% to 31% up through 2008.[3]

In most major paramedic teaching programs in the United States and Canada, students are required to purchase standard undergraduate anatomy and physiology texts.[5,6] Most programs also utilize advanced physiology and pharmacology review books generally developed for exclusive use by medical students. Gould's 1997 publication is the only pathophysiology text written for allied health providers.[7] This book presents a global approach to general pathophysiologic concepts without a specific focus on emergency medicine.

Until now, **no** text has provided both students and experienced providers with an introduction to the basic sciences of emergency prehospital care. Indeed, being able to answer **why** a particular drug is being given, or **how** the natural history of a patient unfolds, greatly facilitates an efficient transfer of prehospital provider care to physician care. It also makes a paramedic a better paramedic.

The information in this book is not solely presented for paramedics. The field of prehospital care is a gateway profession for further training in nursing, medicine, or other allied health professions. Nurses, medical students, physician assistants, and junior residents with an interest in emergency medicine will find the text useful. Since many prehospital providers are also educators (*e.g.*, PALS, ACLS, BTLS), a fundamental understanding of the mechanisms behind disease processes is crucial.

This book is intended for providers of emergency medical care at all levels of training. Its aim is to provide a concise understanding of the known principles behind the science and practice of prehospital care for those not satisfied with the minimal instruction provided in modern paramedic and related emergency medicine courses.

S.M. Galvagno, D.O.

References

1. United States Department of Transportation/ National Highway Traffic Safety Administration. *1998 EMT-Paramedic National Standard Curriculum.* Washington, DC: U.S. DOT, 1998.

2. Bledsoe BE, Porter RS, Cherry RA. *Paramedic Care: Principles and Practice* (Vol 1-5). Englewood Cliffs, NJ: Prentice Hall, 2001.

3. U.S. Department of Labor: Bureau of Labor Statistics. *Occupational Outlook Handbook: 2000-2001 ed.* Washington, DC: U.S. Department of Labor, 2000.

4. Bledsoe BE, Porter RS, Shade BR. *Paramedic Emergency Care.* 2nd ed. Englewood Cliffs, NJ: Brady/Prentice Hall Division, 1994.

5. Boulder County Paramedics. Suggested References. Available online at http://www.bouldercountyparamedic.com/page22.html. Accessed on 7 April, 2001.

6. Loyalist College/ Bancroft Campus. Required Textbook List. Available online at http://www.loyalistcbancroft.on.ca/paramedic_program.htm. Accessed on 7 April, 2001.

7. Gould BE. *Pathophysiology for the Health Related Professions.* Philadelphia: W.B. Saunders, 1997.

Contents

Section I
General Principles

1: CELL PHYSIOLOGY 3

2: BODY FLUIDS AND FLUID THERAPY 11

3: OXYGEN TRANSPORT 21

4: THE AUTONOMIC NERVOUS SYSTEM 29

5: PHARMACOKINETICS 37

Section II
Respiratory Pathophysiology

6: PULMONARY PHYSIOLOGY
AND PHARMACOLOGY 45

7: ASTHMA 59

8: CHRONIC OBSTRUCTIVE PULMONARY DISEASE ...71

9: PULMONARY EMBOLISM 79

Section III
Cardiovascular Pathophysiology

10: BASIC CARDIAC PHYSIOLOGY 89

11: CARDIAC DYSRHYTHMIAS 101

12: ACUTE CORONARY SYNDROMES I: PATHOPHYSIOLOGY OF CORONARY ARTERY DISEASE 113

13: ACUTE CORONARY SYNDROMES II: ANGINA 119

14: ACUTE CORONARY SYNDROMES III: ACUTE MYOCARDIAL INFARCTION 129

15: HEART FAILURE 149

16: HYPERTENSIVE EMERGENCIES AND URGENCIES 169

Section IV
Shock

17: HYPOVOLEMIC SHOCK 185

18: ANAPHYLACTIC SHOCK 197

19: SEPTIC SHOCK 205

Section V
Endocrine Disorders

20: DIABETIC EMERGENCIES 219

21: ADRENAL AND THYROID EMERGENCIES 233

Section VI
Gastrointestinal Emergencies

22: THE ACUTE ABDOMEN 249

23: GASTROINTESTINAL BLEEDING 261

Section VII
Infectious Diseases

24: PNEUMONIA 271

25: INFECTIOUS DISEASE EMERGENCIES 283

Section VIII
Neurological Disorders

26: ACUTE CEREBRAL INFARCTION 303

27: STATUS EPILEPTICUS 319

28: NEUROLOGICAL TRAUMA 329

Section IX
Environmental Emergencies

29: HYPOTHERMIA 351

30: HEAT STROKE AND HEAT EXHAUSTION 361

Appendices

I: PHARMACOLOGY OF RAPID
SEQUENCE INTUBATION 373

II: ESSENTIALS OF 12-LEAD
ELECTROCARDIOGRAPH INTERPRETATION 383

III: ESSENTIALS OF ACID-BASE INTERPRETATION . . .391

Index

Index 397

Section I

General Principles

Cell Physiology

To begin comprehending how medications work and how electrolytes and fluids are distributed, an elementary understanding of cell physiology is essential. In addition to a brief description of cell physiology, this chapter summarizes the processes of diffusion, osmosis, and active transport.

Nearly every basic physiology course begins with a detailed diagram of a cell; however, a detailed description of all the parts of a cell (cellular organelles) is beyond the scope of this book. An understanding of the mechanisms in pharmacology and the physiologic principles behind fluid resuscitation requires a basic appreciation of how cell membranes work.

Cell Membranes

PHOSPHOLIPIDS

Cell membranes are composed mainly of proteins and phospholipids, compounds that hold the cell together while also providing sites for molecules, such as drugs, to bind to for entrance into the cell.[1] Phospholipids have a glycerol backbone that is hydrophilic (water-loving) and fatty acid tails that are hydrophobic (water-hating; Figure 1-1). The hydrophobic sections of a cell membrane are composed of layers of phospholipids and form what is known as a lipid (fat) bilayer. Water cannot pass through this water-hating layer, but fatty molecules can. Following the simple biochemical rule for solubility (ability of a substance to dissolve in another substance) that states "like dissolves like," the hydrophobic portions of the lipid bilayer are able to dissolve compounds composed of fat. This concept has important implications for the absorption of medications because **lipid soluble drugs are readily absorbed into cells.** [2]

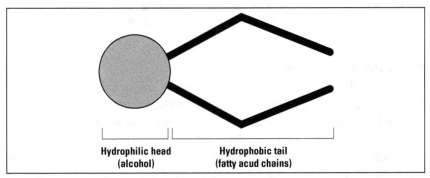

Hydrophilic head
(alcohol)

Hydrophobic tail
(fatty acud chains)

Figure 1-1 The phospholipid molecule.

PROTEINS

Proteins are another class of compounds that comprise the cell membrane. Proteins are embedded in the phospholipid bilayer and play an important role by forming ion channels, or holes in the membrane, through which sodium, potassium, and other minerals and chemicals can pass (Figure 1-2).

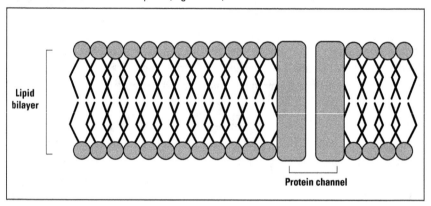

Figure 1-2 Cell membrane structure.

Diffusion

Molecules, such as metabolized drugs, toxins, or electrolytes, move through the body's liquids in random motion, much like a batch of bouncing ping-pong balls. Depending on the concentration, or the number of molecules (bouncing balls) in one area, random thermal motion eventually distributes molecules in such a way as to lead to an eventual **equal** distribution (equilibrium). This process, occurring in and around cells, is known as **diffusion**. Simply stated, molecules behave by moving from areas of **high** to **low** concentrations.

To understand diffusion, think about what would happen if a barrier (semipermeable membrane) were placed in the middle of a tank of water. Different concentrations of glucose are poured into the water on different sides, and on one side, the glucose concentration is 20 mmol/L, while on the other side, the glucose concentration is 10 mmol/L. Assuming that the barrier allows only glucose, not water, to pass through, and applying the principle that molecules move from areas of **higher** concentration to **lower** concentration, eventually both sides of the tank will have equal concentrations of glucose (15 mmol/L).

PASSIVE DIFFUSION

The process of diffusion is especially important for understanding how drugs are transported across biological membranes. Of all the known processes by which drugs cross biological membranes, **passive diffusion is the most common.**[2] Drugs pass through membranes by either dissolving into the membrane or passing through aqueous pores. This process is dependent on the concentration gradient across the membrane. In other words, drugs move across membranes from areas of **higher** to **lower** concentrations.

Osmosis

Osmosis is a process often confused with diffusion. The process of osmosis is essentially the same as the concept of high to low with one important exception: osmosis refers to the diffusion of **water** from an area of higher water concentration to lower water concentration.[3,4] The water concentration is determined by the number of particles in the solution. To understand osmosis, one must be familiar with the concept of **osmolarity.** Osmolarity is the concentration of active particles in a solution. The osmolarity of a body of liquid is determined by the following equation:

Osmolarity = (Number of particles in solution) x (Concentration of solution)

Two solutions with equal osmolarities are said to be **iso-osmotic**. If two solutions have different measured osmolarities, the solution with the higher osmolarity is described as being **hyperosmotic**, and the solution with the lower osmolarity is **hypo-osmotic.**

Consider the following example of osmosis. Picture a tank of water with a barrier (semipermeable membrane) in the middle (Figure 1-3).

As opposed to the previous example provided for diffusion, assume the barrier allows only water to pass through, and nothing else. If one side of the tank is filled with a hyperosmotic solution (remembering the definition of osmolarity) and the other side filled with a hypoosmotic solution, eventually, the water flows from the hyperosmotic side, through the barrier, to the hypo-osmotic side. The end result, over time, is an iso-osmotic solution on both sides of the tank.

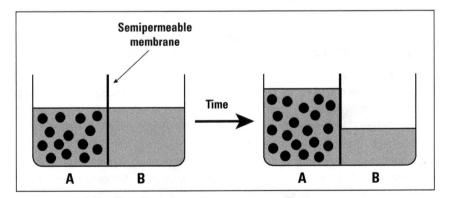

Figure 1-3 Osmosis of water across a semipermeable membrane. Water flows from B to A due to the presence of particles (solute) in A that cannot cross the semipermeable membrane.

Tonicity

Osmolarity is a central concept for understanding the composition of intravenous fluids and how they are distributed when introduced to the fluid compartments of the body. The concept of **tonicity** is similar to osmolarity. Tonicity is the ability of a group of particles or molecules (solute) to cause movement of water from one side of a membrane to the other. For instance, increasing the sodium concentration inside cells (hyperosmolar) causes water to move inside the cell to equalize the concentrations on either side of the cell membrane. Thus, a solution that is **hyperosmolar** is also considered to be **hypertonic;** solutions that are **hypo-osmotic** are **hypotonic,** and solutions that are **iso-osmotic** are **isotonic.** Solutions used in the prehospital care environment are classified as hypotonic, isotonic, or hypertonic. The tonicity of these solutions is compared to the tonicity of human plasma (Table 1-1).

Table 1-1
Tonicities of Selected Intravenous Fluid Preparations.

Intravenous Fluid	Tonicity
Lactated Ringer's	Isotonic
0.9% saline	Isotonic
3 % saline	Hypertonic
5% Dextrose in water (D5W)	Hypotonic

The concepts of osmolarity and tonicity can be understood by considering how red blood cells react when placed in solutions of different osmolarity (Figure 1-4).

If red blood cells are placed in a solution that has the same osmolarity (isotonic) as the cells, the cell volume does not change. That is, the cells do not swell, nor do they shrink. Alternatively, if red blood cells are placed in a solution that has a higher osmolarity than the cells, the cells shrink because the osmotic difference causes water to move from the cells into the solution to equalize the concentration; the cells are hypo-osmotic or **hypotonic** compared to the hyperosmotic (**hypertonic**) solution. Likewise, when cells are placed in a hypo-osmotic solution, the cells rupture since water enters the cells, causing them to swell. The cells swell because they are hyperosmotic or **hypertonic** compared to the solution.

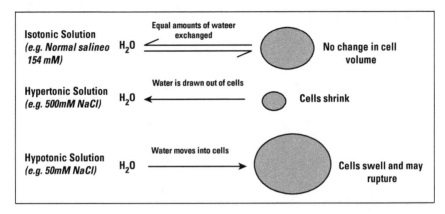

Figure 1-4 The effect of tonicity on red blood cells.

Active Transport

Unlike diffusion where molecules are transported from regions of high to low concentration, in active transport, the molecules move from regions of lower to higher concentration. This uphill movement requires energy, and is supplied in the form of adenosine triphosphate (ATP). ATP can be thought of as the energy currency of the body. Using ATP as an energy source, transport proteins on the surface of cell membranes can function as pumps for molecules too big to diffuse across cell membranes. These pumps move molecules from areas of lower concentrations outside the cell into areas of higher concentrations inside the cell. The sodium-potassium-ATPase pump is one example of active transport (Figure 1-5).[5]

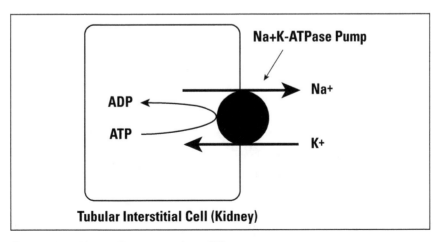

Figure 1-5 The sodium-potassium-ATPase pump.

References

1.   Alberts B, Bray D, Lewis J, Raff M, Roberts K, Watson J. *Molecular Biology of the Cell*. 2nd Ed. New York: Garland Publishing, 1989.

2.   Hardman JG, Limbird LE, eds. *Goodman & Gilman's The Pharmacological Basis of Therapeutics*. 9th ed. New York: McGraw-Hill, 1996.

3.   Vander AJ, Sherman JH, Luciano DS. *Human Physiology: The Mechanisms of Body Function*. 6th Ed. New York: McGraw-Hill, 1994.

4.   Constanzo, L. *Physiology*. Baltimore: Williams and Wilkins, 1995.

5.   Darnell J, Lodish H, Baltimore D. *Molecular Cell Biology*. 2nd Ed. New York: Scientific American Books, 1990.

Review Questions

1. You are on the scene of a farm accident. The patient is trapped in heavy machinery with a prolonged extrication. In addition to having several other serious injuries, the patient has sustained multiple lacerations on the forearms that appear to be grossly contaminated with manure, dirt, and other debris. After properly assessing and stabilizing the patient according to local protocols, medical control orders you to irrigate the lacerations while the rescue team works to extricate the patient. What fluid would theoretically be the most physiologically appropriate for irrigation?
   A. Sterile hypertonic (3%) saline
   B. Sterile isotonic solution (0.9% saline)
   C. Sterile hypotonic solution (5% dextrose in water)
   D. Sterile colloid solution (25% albumin)
   E. Plain tap water

An isotonic solution would be best. Not only is it sterile, but it also has the same tonicity as the tissues. A hypotonic solution could potentially exacerbate edema by causing cells to swell. Tap water, although readily available, would be a viable choice if no other solutions were available, but it is also hypotonic. Colloid preparations are used primarily to temporarily expand the intravascular space and are reserved solely for this purpose. Colloids are infrequently used in the prehospital care setting due to cost. The correct answer is B.

2. All the following statements concerning pharmacokinetics are true EXCEPT:
   A. Lipid insoluble drugs are readily absorbed across cell membranes.
   B. Passive diffusion is the most common process by which drugs cross cell membranes.
   C. Diffusion of drugs into cell membranes generally occurs in the direction of higher concentration to lower concentration.
   D. Uphill transport of drugs across cell membranes occurs through the process of active transport and requires energy.
   E. Active transport ATPase pumps move drugs from areas of lower concentration to higher concentration.

Lipid **soluble** drugs are readily absorbed into cells throughout the body. The correct answer is A.

2

Body Fluids and Fluid Therapy

Selecting the appropriate fluid for resuscitation is of paramount importance. A prerequisite to the understanding of fluid management is knowledge of the various body fluid compartments and the forces affecting the movement of fluids through these compartments.[1]

Total Body Water

Water comprises approximately **60%** of total body weight in males and **50%** in females.[1] Obese individuals tend to have 25% to 30% less body water than a lean individual of the same weight. Likewise, since fat contains little water, a lean individual tends to have a greater proportion of water comprising total body weight than an obese person. The highest proportion of total body water is found in newborns; 75% to 80% of the total body weight is water.[1]

Fluid Compartments

The water of the body is divided into intracellular, intravascular, and extravascular compartments (Figure 2-1).

Of these compartments, 40% of all water is intracellular whereas the remaining 20% (assuming the percentage of water as total body weight for an average male) is located outside cells.[1] The extracellular compartment has two subdivisions: interstitial and intravascular (plasma). The interstitial compartment, the compartment containing fluid outside of cells and blood vessels, is also known as the third space. Fifteen percent of total body water is located in the interstitium. The intravascular compartment is essentially plasma and comprises the remaining 5% of the extracellular fluid.

Water = 60% of total body weight

    40% = Intracellular (First space)

    20% = Extracellular

        5% = Intravascular (plasma) (Second space)
        15% = Interstitial (Third space)

Figure 2-1 Body fluid compartments.

Fluid Distribution

The distribution of body fluids has important clinical implications. For instance, a patient with signs of edema has abnormal redistribution of water from the intracellular and intravascular compartments to the interstitium. A patient with edema, therefore, is said to be **third-spacing**. Therapy would include administration of fluids or other medications to assist with the redistribution of water back into blood vessels and cells.

Forces Affecting Movement of Body Fluids

STARLING'S LAW OF THE CAPILLARY

Movement of body fluids through the various compartments depends on several factors. As mentioned in the previous chapter, molecules and water move across membranes according to different concentration gradients; in general, particles move from areas of high concentration to areas of low concentration to establish equilibrium. This high to low flow of water and its constituents through capillaries is governed by Starling's Law (Figure 2-2).[2]

Starling's Law of the Capillary

$$\text{Flow} = K_f\,[(P_c - P_i) - \sigma(\pi_c - \pi_i)]$$

$(P_c - P_i)$ **Difference in Hydrostatic Pressure**
(driving force for filtration)

$(\pi_c - \pi_i)$ **Difference in Osmotic Pressure**
(driving force for reabsorption)

K_f **Filtration Coefficient** *(Permeability of Membrane)*

σ **Protein Permeability Coefficient**

Figure 2-2 Starling's Law of the capillary.

For a typical capillary anywhere in the body, the flow of fluid is dependent on the pressure differences between the capillary (blood vessel) and the interstitium (tissues). The variables included in Starling's Law are the colloid and interstitial hydrostatic and osmotic pressures as well as a coefficient to estimate the ability of particles to pass through membranes (permeability). Figures 2-3 and 2-4 demonstrate how Starling's equation works in the body's blood vessels (capillaries) .

In Figure 2-3, when the difference between the interstitial and colloid hydrostatic pressure is greater than the difference between the osmotic pressures, fluid flows out of blood vessels into the interstitium (**filtration**).

As demonstrated in Figure 2-4, when the difference between the colloid and interstitial osmotic pressure is greater than the difference between the hydrostatic pressures, fluid flows into blood vessels (**reabsorption**).

Starling's Law can be used to comprehend the reasoning behind the administration of intravenous solutions used in prehospital care. With an understanding of this law, one can better grasp the pathology behind disease states involving fluid overload (third-spacing) as well as the mechanism of action for fluids and medications administered to correct the underlying disorder.

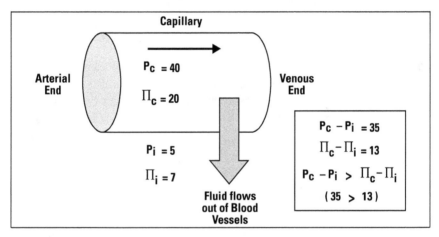

Figure 2-3 Forces affecting movement of water out of blood vessels.

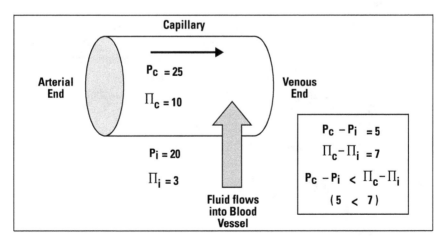

Figure 2-4 Forces affecting movement of water into blood vessels.

Intravenous Fluid Preparations

Fluids used are classified as isotonic, hypotonic, or hypertonic, and are further subdivided into classes of crystalloid or colloid solutions.

ISOTONIC CRYSTALLOIDS

0.9% Saline

Crystalloid fluids are named for the principal ingredient in these fluids: salt.[3] Two commonly used isotonic preparations are .9% sodium chloride (normal saline) and lactated Ringer's. "Normal" saline is somewhat of a misnomer as this solution actually is slightly hypertonic; nevertheless, it is considered **isotonic** because the tonicity closely approximates that of plasma.[3]

Ringer's Lactate

Lactated Ringer's solution contains potassium, calcium, and lactate in addition to sodium and chloride and is an **isotonic** solution. While there is no proven benefit over normal saline, lactated Ringer's has less chloride and slightly less sodium than normal saline solutions, theoretically making it more physiologically compatible.[3]

Table 2-1 lists the electrolyte and buffer composition of several intravenous fluid solutions that are commonly used in prehospital care, comparing them to the composition of normal human plasma.

Both lactated Ringer's and normal saline are presently used to provide immediate expansion of the circulatory volume in conditions of shock or fluid loss (i.e., dehydration, diarrhea, vomiting).[6] Because of their tonicity, both of these fluids eventually distribute to the interstitial space. Therefore, the predominant effect of crystalloid solutions is the expansion of the **interstitial rather than the intravascular** volume.[3] Overzealous administration of these solutions can lead to the development of life-threatening pulmonary edema (discussed further in the chapter on heart failure).

A final word of caution regarding the use of lactated Ringer's. Table 2-2 lists several commonly used prehospital care medications that are likely to be incompatible with Ringer's solution.[3] Lactated Ringer's is contraindicated in patients receiving blood transfusions because the calcium binds the anticoagulants added to blood products and may cause the transfused blood to clot.[12,13] One study showed that blood clots do not form when lactated Ringer's is used, as long as the transfusion is infused rapidly.[14] Nevertheless, in patients with profound hemorrhagic shock, the use of this solution should be carefully considered for resuscitation if the patient is likely to need a blood transfusion.

Table 2-1

Compositions of Commonly Used Intravenous Fluid Preparations.

Fluid	Sodium	Chloride	Potassium	Calcium	Magnesium	Buffers
Normal human plasma	141	103	4-5	5	2	Bicarbonate (26)
0.9% Sodium Chloride	154	154	0	0	0	0
Lactated Ringer's	130	109	4	3	0	Lactate (28)
Plasma-lyte	140	98	5	0	3	Acetate (27) Gluconate (23)

* All values are expressed as mEq/L

Table 2-2

Emergency Medications Incompatible with Lactated Ringer's Solution

Nitroglycerin
Nitroprusside
Norepinephrine
Mannitol
Procainamide
Propranolol
Methylprednisolone

HYPOTONIC CRYSTALLOIDS

5% Dextrose

In medical patients without evidence of fluid loss or hemorrhage, a 5% dextrose-in-water (D5W) solution is commonly used to provide a route for medication administration and to keep a cannulated vein open.[7] This choice of fluid administration in critically ill patients should be avoided for several reasons. First, the addition of glucose can create an undesirable osmotic force (D5W is a **hypotonic** solution) that can cause shrinkage of cells. Use of this fluid for resuscitation can lead to volume overload and can be fatal, especially in pediatric populations.[8] Moreover, critically ill patients have abnormal glucose metabolism; therefore, administrating a glucose-containing solution such as D5W can promote the formation of lactate, a toxin.[9] Dextrose solutions, when administered without thiamine, can precipitate Wernicke's encephalopathy.[10,11] Thiamine is needed for the conversion of pyruvate, which is the end product of the breakdown of glucose (dextrose).

COLLOIDS

Colloid solutions are a class of intravenous fluid preparations used for patients in need of immediate volume expansion. According to Starling's Law, the driving force for reabsorption of fluids into the intravascular space depends on the **osmotic pressure**. Since colloids, large molecules that do not pass through membranes as readily as crystalloids, increase the osmotic pressure, they cause absorption of fluids into the blood vessels, thereby expanding the plasma volume.[12] Common colloid preparations include 5% and 25% albumin and hetastarch.[4]

There are several reasons why colloid solutions are not frequently used in most EMS systems. Colloids have a relatively short duration of action despite having a long half-life.[4] These fluids can theoretically cause a secondary increase in interstitial fluid (i.e., edema) as they are eventually redistributed from the intravascular space to the interstitial space. Furthermore, colloids are up to three times more expensive than crystalloid solutions.[3,4]

References

1. Shires GT, Canizaro PC. *Fluid and Electrolyte Management of the Surgical Patient.* In Sabiston DC (ed.). *Sabiston Textbook of Surgery: The Biological Basis of Modern Surgical Practices.* 15th ed. New York: McGraw-Hill, 1999.

2. Cogan MG. *Fluid and Electrolytes: Physiology and Pathophysiology.* New York: Appleton and Lange, 1991.

3. Marino P. *The ICU Book.* 2nd Ed. Baltimore: Williams and Wilkins, 1998.

4. Giffel MI, Kaufman BS. Pharmacology of colloids and crystalloids. *Critical Care Clinics* 1992; 8:235-254.

5. Brenner BM, Rector RC (editors). *The Kidney.* 4th Ed. New York: Saunders, 1991.

6. Imm A, Carlson RW. Fluid resuscitation in circulatory shock. *Critical Care Clinics* 1993; 9:313-333.

7. Bledsoe BE, Porter RS, and Shade BR. *Paramedic Emergency Care.* 2nd Ed. Englewood Cliffs, NJ: Brady/Prentice Hall, 1994.

8. Jackson J, Bolte RG. Risks of intravenous administration of hypotonic fluids for pediatric patients in ED and prehospital settings: let's remove the handle from the pump. *Amer J Emer Med* 2000; 18(3): 269-270.

9. Degoute CS, Ray MJ, Manchon M, et al. Intraoperative glucose infusion and blood lactate: endocrine and metabolic relationships during abdominal aortic surgery. *Anesthesiology* 1989; 71(3): 355-361.

10. Penland B, Mawdsley C. Wernicke's encephalopathy following "hunger strike." *Postgraduate Med J* 1982; 58(681): 427-428.

11. Lavin PJ, Smith D, Kori SH, et al. Wernicke's encephalopathy: a predictable complication of hyperemesis gravidarum. *Obstet Gyn* 1983; 62(3 Suppl): 13s-15s.

12. Kaminiski MV, Haase TJ. Albumin and colloid osmotic pressure: implications for fluid resuscitation. *Critical Care Clinics* 1992; 8:311-322.

13. *American Association of Blood Banks Technical Manual.* 10th Ed. Arlington, VA: American Association of Blood Banks, 1990.

14. Lorenzo M, Davis J, Negin S, et al. Can Ringer's lactate be used safely with blood transfusions? *Amer J Surg* 1998; 175(4): 308-310.

Review Questions

1. You are called to the scene of a motor vehicle accident. The patient is a 23-year-old male with extensive multi-system trauma including a lower extremity amputation with active bleeding. Vital signs are as follows: BP 90/palpation HR 122 RR 24. Which intravenous fluid would be the most physiologically appropriate for resuscitation?
   A. 5% dextrose in water
   B. 0.9% saline
   C. 0.45% saline
   D. lactated Ringer's solution
   E. 5% dextrose in lactated Ringer's solution

An isotonic solution is the most physiologically sound choice in a patient with active hemorrhage and anticipated transfusion. Lactated Ringer's solution is incompatible with blood transfusions due to the effect of calcium binding to the anticoagulants added to blood products, although this effect may not be as common as was once thought if fluids are rapidly infused. Hypotonic solutions such as 5% dextrose are absolutely contraindicated in hemorrhaging patients because they contribute to edema and do not replete the intravascular space. The answer is B.

2. What would happen if a colloid solution was used for resuscitation in the patient above?
   A. Lactate formation would be promoted, leading to build-up of toxic substrates.
   B. The fluid would distribute to the interstitial space since the osmotic pressure would be decreased.
   C. Fluid would be absorbed into the blood vessels because the osmotic pressure would increase.
   D. The intravascular volume would become further depleted because the osmotic pressure would increase.
   E. The patient would not be able to receive crystalloid fluids because they are incompatible with colloids and lead to severe anaphylactic reactions.

According to Starling's law of the capillary, when the osmotic pressure increases, fluid is reabsorbed into blood vessels. Colloid preparations are large molecules that do not pass through cell membranes as readily as crystalloids. Colloids promote intravascular volume expansion by increasing the osmotic pressure. Lactate formation only occurs when glucose-containing fluids such as 5% dextrose in water are used due to abnormal glucose metabolism in critically ill patients. The answer is C.

3. All of the following are reasons to avoid glucose-containing solutions in a trauma patient EXCEPT:
   A. Hypotonic glucose solutions such as 5% dextrose in water create undesirable osmotic forces that favor shrinkage of cells and edema rather than intravascular volume repletion
   B. Glucose-containing solutions can promote the formation of toxins in critically ill patients
   C. In pediatric patients, boluses of 5% dextrose in water are the fluid of choice for hypovolemic trauma patients
   D. When given without thiamine in known alcoholic trauma patients, Wernicke's encephalopathy can occur
   E. All of the above are reasons to avoid glucose-containing solutions in trauma patients

5% dextrose in water should never be used as a resuscitation fluid for pediatric patients; use of this preparation in the pediatric patient can be fatal because of undesirable osmotic forces that can exacerbate edema. Lactate production is promoted in critically ill patients given glucose-containing fluids due to the abnormal metabolism of glucose. In known alcoholics, 5% dextrose should be given with thiamine because thiamine is necessary for the conversion of glucose to pyruvate. The answer is C.

Oxygen Transport

Most of the energy required by the human body is obtained from chemical reactions involving oxygen. Oxygen is capable of releasing the energy stored in organic fuels through the process of aerobic metabolism. The features of this system must be recognized in order to understand how abnormalities in the normal transport of oxygen can be corrected.

Hemoglobin

Although oxygen is the most abundant element on the surface of the earth, it does not dissolve readily in water and cannot be utilized without the presence of other molecules.[1] Hemoglobin, a protein composed of four iron-containing polypeptide chains, can reversibly bind oxygen and is directly responsible for oxygen distribution to cells (Figure 3-1). Hemoglobin generally exists in one of two forms, deoxyhemoglobin and oxyhemoglobin.

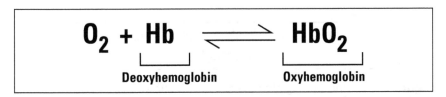

$$O_2 + Hb \rightleftharpoons HbO_2$$

          Deoxyhemoglobin   **Oxyhemoglobin**

Figure 3-1 Reversible reactions of oxygen and hemoglobin.

Hemoglobin-Oxygen Dissociation Curve

The reversible combination of hemoglobin with oxygen is defined by the hemoglobin-oxygen dissociation curve.[2] This curve is a plot of the partial pressure of oxygen (PO_2) versus the percent saturation of hemoglobin. The majority of oxygen in the human body is transported in the blood bound to hemoglobin, although a small percentage is dissolved in the blood.[2] The PO_2, also abbreviated as PaO_2, describes the partial pressure of oxygen because the air in the atmosphere is composed of several different gases, each having its own pressure, with each contributing to a single overall pressure. This pressure determines the movement of oxygen because gases, like particles in liquid solutions, move from regions of **higher** pressure to **lower** pressure. As long as the PO_2 of oxygen in the gas phase (*i.e.*, air) is greater than the PO_2 in liquid (*i.e.*, blood), a net diffusion of oxygen into blood takes place. The percent saturation (SpO_2) describes the amount of oxygen molecules bound to hemoglobin.

Since each hemoglobin molecule contains four polypeptide chains, each with one oxygen-binding iron molecule, the hemoglobin-oxygen dissociation curve demonstrates how oxygen can associate (combine) and dissociate (separate) from hemoglobin. The sigmoid or "S" shape of the curve is the result of a change in binding ability of oxygen to hemoglobin. After the first oxygen molecule binds hemoglobin, each additional molecule binds with less difficulty. This is known as the **affinity** of hemoglobin for oxygen. The final oxygen molecule to bind hemoglobin binds with the greatest affinity. Figure 3-2 demonstrates a normal hemoglobin-oxygen dissociation curve.

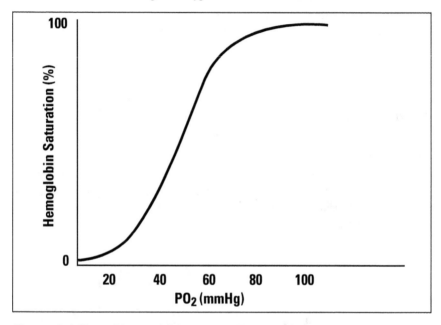

Figure 3-2 Normal hemoglobin-oxygen dissociation curve.

SHIFTING OF OXYGEN DISSOCIATION CURVE TO RIGHT

Several variables can affect the hemoglobin-oxygen dissociation curve and the distribution of oxygen to the cells of the body.

When the curve shifts to the right, the affinity of hemoglobin for oxygen is **decreased**, making it easier for the hemoglobin molecule to unload oxygen.[2] This leads to hypoxia because less oxygen is supplied to the body's cells as a result of hemoglobin's refusal to bind oxygen appropriately. Acidotic patients demonstrate hemoglobin-oxygen dissociation curves that shift to the right. For example, when the byproduct of respiration (CO_2) increases, the pH decreases (acidosis). This increase in CO_2 commonly occurs during exercise or in various disease states (*e.g.*, metabolic acidosis). Since hemoglobin has less of an affinity for oxygen in an acidic environment; this mechanism is protective because O_2 can rapidly be unloaded (dissociated) to meet the increased metabolic demands (this is known as the **Bohr effect**).[2,3] Other causes of a right shift of the curve include temperature increases and increases in the molecule [2,3]-DPG, a substance that binds reversibly to hemoglobin so that oxygen can be released more easily.[2] Individuals living at high altitudes are exposed to chronic hypoxemia. An adaptive response for this population is the synthesis of more [2,3]-DPG to allow what little oxygen that does bind hemoglobin to be released more rapidly for cellular uptake.

SHIFTING OF CURVE TO LEFT
Left shifts in the hemoglobin-oxygen dissociation curve occur as the result of conditions that cause hemoglobin to have a **greater** affinity for oxygen.

Conditions that are the opposite of those known to cause right shifts in the curve can cause left shifts (*i.e.,* temperature decreases, increased pH, decreased CO_2, decreased [2,3]-DPG production). Carbon monoxide poisoning is another important cause for left shifts in the curve. Carbon monoxide binds hemoglobin with a far greater affinity than oxygen. Thus, the curve is shifted to the left in cases of carbon monoxide intoxication, causing impaired ability of oxygen unloading in the cells and decreased total body oxygen.

Hypoxia

There are five main mechanisms for the development of decreased oxygen delivery to the tissues (hypoxia): **decreased PO_2, hypoventilation, ventilation-perfusion inequality, shunting, and decreased oxygen-carrying capacity** (Table 3-1).[4] A decreased PO_2, as occurs with individuals living at high altitudes, is one cause of hypoxia. Another cause is hypoventilation. Conditions causing hypoxia as a result of hypoventilation include excessive use of sedatives (*e.g.,* morphine, diazepam), chronic obstructive pulmonary disease (*e.g.,* emphysema), or neuromuscular disease (*e.g.,* myasthenia gravis). Ventilation-perfusion mismatches are probably the **most common cause of hypoxia.**[4] Lung segments that are ventilated but not perfused with blood (*e.g.,* pulmonary embolus, COPD) fail to deliver adequate amounts of oxygen to the body. Other causes of ventilation-perfusion inequalities include pulmonary edema and pulmonary fibrosis. Patients with abnormalities in the lungs or cardiovascular system that cause blood to not pass through areas of ventilation (oxygen uptake) represent another class of conditions that can cause hypoxia (*i.e.,* right-to-left cardiac shunts). Conditions that decrease the oxygen-carrying capacity of the blood (*e.g.,* anemia, carbon monoxide poisoning) can also cause hypoxia.

Table 3-1
Causes of Hypoxia
1. Decreased PO_2
2. Hypoventilation
3. Ventilation-perfusion (V/Q) inequality
4. Shunting
5. Decreased oxygen-carrying capacity

Carbon Dioxide Transport

CO_2 is produced in the tissues and carried to the lungs through venous blood. Some CO_2 molecules dissolve in plasma since CO_2 is much more soluble in water than O_2, while others form carbamino compounds. The majority of carbon dioxide molecules are transported for elimination via the bicarbonate-buffer system. The reaction wherein CO_2 forms bicarbonate is illustrated in Figure 3-3. The rate of this reaction is limited by carbonic anhydrase, an enzyme found only in red blood cells. The formation of bicarbonate allows CO_2 to be carried to the lungs in red blood cells where it can then be expired.

$$CO_2 + H_2O \underset{\text{Carbonic anhydrase}}{\rightleftharpoons} H_2CO_3 \rightleftharpoons H^+ + HCO_3^-$$

Carbonic acid   Bicarbonate

Figure 3-3 The formation of bicarbonate from carbon dioxide.

Pulse Oximetry

Using optical detection methods, the concentration of oxygenated and deoxygenated blood can be determined with noninvasive techniques. These techniques include pulse oximetry, a procedure now commonly used in many emergency medical services systems. By recording reflected light from the red (660 nm) and infrared (940 nm) spectrums, the saturation of hemoglobin by oxygen can be determined (SpO_2), usually within a 3% margin of error compared to the actual arterial hemoglobin saturation (SaO_2).[1,2] Patients with hypovolemia, hypotension, and anemia can still be monitored with this technique.[5,6] Pulse oximetry can help estimate the PO_2. Figure 3-4 shows the approximate PO_2 value for the measured SpO_2.

Downfalls include inaccurate (falsely low) readings in carbon monoxide poisoning, darkly pigmented individuals, and patients wearing nail polish.[7,8] Pulse oximetry is but one measure that can be used to assess oxygen transport. Over-reliance on this fifth vital sign is discouraged; every prehospital care provider should only consider the information provided by pulse oximetry after a thorough patient assessment.

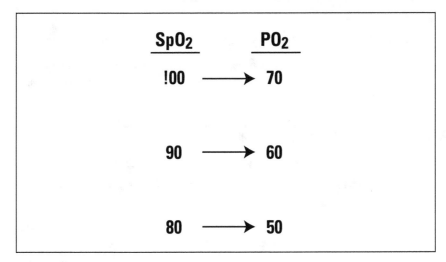

Figure 3-4 Approximate values of PO_2 for measured SpO_2.

End-Tidal CO_2 Measurement

The most popular device used in prehospital care for measuring CO_2 is the end-tidal CO_2 colorimetric detector. These devices measure exhaled CO_2 (end-tidal) as a function of color changes that occur as a function of pH. When attached to an ET tube immediately after intubation, a yellow color change indicates a successful tracheal intubation whereas a purple change suggests probable esophageal intubation.[9] In patients intubated for reasons other than cardiac arrest, these devices are approximately 100% sensitive for detecting the correct end-tidal CO_2. However, in instances of cardiac arrest, they are less accurate, and less sensitive for detecting the correct end-tidal CO_2.

References

1. Marino PL. *The ICU Book.* 2nd ed. Philadelphia: Williams and Wilkins, 1998.

2. White AC. Prolonged critical illness management of long term acute care: The evaluation and management of hypoxemia in the chronic critically ill patient. *Clinics in Chest Medicine.* 2001; 22(1).

3. Vander AJ, Sherman JH, and Luciano DS. *Human Physiology: The Mechanisms of Body Function.* 6th Ed. New York: McGraw-Hill, 1994.

4. Mines AH. *Respiratory Physiology.* 3rd ed. New York: Raven, 1992.

5. Jay GD, Hughes L, Renzi FP. Pulse oximetry is accurate in acute anemia from hemorrhage. *Ann Emerg Med.* 1994;24:32-35.

6. Severinghaus JW, Spellman MJ. Pulse oximeter failure thresholds in hypotension and vasoconstriction. *Anesthesiology.* 1990;73:532-537.

7. Ries AI, Prewitt LM, Johnson JJ. Skin color and ear oximetry. *Chest.* 1989;96:287-290.

8. Rubin AS. Nail polish color can affect pulse oximeter saturation. *Anesthesiology.* 1988;68:825.

9. MacLeod BA, Heller MB, Gerard J, et al. Verification of endotracheal tube placement with colorimetric end-tidal CO_2 detection. *Ann Emerg Med.* 1991;20:267-270.

Review Questions

1. Which of the following can cause a shift of the oxygen-hemoglobin dissociation curve to the right?
   A. Metabolic acidosis
   B. High fever
   C. Living at high altitude
   D. Strenuous exercise
   E. All of the above

All of the above. The answer is E.

2. All of the following are known mechanisms for the development of hypoxia EXCEPT:
   A. Living at high altitude
   B. Hyperventilation
   C. Severe anemia
   D. Pulmonary embolism
   E. Heart chamber defects

High altitude results in a lower PO_2. **Hypo**ventilation, not **hyper**ventilation, can cause hypoxia. Severe anemia can lead to decreased oxygen-carrying capacity of the blood. Ventilation-perfusion inequality is the pathophysiologic hallmark for pulmonary embolism. Abnormalities in the valves and chambers of the heart can lead to the circulation of deoxygenated blood as the lungs may be bypassed. The answer is B.

3. Which of the following is FALSE with regards to pulse oximetry?
   A. The saturation of oxygen can be measured within a 3% margin of error
   B. An SpO_2 of 100% corresponds roughly to a PO_2 of 70
   C. Pulse oximetry is a useful adjunct for assessing oxygen transport
   D. Patients with hypovolemia, hypotension, and anemia can still be monitored with a pulse oximeter
   E. Pulse oximetry can reveal unsuspected hypoxemia in cases of carbon monoxide poisoning

Pulse oximetry is inaccurate in carbon monoxide poisoning, darkly pigmented individuals, and patients wearing nail polish. Falsely low readings are often obtained in these situations. The answer is E.

4. You are called to the scene to intubate a pulseless, apneic patient. After intubation, you notice fogging of the ET tube, breath sounds by 5-point auscultation, and absence of abdominal distention. What else would help to confirm proper tube placement in the field?
   A. A chest x-ray
   B. Pulse oximetry
   C. A yellow color change on a colorimetric end-tidal CO_2 detector
   D. Presence of breath sounds heard over the trachea
   E. An arterial blood gas

End-tidal CO_2 detectors are an excellent means of detecting successful ET tube placement, but are less accurate for patients intubated with cardiac arrest. Neither a chest x-ray or arterial blood gas are available in the field, and neither are used in the emergency department for the initial assessment of proper tube placement. Pulse oximetry is an indicator of oxygen saturation, and is not the adjunctive measure of choice for determining successful intubation. Tracheal breath sounds are difficult to assess in the field and are an unreliable sign of successful intubation. The answer is C.

The Autonomic Nervous System

The autonomic nervous system consists of a set of pathways derived from the central nervous system that controls and regulates cardiac muscle, smooth muscle (*e.g.*, the gastrointestinal tract), and various glands. Although the autonomic nervous system has three essential divisions, sympathetic, parasympathetic, and enteric, this chapter is limited to a focused discussion of only the sympathetic and parasympathetic divisions. Comprehending the organization, receptor types, and effects on various organ systems is crucial for determining the appropriate pharmacologic therapy to correct imbalances within this system.

Organization of the Autonomic Nervous System

The innervation of most tissues other than skeletal muscle is derived from the autonomic nervous system.[1] The autonomic nervous system is comprised of millions of efferent pathways (neurons directed from the central nervous system to the tissues) and is divided into three divisions: sympathetic, parasympathetic, and enteric. The neurons of each division connect outside the CNS in cell clusters known as ganglia. Parasympathetic ganglia are located in the innervated organs whereas sympathetic ganglia are located closer to the spinal cord. The nerve fibers of the parasympathetic and sympathetic nervous system leave the CNS at different levels.[2] Sympathetic neurons leave the CNS at the thoracic and lumbar spinal cord levels; accordingly, this division is also known as the **thoracolumbar** division. Parasympathetic neurons exit from different regions of the brain and sacrum; hence, this division is referred to as the **craniosacral** division.

Synapses

Between each of the neurons of the autonomic nervous system, neurotransmitters function as chemical bridges to relay signals from neuron to neuron.[3] In both sympathetic and parasympathetic divisions, the major neurotransmitter is acetylcholine (ACh; Figure 4-1).

This neurotransmitter also functions in the **post**ganglionic fibers leading to the innervated tissue in the parasympathetic division. For sympathetic neurons, norepinephrine (NE) is the major neurotransmitter released in **post**ganglionic fibers. Various **co-transmitters** help carry the neural impulse from neuron to neuron.

Co-transmitters released between neurons include dopamine and ATP. Figure 4-1 illustrates how the sympathetic and parasympathetic neurons are organized as they leave the CNS.

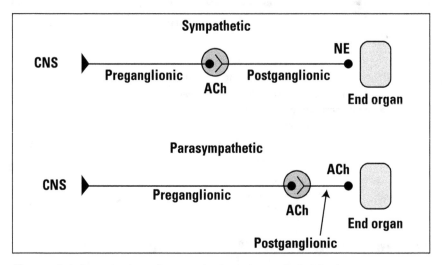

Figure 4-1 Organization of sympathetic and parasympathetic neurons.

CLINICAL CORRELATION

After synapsing in the pre- and postganglionic neurons, both divisions reach various receptors at the tissue level. **In prehospital care, many of the medications administered work at the receptor level of the sympathetic and parasympathetic divisions of the autonomic nervous system.** These receptors are either adrenergic or cholinergic and the action of the receptor is determined by which division is affecting it.

Adrenergic Receptors

Adrenergic receptors are composed of alpha and beta receptors.[4] Each class is further subdivided in to two additional classes of receptor types: alpha-1, alpha-2, and beta-1, beta-2. Cholinergic receptors are classified as nicotinic and muscarinic receptors.

ALPHA RECEPTORS

The alpha-1 (α-1) receptors are generally located on smooth muscle and depend on the formation of inositol triphosphate and an increase in intracellular calcium to function properly.[5] These receptors are very sensitive to norepinephrine and epinephrine, and usually elicit an excitatory response (*e.g.*, vasoconstriction). Alpha-2 (α-2) receptors are located in smooth muscle as well as various other nerve terminals, platelets, and even fat cells. These receptors function when the enzyme adenylate cyclase is inhibited and cyclic adenosine monophosphate is decreased (cAMP).[4] When activated, these receptors normally produce an inhibitory response (*e.g.*, lowered blood pressure).

BETA RECEPTORS

Beta receptors are divided into two classes. Beta-1 (β-1) receptors are located primarily in the heart and produce an excitatory response when stimulated (*e.g.*, increased heart rate). These receptors work when adenylate cyclase is activated and cAMP is increased. The Beta-2 (β-2) receptors are located in vascular smooth muscle, the gastrointestinal tract, and in bronchial smooth muscle. The mechanism of action of these receptors involves an increase in cAMP. The result of β-2 stimulation is usually relaxation (*e.g.*, bronchodilation).[4] Table 4-1 summarizes some of the effects of each division of the autonomic nervous system on the various adrenergic receptors in the respiratory and cardiovascular systems.[6]

Cholinergic Receptors

Cholinergic receptors consist of nicotinic and muscarinic receptors.[4] Nicotinic receptors can be found at the neuromuscular junction and in autonomic ganglia. These receptors are ion channels that allow cells to exchange sodium and potassium and to produce excitation when stimulated. Muscarinic receptors are located in the tissues of the heart and various smooth muscles. In the heart, these receptors evoke an inhibitory response (*e.g.*, slowed the heart rate) by inhibiting the action of adenylate cyclase and by opening ion channels. These receptors paradoxically cause an excitatory response in smooth muscle by increasing the formation of inositol triphosphate and increasing intracellular calcium.

Neurotransmitters

The receptors in the nervous system interact with a variety of chemical compounds known as neurotransmitters. Neurotransmitters function to complete the chemical bridge between individual neurons. Extensively studied neurotransmitters include norepinephrine, 5-hydroxytryptamine (serotonin), glutamic acid, gamma aminobutyric acid (GABA), glycine, and acetylcholine.[3] Many drugs used in emergency care act immediately on the synapses between neurons, functioning to either block postsynaptic effects (antagonists) or expedite them (agonists).

SYNAPTIC TRANSMISSION

Neurotransmitters are synthesized by a series of complex chemical reactions controlled by various enzymes in the neuron. Once the neurotransmitter is formed, it is stored in a vesicle for later release. When an action potential occurs, the vesicles release the neurotransmitter into the synapse, the area between two adjacent neurons. Receptors on the adjacent neuron (postsynaptic membrane) receive the neurotransmitter and ion channels are opened. Each of the steps necessary for synaptic transmission of neural impulses can be blocked by pharmacological agents. A brief summary of the ways synaptic transmission can be altered is outlined in Figure 4-2.

Table 4-1

Division of the Autonomic Nervous System

Organ	Receptor Type	Sympathetic Effect	Parasympathetic Effect
Heart			
SA node	Beta-1	Increases heart rate	Decreases heart rate
Atria	Beta-1	Increases contractility	Decreases contractility
AV node	Beta-1	Increases conduction velocity	Decreases conduction velocity
Ventricles	Beta-1	Increases contractility	Decreases contractility
Lungs			
Bronchial smooth muscle	Beta-1	Relaxes	Constricts
Bronchial glands	Beta-2	Inhibits secretion	(No effect)
	Alpha-1	Inhibits secretion	Stimulates secretion
Arterioles			
Coronary	Alpha-1,2 Beta-2	Vasoconstriction Vasodilation	Vasodilation (No effect)
Skin	Alpha-1,2	Vasoconstriction	(No effect)
Skeletal muscle	Alpha (?) Beta-2	Vasoconstriction Vasodilation	(No effect) (No effect)
Abdominal viscera	Alpha-1 Beta-2	Vasoconstriction Vasodilation	(No effect) (No effect)
Veins	Alpha-1 Beta-2	Vasoconstriction Vasodilation	(No effect) (No effect)
Eyes			
Iris muscle	Alpha-1	Widens pupil	Makes pupil smaller
Ciliary muscle	Beta-2	Changes lens for distant vision	Changes lens for near vision
Skin (piloerection)	Alpha-1	Contracts	(No effect)

Adapted from Goodman and Gilman's *The Pharmacological Basis of Therapeutics.*
Gilman AG, Rall TW, Nies AS, and Taylor P, eds. 8th ed. New York: Pergamon Press, 1990.

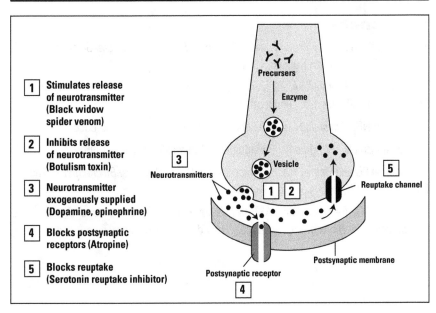

Figure 4-2 Synaptic transmission and selected sites of drug action.
Adapted from Carlson NR. *Physiology of Behavior.* Boston: Allyn & Bacon, 1994.

References

1. Kandel KL, Schwartz JH, and Jessel TM, eds.. *Principles of Neural Science.* 3rd ed. New York: Elsevier/North Holland, 1991.

2. Barr ML and Kierman JA. *The Human Nervous System: An Anatomical Viewpoint.* 6th ed. Philadelphia: J.B. Lippincott Co., 1993.

3. Carlson NR. *Physiology of Behavior.* 5th ed. Boston: Allyn and Bacon, 1994.

4. Constanzo LS. *Physiology.* Philadelphia: Williams & Wilkins, 1995.

5. Champe PC and Harvey RA. *Lippincott's Illustrated Reviews: Biochemistry.* 2nd ed. Philadelphia: J.B. Lippincott Co., 1994.

6. Gilman AG, Rall TW, Nies AS, and Taylor P, eds. *Goodman and Gilman's The Pharmacological Basis of Therapeutics.* 8th ed. New York: Pergamon Press, 1990.

Review Questions

1-7. Match the end-organ action with the appropriate receptor type.
   A. Beta-1
   B. Beta-2
   C. Alpha-1
   D. Alpha-2
   E. Alpha-1 & -2

   1. Increased or decreased heart rate
   2. Bronchodilation or bronchoconstriction
   3. Arteriolar vasoconstriction in skin
   4. Piloerection
   5. Pupillary dilation
   6. Pupillary constriction
   7. Increased or decreased conduction velocity at the A-V node

1. A.

2. B.

3. E.

4. C.

5. C. Sympathetic effect on iris.

6. C. Parasympathetic effect on iris.

7. A.

Pharmacokinetics

The study of pharmacokinetics attempts to define the dynamics of drug behavior in the living body (Figure 5-1).

The biological fate of a drug after it has been administered depends on four essential processes: absorption, distribution, metabolism, and elimination.[1] These processes occur simultaneously until the entire drug is fully absorbed and metabolized. Understanding these concepts enables one to make better choices about what drugs to administer while assessing the variability in drug response.

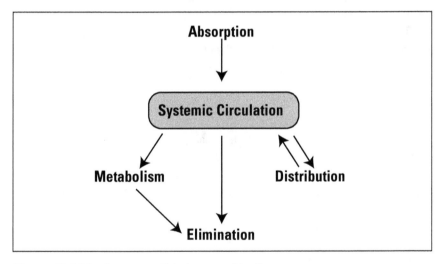

Figure 5-1 The four essential pharmacokinetic processes.

Absorption

Absorption refers to the rate and quantity of a drug that is introduced to the fluids of the body. Several factors affect the rate of absorption. For orally administered drugs, the solubility in the stomach and intestinal fluids is an important factor.[1] The rate of dissolution in the stomach or gastrointestinal tract is equally important and may be affected by the presence or absence of food in the stomach. The presence of other drugs or preexisting conditions that alter the motility of the gastrointestinal tract can interfere with oral absorption of drugs. For intravenous, subcutaneous, or intramuscularly administered drugs, absorption is dependent on how quickly the drug can be introduced to the body fluids. For example, in an obese or edematous patient, drug absorption by the subcutaneous route may potentially be delayed.

Distribution

The process of distribution refers to the movement or temporary storage of a drug once introduced to the body fluids. Drugs that are absorbed circulate to areas of the body where there is blood flow. Most drugs have target organs or tissues that preferentially take up or release drugs at varying rates. In general, organs with higher blood flow (i.e., heart, brain, kidneys) tend to accumulate drugs more rapidly.[1] As the dose of a given drug increases, so does the concentration. When given by most routes, with the exception of intravenously administered drugs, several semipermeable cell membranes must be traversed by the processes of diffusion or active transport before a drug reaches the intended site of action.

Metabolism

Metabolism is the process of chemical conversion of the original drug to an active or inactive metabolite. Indeed, many drugs must first be converted to a metabolite before being eliminated from the body.[1] Most metabolites are formed in the liver, filtered by the kidney, and excreted in the urine. Drugs that are metabolized may form pharmacologically active or inactive metabolites, depending on the drug.

Elimination

Elimination involves the various pathways for removal of a drug from the body. Pathways for elimination include the kidney, lungs, and liver as well as the body fluids (urine, bile, sweat). The rate at which a drug is excreted is referred to as its half-life (t/2). The half-life is the amount of time required for removal of 50% of a drug from the body. Six half-lives are generally required to remove 98% of a drug from the body; a total of ten half-lives completely eliminates a drug.[2]

Bioavailability

When treating patients with drugs, the goal is to provide enough drug to achieve the desired therapeutic effect while minimizing toxicity (Figure 5-2).

The amount of drug in systemic circulation is usually a fraction of the original dose; this fraction is referred to as bioavailability. Bioavailability is mathematically expressed as the area under the curve for a plot of drug concentration versus time. For drugs given intravenously, bioavailability is approximately 100%.[2] For drugs given orally, bioavailability depends on a drug's individual rate of absorption, distribution, metabolism, and elimination. Over time, a drug's rate of bioavailability equals the rate of elimination. This is known as the steady state. It typically takes about four half-lives for most drugs to reach steady state.[1] Once the steady-state is achieved, maintenance doses must be administered.

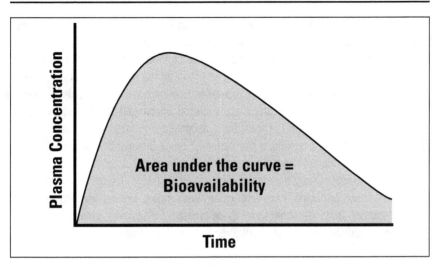

Figure 5-2 A bioavailability curve. See text for explanation.

Protein Binding

Most drug molecules exist in the body fluids bound to large proteins, such as albumin, alpha-1-glycoprotein, and lipoproteins.[1] Acidic drugs are generally bound more extensively to albumin, and basic drugs to 1-acid glycoprotein or lipoproteins. Examples of highly protein-bound drugs include warfarin (Coumadin®), diazepam (Valium®), furosemide (Lasix®), and phenytoin (Dilantin®).[3]

The amount of free drug versus bound drug is important in determining the onset and duration of action. Drugs that remain unbound to plasma proteins can travel freely throughout the body, delivering the desired pharmacological effect. Only unbound drugs are thought to be available for distribution to the fluid compartments within the body where pharmacologic effects occur.[3] Therefore, the unbound drug concentration is closely related to drug concentration at the active site and drug effects. Unbound drugs may be metabolized and eliminated more rapidly than bound drugs. Bound drugs tend to have a lower volume of distribution throughout the body and a longer duration of action. Patients often have to take a higher dose to achieve the desired therapeutic response. The concept of protein binding is especially important when two plasma protein bound drugs are co-administered. Both drugs compete for plasma protein binding sites; the less competitive drug remains displaced, and increases the level of unbound or free drug.

Organ Impairment

Once a drug enters the body, it is eventually eliminated either by excretion or metabolism. Most drugs are eliminated as unchanged drug by the kidney or liver.[1] Renal or hepatic impairment can lead to drug accumulation, failure to form metabolites, diminished efficacy, and increased toxic effects. The relationship between hepatic disease and drug metabolism is complex; however, since many drugs are metabolized via the liver, in patients with liver disease (*e.g.*, cirrhosis, hepatocellular carcinoma) significant dosage adjustments and close observation are often required.[4] Thyroid disease can have an effect on the metabolism of drugs. The hepatic metabolism of some drugs is increased in hyperthyroidism and decreased in hypothyroidism. A number of drugs are excreted unchanged by the kidneys (*e.g.*, digoxin, lithium, gentamicin).[5] These drugs accumulate in renal impairment. Heart failure can affect pharmacokinetic properties of drugs by several mechanisms. The congestion associated with heart failure can lead to impaired absorption due to edema of the intestinal mucosa and decreased splanchnic circulation. Hepatic congestion and decreased renal perfusion can also occur with heart failure, leading to toxic accumulation of drugs metabolized by these organs. Furthermore, some cardioactive drugs have a reduced volume of distribution in heart failure patients.[1]

First Pass Hepatic Effect

Drugs absorbed from the gastrointestinal tract have to pass first through the liver via the hepatic portal vein before entering the systemic circulation. If the liver removes or metabolizes a percentage of the drug, this action is referred to as the first pass hepatic effect. Some examples of drugs metabolized by the first pass hepatic effect include aspirin, morphine, and propranolol.[1] Drugs with an extensive first pass effect may be completely destroyed by the liver's enzymes and never reach the circulation in sufficient amounts to produce the desired pharmacologic effect.

References

1. Hardman JG, Limbird LE, eds. *Goodman & Gilman's The Pharmacological Basis of Therapeutics.* 9th ed. New York: McGraw-Hill; 1996.

2. Peck CC, Conner DP, Murphy MG. *Bedside Clinical Pharmacokinetics: Simple Techniques for Individualizing Drug Therapy.* Vancouver, WA: Applied Therapeutics, Inc.; 1989: 3-11.

3. Rowland M, Tozer TN, eds. *Clinical Pharmacokinetics: Concepts and applications.* 3rd ed. Philadelphia, PA: Lippincott, Williams & Wilkins; 1995.

4. Draft Guidance for Industry: *Pharmacokinetics in patients with impaired hepatic function--study design, data analysis, and impact on dosing and labeling.* US Food and Drug Administration, Center for Drug Evaluation and Research, Center for Biologics Evaluation and Research, November 1999.

5. Draft Guidance for Industry: *Pharmacokinetics in patients with impaired renal function--study design, data analysis, and impact on dosing and labeling.* US Food and Drug Administration, Center for Drug Evaluation and Research, Center for Biologics Evaluation and Research, May 1998.

Review Questions

1. You are called to a remote location to assess a pediatric patient with an accidental ingestion of one tablet of his mother's pain medication (drug X). Poison control and medical control are unavailable. After performing an appropriate assessment and providing supportive measures, the patient is determined to be stable. En route, you read an information file on drug X. The half life is listed as 1 hour. When would 98% of the drug be eliminated from the patient's body?

   A. 2 hours
   B. 4 hours
   C. 6 hours
   D. 24 hours
   E. 36 hours

For this theoretical case, 6 half lives would have passed in 6 hours, and for most drugs, this is the number of half-lives generally required to remove 98% of a drug from the body. The half-life is defined as the amount of time required for removal of 50% of a drug from the body. Ten half-lives are usually required for complete elimination. The answer is C.

2. Which of the following medications used in emergency care has the most extensive first-pass hepatic effect?

   A. Amiodarone
   B. Epinephrine
   C. Furosemide
   D. Diazepam
   E. Morphine

Morphine is an example of a medication with the first-pass hepatic effect. The answer is E.

3. Drugs must be carefully administered to patients with which of the following medical conditions?

   A. Heart failure
   B. Hyperthyroidism
   C. Hypothyroidism
   D. Cirrhosis
   E All of the above

Since most drugs are eliminated as unchanged drug by the kidney or liver, any organ impairment can lead to drug accumulation, diminished efficacy, and toxic effects. The answer is E.

Section II

Respiratory Pathophysiology

6

Pulmonary Physiology and Pharmacology

The overall goal of the respiratory system is to provide oxygenated blood for body tissues while removing carbon dioxide, the byproduct of the cellular use of oxygen. Although the lung is the lightest organ in the human body, it receives 100% of the cardiac output, taking in desaturated arterial blood and returning oxygenated pulmonary venous blood. Attaining an appreciation of basic respiratory physiology and pathophysiology demonstrates how the lung is pivotal for the proper function of other organ systems.

Airways

The airways consist of a series of passages for airflow that become progressively smaller and more numerous while branching into the different areas of the lung. This progressive narrowing and branching of the airways is known also as arborization, and is demonstrated in Figure 6-1.[1]

AIRWAY ZONES

The respiratory system begins with the nostrils and the mouth, both of which conduct air into the larynx and trachea. The nose plays an important role as it allows inhaled air to become warm, clean, and moist, and prevents crusting of lung tissue and infection. This system of filtration is bypassed in patients with tracheostomies or

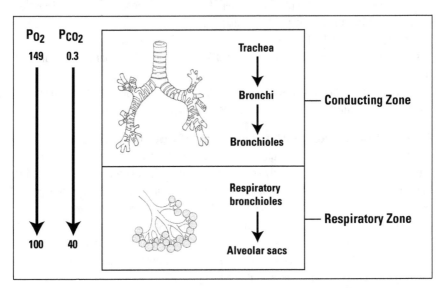

Figure 6-1 The arborization of airway zones.

endotracheal tubes. Air passes through the trachea and into the right and left mainstem bronchi, both of which are divided at a bifurcation known as the carina, and further subdivided into smaller bronchi, bronchioles, and ultimately, into small air sacs known as alveoli. Since the air passing through the larger airways (*e.g.*, trachea, bronchi) is not exchanged with tissues, these airways are defined collectively as the **conducting zone.** Once air reaches the terminal airways (*e.g.*, bronchioles and alveoli), oxygen and carbon dioxide is being exchanged; this area of the lung is defined as the **respiratory zone.**

Respiratory Dynamics

INSPIRATION AND EXPIRATION

The passage of air into the lungs is governed by pressure differences caused by changes in lung volume. Changes in volume are caused by contraction of the diaphragm as well as the inherent elasticity (compliance) of the chest, lungs, abdomen, and the action of additional muscles of inspiration and expiration. The thoracic diaphragm is the principle muscle of respiration. This dome-shaped musculotendinous structure is innervated by the phrenic nerves that are derived from the ventral rami of cervical segments 3 to 5 of the spinal cord.[2] When the diaphragm contracts, the vertical diameter of the thoracic cavity is increased. Since increases in volume cause decreases in pressure according to **Boyle's law** (an increase in the volume of a gas is inversely proportional to the change in pressure), when the thoracic cavity expands, the intrathoracic pressure decreases and air moves into the lungs (high to low).[1] The expansion of the lungs during respiration is a passive process; the lungs rely on other muscles such as the diaphragm to expand. In certain disease states, the inspiratory effort is dependent on a number of additional accessory muscles. Muscles of **inspiration**, in addition to the diaphragm, include the following: external intercostals, sternocleidomastoids, scaleni, anterior serrati, trapezius, and the posterior neck muscles.[2] Muscles of **expiration** include the internal intercostals, the posterior inferior serrati, and the abdominal muscles (rectus abdominus, transversus abdominus, external and internal obliques). Under normal conditions, only the diaphragm and intercostals muscles are used for inspiration and expiration.

Clinical Correlation: Pathophysiology of Pneumothorax

Since inflation of the lung occurs as the result of simple changes in intrathoracic pressures, the lung spontaneously collapses whenever the force to keep it inflated is absent. To keep the lung from expelling air and collapsing when deflated, a negative pressure exists between the lung and the thoracic wall. This negative pressure, known as the intrapleural pressure, is maintained in a narrow space between the lung pleura and chest wall pleura, allowing the lung to float within the thoracic cavity. In a patient with a pneumothorax, the lung collapses when the intrapleural space is violated and the negative pressure no longer maintained (Figure 6-2).

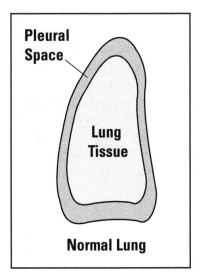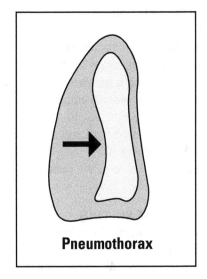

Figure 6-2 The pathophysiology of pneumothorax.

Respiratory Physiology

THE SPIROGRAM
Respiratory excursions during normal breathing, maximal inspiration, and maximal expiration can be visualized with a spirogram. A spirogram is generated as a patient breathes into a device that measures the volume of air inspired and expired over a given period of time (Figure 6-3).

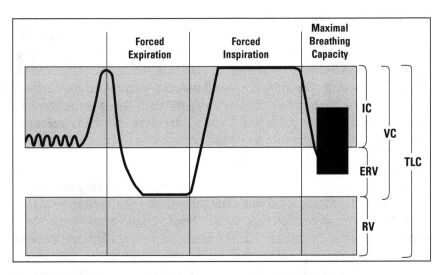

Figure 6-3
A representative spirogram for a patient without respiratory disease.

LUNG VOLUMES

The **tidal volume** (TV) is the volume of air that enters the lungs during a single inspiration and is roughly equal to the volume leaving the lungs during a subsequent exhalation. This volume is equal to approximately 500 cc (500 mL). After exhalation, the tidal volume is released, but the lungs still contain air. This volume is known as the **expiratory reserve volume** (ERV) and is the volume that can be expired after the expiration of a tidal volume. During maximal inspiration, a volume of air can be inspired that is over and above the tidal volume. This is known as the **inspiratory reserve volume** (IRV). The volume that remains in the lungs after a maximal expiration is known as the **residual volume** (RV). This volume cannot be measured with spirometry.

LUNG CAPACITIES

The measurements of two lung capacities, the vital capacity (VC) and the total lung capacity (TLC) can provide useful clinical information. The vital capacity is the sum of the IRV, TV, and ERV. This measurement represents the total volume that is expired after a maximal inspiration. The **total lung capacity** is the sum of **all** lung volumes (TV, IRV, ERV, IC). Since capacity includes the residual volume, it cannot be measured by spirometry.

Clinical Correlation: Asthma

Patients with asthma have narrowed air passages due to smooth muscle contraction, mucus plugging, and inflammation. Although the pathogenesis of airway narrowing in asthma is principally related to inflammation, this disorder results in a progressive obstruction of the airways. Since air cannot be expired, the residual volume **increases** and the vital capacity and ERV **decreases**. Therapy is aimed at reversing airway obstruction by increasing the diameter of the bronchi and decreasing inflammation.

Clinical Correlation: Emphysema

In patients with emphysema, lung tissue is destroyed and weakened airway walls collapse during expiration. Because of chronic lung tissue inflammation and swelling, the airway walls have decreased recoil and elasticity. Thus, although the pathogenesis is different, emphysema, like asthma, is an **obstructive** pulmonary disease because patients with this disorder have difficulty with expiration. Air cannot escape from collapsed airway segments, and both the IC and ERV **decrease** while the RV **increases**. Figure 6-4 shows a spirogram for a patient with an obstructive lung disorder.

ALVEOLI AND SURFACTANT

The terminal air spaces (alveoli) are also affected by physical forces that cause them to shrink or expand. According to **LaPlace's law**, the surface tension (tendency to collapse) of smaller alveoli is greater than large alveoli.[1] Therefore, small alveoli have a greater tendency to collapse. The problem of surface tension is solved by a substance known as surfactant, a phospholipid made by type II alveolar cells. Surfactant decreases surface tension in alveoli in addition to helping minimize the pressure needed to expand the lungs and hold them open. Neonatal respiratory distress syndrome can occur in infants born only 1 week premature due to lack of surfactant. Lack of surfactant causes collapse of alveoli (atelectasis) upon expiration. Hypoxemia results as the lungs become less compliant and difficult to re-inflate.

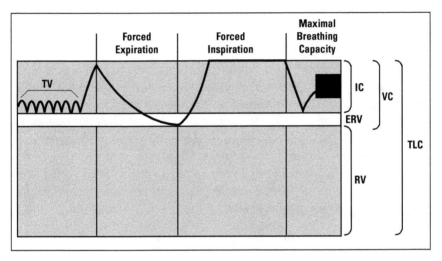

Figure 6-4
A representative spirogram for a patient with obstructive lung disease.

STARLING'S LAW
The factors affecting movement of fluid through the alveolar capillaries are similar to those in the systemic circulation and are described by Starling's Law. Normally, the forces driving fluid out of the capillaries surrounding alveoli are greater than the forces driving fluid in. Excess fluid is usually removed by the lymphatics in the lung. In pulmonary edema, an imbalance in the normal forces at the alveolar capillary membrane causes fluid to accumulate in the pulmonary interstitial space and alveoli. For fluid to accumulate, the pressure in the pulmonary capillaries must be equal to or greater than the plasma colloid osmotic pressure. This can be induced by damage to the capillary membrane (*i.e.*, infections, chemicals, inflammation) or from heart failure or valvular disease. The various causes and treatment of pulmonary edema are discussed in Chapter 15.

RESPIRATORY NEUROPHYSIOLOGY
The regulation of ventilation is controlled by different nervous pathways. Central and peripheral chemoreceptors, lung stretch receptors, irritant receptors, J receptors, and the sympathetic and parasympathetic nervous system all contribute by interpreting stimuli and sensory input and increasing or decreasing the breathing rate.[1]

Airway diameter and secretions are controlled primarily by the sympathetic and parasympathetic nervous systems. The airways are lined with layers of smooth muscle from the trachea to the alveoli; however, **the largest proportion of muscle is found at the end of the conducting zone in the terminal bronchioles.**[1] Beta-2 receptors function to dilate the bronchioles when activated by adrenergic agonists such as epinephrine and norepinephrine. Stimulation of beta-2 receptors also helps decrease the secretions of mucous and serous glands. Alternatively, parasympathetic fibers derived from the vagus nerve stimulate muscarinic cholinergic receptors embedded in the bronchial musculature. Activation of these receptors leads to constriction of the bronchioles in addition to increased amounts of secretions.

NEUROREGULATORY MECHANISMS

Information regarding the PCO_2 and other factors is received by various parts of the brainstem and cortex. The medullary respiratory center, located in the reticular formation of the brainstem, is responsible for generating nervous impulses to the phrenic nerve, regulating inspiration. Additional inspiratory regulators exist as the apneustic and the pneumotaxic centers of the pons.[1] The ventral respiratory group is responsible for expiration and is usually only activated during exercise or with certain disease processes where expiration becomes an active process (e.g., COPD). Since breathing can also be controlled voluntarily, the cortex becomes activated when a person voluntarily hyper- or hypoventilates.

Central Chemoreceptors

Chemoreceptors also play an important role in the regulation of respiration. Central chemoreceptors in the medulla are sensitive to the pH of cerebrospinal fluid (CSF). CO_2 is lipid soluble and readily diffuses into the CSF, combining with water to form bicarbonate and hydrogen ions. When excess CO_2 and hydrogen ions are produced, the ventilatory rate is increased (to blow off the CO_2). Similarly, when the PCO_2 and hydrogen concentration is low, **the ventilatory rate decreases**. This is why hyperventilating patients lose consciousness.

Peripheral Chemoreceptors

Additional peripheral chemoreceptors exist in the carotid and aortic bodies and also affect the respiratory rate. The carotid bodies, as opposed to the central chemoreceptors, are sensitive to decreases in oxygen. Thus, in a patient with a low PO_2, the respiratory rate increases. **The PO_2 must fall to very low levels ($PO_2 <$ 60 mm Hg) for this mechanism to be stimulated.**[4] Since patients with chronic obstructive pulmonary disease (e.g., emphysema) often have a sustained low PO_2, the carotid bodies regulate the breathing rate, not the central chemoreceptors. This is known as the **hypoxic drive** for respiration. This concept is important to comprehend because high volumes of supplemental oxygen administered haphazardly have the potential to suppress respiration completely in patients who are otherwise dependent on a low PO_2 to regulate their respiratory rate. Figure 6-5 depicts the relationship between ventilation and PO_2 levels in a patient with hypoxic drive.

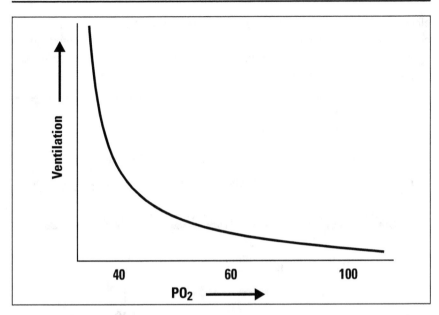

Figure 6-5 The relationship of ventilation to PO_2 in hypoxic drive. As PO_2 increases, ventilation decreases; as PO_2 decreases, ventilation increases.

Pulmonary Pharmacology

Medications for respiratory disease generally work at the level of the autonomic nervous system or locally. The specific therapies for asthma and COPD are discussed in the next two chapters. The following is a brief description of the mechanisms and rationale for commonly used respiratory medications.

PHARMACOLOGY OF BETA-2 RECEPTOR ACTIVATION

Pharmacologic agents can induce relaxation of the bronchial musculature by activating beta-2 receptors. These receptors are located on the cell membranes of bronchial smooth muscle, bronchial epithelium (lining of bronchi), and mast cells.[5] When the receptor is activated by a drug or endogenous hormone (*e.g.*, epinephrine), a cascade of chemical reactions is set in motion. Activation of adenylate cyclase causes cyclic adenosine monophosphate (cAMP) levels to become elevated. This elevation of cAMP allows specific proteins to become phosphorylated by ATP. Phosphorylation activates these proteins and allows them to produce specific intracellular effects (*e.g.*, relaxation of bronchial smooth muscle). Figure 6-6 illustrates this cascade of biochemical reactions.

Beta-2 Agonists

Beta-2 agonists used in asthma and COPD include **albuterol** (Ventolin®, Proventil®), **bitolterol** (Tornalate®), **levalbuterol** (Xopenex®), **metaproterenol** (Alupent®, Metaprel®, ProMeta®), **pirbuterol** (Maxair®), **salmeterol** (Serevent®), and **terbutaline** (Brethine®, Bricanyl®, Brethaire®). These medications are typically given as inhaled aerosols or by nebulizer. Each agent has a different duration of action;

albuterol is generally active for 4 to 6 hours while salmeterol is longer acting (12 hours). Even though beta-2 agonists are fairly specific for beta-2 receptors, these agents can also activate beta-1 receptors in some patients, causing increases in heart rate and other beta-1 effects.

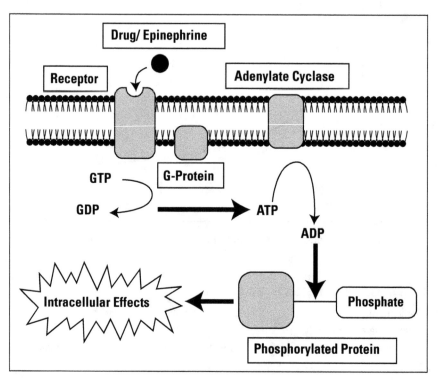

Figure 6-6 Activation of adenylate cyclase by cyclic AMP. This is the common pathway activated by agents such as albuterol, epinephrine, and other beta agonists.

Other Bronchodilators

The methylated xanthines, of which theophylline is the prototype, represent another class of agents capable of relaxing bronchial smooth muscle. Methylated xanthines have numerous mechanisms of action that have been proposed. These agents increase cAMP, but by inhibiting phosphodiesterase, the enzyme that degrades cAMP, rather than activating adenylate cyclase. Smooth muscle relaxation is achieved by direct mobilization of intracellular calcium and inhibition of extracellular adenosine, which is a bronchoconstrictor. Methylated xanthines inhibit prostaglandins and decrease the metabolism of catecholamines.[4] These preparations also increase the force of contraction of the diaphragm.

Both theophylline and aminophylline have fallen out of popular use in many systems due to an extensive toxicodynamic profile and numerous drug-drug interactions. At serum concentrations of theophylline greater than 35 mcg/mL, seizures, cerebral hypoxia, arrhythmias, and death occur.[4] At lower levels of intoxication, tremors, headache, gastrointestinal disturbances, and tachycardia are commonly reported.

ANTICHOLINERGIC AGENTS

Ipratropium bromide (Atrovent®) is another agent that works to reverse overstimulation of the autonomic nervous system. A derivative of atropine, ipratropium is a parasympathetic blocker used by patients with chronic obstructive pulmonary disease (COPD) and asthma. Administered via inhaler, it has a duration of action of approximately 4 to 6 hours (Figure 6-7).

Steroids

Glucocorticoids, also referred to as **corticosteroids**, are compounds synthesized to resemble the natural glucocorticoids, as opposed to other steroid hormones such as testosterone that are synthesized by the gonads and other histological layers of the adrenal gland (Figure 6-8).

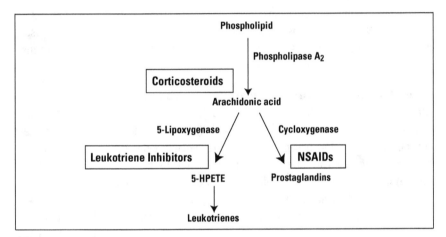

Figure 6-7 The pathways of leukotriene and prostaglandin synthesis and sites of pharmacologic inhibition.

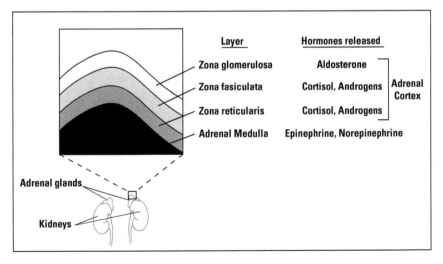

Figure 6-8 The histological layers of the adrenal gland.

Glucocorticoids are naturally synthesized from the zona reticularis and zona fascicularis of the adrenal cortex. Inhaled preparations include **beclomethasone** (Vanceril®, Beclovent®), **budesonide** (Pulmicort®), **flunisolide** (AeroBid®), **fluticasone** (Flovent®), and **triamcinolone acetonide** (Azmacort®). The intravenous preparation used for severe asthma exacerbations is **methylprednisolone** (Solu-Medrol®). All of these compounds possess potent anti-inflammatory properties because of an ability to inhibit phospholipase A2, the enzyme leading to the formation of prostaglandins and other inflammatory mediators. Steroids cause increased amino acid metabolism and gluconeogenesis, increased production of platelets, increased breakdown of collagen, decreased numbers of circulating lymphocytes and eosinophils, and numerous other effects. Although inhaled preparations have relatively few proven side effects, intravenous steroids can cause metabolic disturbances, immunosuppression, ulcers, electrolyte imbalances, skin changes, ocular problems, CNS complications, and a variety of other side effects. For this reason, intravenous preparations are reserved exclusively to treat the late response component of an asthma exacerbation.

Leukotriene Inhibitors and Mast Cell Stabilizers

Other respiratory medications include the leukotriene inhibitors and mast cell stabilizers. Leukotriene inhibitors work by inhibiting the formation of leukotrienes, substances derived from phospholipids and arachidonic acid that cause smooth muscle contraction, vasoconstriction, and inflammation. Common preparations include **montelukast** (Singulair®), **zafirlukast** (Accolate®), and **zileuton** (Zyflo®). Mast cell stabilizers include **cromolyn sodium** (Intal®) and **nedocromil** (Tilade®). These agents are used strictly as a prophylactic measure to prevent mast cells from releasing histamine and other bronchoconstrictors during an asthma exacerbation. Mast cell stabilizers currently have no role in the management of an acute asthma or COPD episode.

References

1. West JB. R*espiratory Physiology: The Essentials.* 5th Ed. Philadelphia: Williams & Wilkins, 1995.

2. Moore KL. *Clinically Oriented Anatomy.* 3rd Ed. Philadelphia: Williams & Wilkins, 1992.

3. Champe PC, Harvey RA. *Biochemistry.* 2nd Ed. Philadelphia: J.B. Lippincott Co., 1994.

4. Fauci AS, Braunwald E, Isselbacher KJ, et al. *Harrison's Principles of Internal Medicine.* 14th Ed. New York: McGraw-Hill, 1998.

5. Bulger EM, Maier RV. *Lipid mediators in the pathophysiology of illness. Crit Care Med* (Supplement). 2000; 28(4): N27-31.

6. Vander AJ, Sherman JH, Luciano DS. *Human Physiology: The Mechanisms of Body Function.* 6th Ed. New York: McGraw-Hill, 1994.

Review Questions

1. Your unit is called to the scene of a 33-year-old asthmatic patient complaining of severe shortness of breath. Vital signs on scene are: BP 140/90 RR 28 HR 110. Accessory muscle use is evident. Lung sounds are decreased with diffuse wheezing and a prolonged expiratory component. All of the following are muscles of expiration EXCEPT:
   A. Internal intercostals
   B. Posterior inferior serrati
   C. Rectus abdominus
   D. Sternocleidomastoids
   E. External obliques

The scalenes, sternocleidomastoids, anterior serrati, trapezius, posterior neck muscles, and diaphragm are all muscles of inspiration. The abdominal muscles, including the internal and external obliques, as well as the intercostals and posterior serrati, are muscles of expiration. The answer is D.

2. For the patient in the question above, what would pulmonary function testing likely show?
   A. Increased residual volume
   B. Increased expiratory reserve volume
   C. Increased vital capacity
   D. Decreased inspiratory capacity
   E. Little change in total lung capacity

One of the hallmarks of asthma is an increased residual volume due to air trapped in the inflamed bronchioles. Vital capacity and expiratory reserve volume decrease. The answer is A.

3. You are assessing a 74-year-old female complaining of dyspnea with a history of heavy tobacco use for over 30 years. After a focused physical exam, you believe the patient is suffering from COPD. Patients with this disorder are expected to have which of the following?
   A. Difficulty with inspiring air due to bronchial narrowing
   B. A decreased residual volume due to air trapped in dilated alveoli
   C. Increased inspiratory capacity and decreased expiratory reserve volume
   D. Increased elastic recoil of lung segments
   E. Difficulty with expiration due to chronic lung tissue inflammation and swelling

Patients with COPD have difficulty with expiration due to damaged airways. Both the inspiratory capacity and expiratory reserve volume decrease while the residual volume increases. Elastic recoil is decreased due to chronic inflammation and swelling of the airways. The answer is E.

4. During a critical care aeromedical transport, you notice the 4-day-old prema-
ture neonate that you are transporting becoming more tachypneic. Neonatal res-
piratory distress syndrome occurs in certain infants as a result of:
   A. Chronic airways inflammation
   B. Hypertrophy of type II alveolar cells
   C. Hyperactivity of type I alveolar cells
   D. Collapse of alveoli during expiration due to lack of surfactant
   E. Bronchoconstriction due to hyperresponsiveness to supplemental oxygen

Infants born only 1 week premature can have neonatal respiratory distress syndrome. The
pathogenesis is related to lack of surfactant. Without surfactant, the surface tension of
small alveoli have a greater tendency to collapse. The answer is D.

5. You are assisting a pediatric asthmatic patient in the emergency room with
her nebulizer treatment. The mechanism of beta-2 agonists in asthma is:
   A. Activation of parasympathetic neurons to provide bronchodilation
   B. Stimulation to increase the secretions of the mucus glands to rid the lungs
      of irritants
   C. Stimulation of beta-2 adrenergic receptors on cells in the
      terminal bronchioles
   D. Stimulation of beta-2 adrenergic receptors on cells in the proximal bronchi
   E. Disinhibition of the medullary respiratory center located in the brainstem

Beta-2 agonists have the greatest bronchodilatory effect in the terminal bronchioles since
the largest proportion of muscle is found there. These agents also help decrease the
secretions of mucus and serous glands within the airways. The answer is C.

6. A patient is hyperventilating and loses consciousness. What is the
pathologic mechanism responsible for this disorder?
   A. Increased carbon dioxide levels in the cerebrospinal fluid
   B. Decreased carbon dioxide and hydrogen concentrations in the
      cerebrospinal fluid
   C. Increased oxygen levels in the cerebrospinal fluid
   D. nhibition of central chemoreceptors in the medulla
   E. Activation of the carotid bodies in response to decreased inhaled
      carbon dioxide

As the PCO_2 and hydrogen ion concentrations in the cerebrospinal fluid decrease, the
respiratory rate decreases. Central chemoreceptors in the medulla respond to these
concentrations by decreasing the ventilatory rate to reestablish normal levels. The
answer is B.

7. A 69-year-old with emphysema becomes less responsive with decreased respirations while on 4 liters of oxygen during a prolonged inter-facility transport.
What is the likely mechanism for these findings?

   A. Lowering of the PO_2 to very low levels causing a hypoxic drive, stimulated
      by the peripheral chemoreceptors in the carotid bodies, and suppressed
      by administration of oxygen
   B. Lowering of the PO_2 to very low levels causing suppression of the hypoxic
      drive, stimulated by the peripheral chemoreceptors in the carotid bodies
   C. Build-up of CO_2 and hydrogen ions in the cerebrospinal fluid, causing
      activation of the central chemoreceptors to suppress ventilations
   D. Lowering of the PO_2 to very low levels causing suppression of the hypoxic
      drive, stimulated by the central chemoreceptors in the medulla
   E. Lowering of the PCO_2 to very low levels causing suppression of the
      hypoxic drive, stimulated by the central chemoreceptors in the medulla

When the PO_2 falls to very low levels, the carotid bodies become sensitive to decreased
oxygen and stimulate respiration. Patients with COPD or other chronic lung disorders are
likely to have sustained low PO_2 levels and become dependent on the hypoxic drive for
regulation of respirations. High volumes of oxygen have the potential to suppress the respiratory drive in patients dependent on the peripheral rather than central chemoreceptors
for control of ventilation. The answer is A.

Despite advances in understanding the pathophysiology, diagnosis, and treatment of asthma, an increased prevalence is noted throughout the world.[1] **Bronchial asthma affects nearly 5% of the population in the United States**.[1,12] Asthma frequently takes a toll in the most vulnerable patient populations. Asthma-related mortality is especially high in the elderly and the incidence in children has increased by approximately 40% over the past 20 years.[2,3] Prehospital providers must be prepared to recognize and manage this clinical challenge as increasing numbers of patients continue to present with asthma: a disease with an immense potential for clinical deterioration.

Definitions

The National Heart, Lung, and Blood Institute defines asthma as a chronic inflammatory disorder of the airways.[3] In the past, asthma was regarded as a chronic obstructive pulmonary disease; however, since airway inflammation is the predominant feature, asthma is no longer classified primarily as an obstructive disease. For clinical purposes, patients with asthma are generally classified as having **extrinsic** or **intrinsic** asthma although most patients exhibit features of both.[2]

EXTRINSIC ASTHMA
Extrinsic asthma is believed to be caused by an antibody-dependent (IgE) activation of cells that release inflammatory mediators; for that reason, it is known also as **allergic asthma.** Usually beginning in childhood, patients with extrinsic asthma typically have a family history of allergies and a history of signs and symptoms of asthma after exposure to an allergen. This type often responds well to treatment and may improve in adolescence although reactivation in adulthood is possible.

INTRINSIC ASTHMA
Intrinsic asthma is more common in adults, is not related to antibody activation, tends to be more chronic and severe than extrinsic asthma, and is often controlled only with corticosteroids. Triggers for intrinsic asthma include exercise or infections rather than exposure to allergens. The pathophysiology of intrinsic asthma is currently poorly understood.

Pathogenesis

TRIGGERS
The hallmarks of asthma (dyspnea, chest tightness, wheezing, and cough) are related to airway obstruction caused by inflammation. In patients with intrinsic or allergic asthma, the disease process begins when a trigger (allergen) binds with an antibody (IgE) that is capable of stimulating mast cells.[4] Triggers include infections, pollens, dust mites, and other factors, many of which are listed in Table 7-1.

BRONCHIAL HYPERRESPONSIVENESS
When mast cells are stimulated by IgE antibodies, numerous mediators (*i.e.*, cytokines) are released causing smooth muscle constriction in the bronchioles, edema, and increased mucus secretion. Mediators such as leukotrienes, histamine, prostaglandins, and platelet-activating factor produce an inflammatory response and contribute to what is known as a generalized state of **bronchial hyperresponsiveness**.[2] In some instances, complete airway narrowing and severe airflow limitation can occur.

Figure 7-1 illustrates the events leading to inflammation, edema, and smooth muscle contraction in the early asthmatic response.

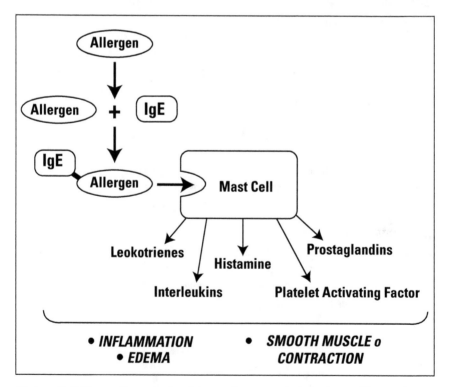

Figure 7-1 The pathogenesis of the early response in asthma. The end result is airway inflammation, edema, and smooth muscle contraction.

Table 7-1
Triggers for Asthma

Infections	Allergens	Irritants	Drugs	Food	Exercise
Chest cold	Pollens	Resins	Aspirin	Sulfites (wine)	Hyperventilation
Sinusitis	Dust	Chemicals	Beta-blockers	Shellfish	
Bronchitis	Fungal spores	Inhalants	ACE-inhibitors	MSG	
Bronchiolitis	Feathers	Tobacco smoke	NSAIDs	Food coloring	
	Animal dander	Indoor heaters	Morphine		
	Cockroaches	Cold air	Antibiotics		
		Air pollutants			

Adapted from: Williams PV. Management of asthma. *Clinical Symposium.* 1997; 49(3): 6.

THE LATE RESPONSE

The **late** response represents the secondary phase of an asthma episode, typically occurring 4 to 12 hours after the initial allergen induction in approximately 50% of all adults with extrinsic asthma and in 30% to 40% of patients with intrinsic asthma.[5] Cytokines and other mediators cause adhesion molecules to form on the inner surface of bronchi and bronchioles, allowing inflammatory cells to attach to and enter the airway tissues. As early as 15 minutes after the initial insult, T-cells enter the airway tissue followed by eosinophils and basophils.[1] These cells release mediators that are very similar to mast cells, causing airway narrowing secondary to progressive inflammation and mucus secretion. Inflammation causes the leakage of proteins into the airway tissues while the parasympathetic nervous system releases acetylcholine and causes bronchoconstriction. Once a late response is initiated in a patient with asthma, the patient is primed for future severe exacerbations as the inflammatory damage to the surface of airway cells exposes sensitive irritant receptors that can later be activated more easily upon future exposures to allergens or other stimuli.[5] Some patients with recurring signs and symptoms may also develop fibrosis below the basement membranes of the airway cell layers, a condition that can lead to chronic lung function abnormalities.

EPISODIC ASTHMA

Asthma can also be described as **episodic** if there are symptom-free intervals between symptomatic episodes, but this does not imply a different type of asthma.[2] Asthma that is initially episodic may become persistent with time. Variation of symptoms over a 24-hour period is common, with most patients developing the greatest airway narrowing in the very early morning hours (3-5 AM), resulting in wakening (nocturnal asthma) or morning tightness.[2] These patterns are manifestations of asthma severity rather than particular variants of asthma.

Clinical Assessment

CLINICAL EXAM

Asthma is a disease of airway inflammation and airflow obstruction; as such, the signs and symptoms can be highly variable, owing to the degree of severity and progression of the disease.

Wheezing occurs as airways narrow due to smooth muscle contraction. Superimposed respiratory infections can also lead to inflammation and wheezing and the intensity of wheezing does not correlate well with the severity of the asthma attack.[6] In some instances, airflow may be limited so as to produce the silent chest, a late and ominous finding in patients with asthma. The axiom that "not all that wheezes is asthma" and "not all asthma wheezes" is an appropriate clinical characterization of this disease.

A host of various nonspecific symptoms and signs can accompany an acute exacerbation of asthma. The work of breathing increases when hyperinflation occurs from air trapping in the inflamed and narrowed distal airways, leading to dyspnea and tachypnea.   Airway narrowing and mucus hypersecretion results in cough and progressive chest tightness. A fall of more than 10 mm Hg in systolic arterial pressure during inspiration, an abnormal response known as **pulsus paradoxus**, may occur as a consequence of lung hyperinflation and compression of the left ventricle. When an asthmatic patient takes a deep breath, the right ventricular end-diastolic volume temporarily increases, compressing the intraventricular septum into the left ventricle, leading to decreased cardiac output. Increased ventilation-perfusion mismatching leads to hypoxemia (*i.e.*, low SpO_2) with airway obstruction. This in turn causes decreased ventilation to airway segments while blood perfusion to these segments stays the same.

PEAK EXPIRATORY FLOW
The peak expiratory flow rate (PEF) is the highest flow rate that occurs during a forced exhalation from total lung capacity.[7] This measure can be used to provide a relatively accurate prediction of the forced expiratory volume in 1 second (FEV1) by multiplying the PEF by 9.[8] The PEF is abnormally low in asthma, although readings are highly dependent on the effort of the patient and must be interpreted prudently. Charts are available for the relative age-specific normal values; however, the PEF is best interpreted by asking the patient her or his best previous PEF, with comparison to the present value.

CLINICAL CLASSIFICATION
A classification for asthma severity was published in 1997 and is useful for guiding long-term treatment[3] (Table 7-2).

Table 7-2

The 1997 Expert Panel Report Classification of Severity of Asthma.

These clinical features are present before treatment.
Asthma Classification

Step I (Mild Intermittent)
Symptoms <2x/wk., brief exacerbations; PEF >80% predicted (+/- 20%)

Step II (Mild Persistent)
Symptoms >2x/wk., night symptoms >2x/mo., exacerbations may affect activity; PEF >80% predicted (+/- 20-30%)

Step III (Moderate Persistent)
Symptoms daily, daily use of albuterol, exacerbations > 2x/wk., night symptoms >1x/wk.; PEF>60-<80% predicted (+/- 30%)

Step IV (Severe Persistent)
Continual symptoms, limited physical activity, frequent night symptoms; PEF <60% predicted (+/- 30%)

(Source: National Asthma Education Program. *Expert Panel Report : Guidelines for the diagnosis and management of asthma.* 1997. Bethesda, MD: National Institutes of Health)

Management

While asthma is not curable, the goal of therapy in acute exacerbations is stabilization and control of symptoms with existing pharmacologic therapies. Recognizing the different stages of asthma can help direct appropriate therapy. The early asthmatic response is usually responsive to bronchodilators (*e.g.*, beta-2 agonists) save for the severe inflammation associated with the late response that can often only be controlled with corticosteroids.

BETA-ADRENERGIC AGONISTS

Beta-adrenergic agonists represent the first-line class of medications used to relieve acute symptoms in mild to moderate asthma.[11] These medications are given by inhalation and act to relax smooth muscle while also decreasing the release of mediators from mast cells and basophils. Commonly used preparations for acute exacerbations include albuterol (Ventolin®, Proventil® 0.5% solution , 5 mg/mL) and terbutaline (Brethine® 0.1% solution, 1mg/mL).

Albuterol is currently the beta-2 agonist of choice because of its relatively quick onset (within a few minutes) and duration of action (3-6 hours). Although usually administered via nebulizer, recent studies show comparable rates of symptom improvement in patients using metered dose inhalers with spacers.[7,10] For patients in severe distress, albuterol treatments can be given every 15 to 20 minutes or continuously up to three doses.

Terbutaline is another beta-2 adrenergic agonist that is usually given subcutaneously although it can also be inhaled. Its onset of action is slower than albuterol (30 minutes) with a slightly shorter duration of action (3-4 hours).

Epinephrine, a potent alpha and beta adrenergic agonist, can be administered subcutaneously although its efficacy is less than inhaled beta-2 agonists. The use of epinephrine for anaphylaxis is discussed in Chapter 18.

ANTI-INFLAMMATORY AGENTS

Since asthma is primarily an inflammatory disorder, patients should be expected to respond well to anti-inflammatory therapies. As discussed in the previous chapter, corticosteroids exert an inhibitory effect on the formation of inflammatory mediators formed in the arachidonic acid pathway. By inhibiting phospholipid A_2, these medications prevent the formation of the bronchoconstricting leukotrienes and prostaglandins. Inhaled steroids are not typically used for acute exacerbations. Oral prednisone or prednisolone is rarely given in the field and is used only when patients do not respond well to a course of bronchodilator therapy. For patients on multiple asthma medications, recent courses of steroids, or those presenting with an asthma episode of prolonged duration, **failure to initiate steroids in a timely manner could result in death.**[2,4,9] Although several studies in hospitalized patients have failed to demonstrate an advantage of IV steroids (*e.g.*, methylprednisolone) over oral steroids (e.g., prednisone), the IV route is generally preferred in most EMS systems and emergency departments.[9]

SECONDARY AGENTS
Other agents used in the chronic management of asthma include the methylated xanthines (theophylline, aminophylline), anticholinergics (ipratropium), mast cell stabilizers (cromolyn, nedocromil), and leukotriene inhibitors (zafirlukast, zileuton).[3] None of these agents, with the exception of ipratropium that can be administered with a beta-2 agonist, are currently recommended for use in acute exacerbations of asthma.[3]

Magnesium
Small studies and several case reports suggest that magnesium sulfate, a calcium channel blocker and smooth muscle relaxant, may be beneficial in the treatment of acute severe asthma.[12] This medication causes rapid but short-lived bronchodilation in human subjects. Although the medical literature has not been able to consistently affirm the possible positive effect of this drug, when administered for severe asthma, it has not been shown to be harmful.[12]

Monitoring Clinical Response

PEAK EXPIRATORY FLOW MEASUREMENTS
In the emergency department, peak expiratory flow (PEF) monitoring is frequently used to assess a patient's response to treatment. Although this technique should never be used to make the diagnosis of asthma, if the baseline PEF level is known, the severity of an acute episode can be estimated. A severe exacerbation of asthma can be correlated with a PEF value less than 50% of the patient's personal best or predicted PEF value. Unfortunately, children under 5 cannot reliably perform PEF tests and cooperation can be difficult in overly anxious and agitated patients. Therefore, while PEF provides a rapid objective assessment of a patient's condition, it should be reserved to serve as a guide to the effectiveness of therapy rather than as a diagnostic tool during acute asthma episodes.

Pulse oximetry, described in Chapter 3, is a noninvasive method for measuring oxygen saturation in patients with suspected acute exacerbations of asthma. As with PEF tests, this technology can be used to monitor responses to therapy.

Chronic Management
A stepwise approach for managing asthma in adults and children is outlined in Table 7-3.

Table 7-3
A Stepwise Approach for Managing Asthma
in Adults and Children.

Step	Quick Relief	Long-Term Control
Step 4 **Severe persistent**	Short-acting bronchodilator (a)	High dose inhaled corticosteroid AND Long-acting bronchodilator AND Corticosteroid tablets or syrup
Step 3 **Moderate persistent**	Short-acting bronchodilator (a)	Medium dose inhaled corticosteroid OR Low to medium dose inhaled corticosteroid AND Long-acting bronchodilator
Step 2 **Mild persistent**	Short-acting bronchodilator	Low dose inhaled corticosteroid OR Mast cell stabilizer (b) OR Leukotriene inhibitor
Step 1 **Mild intermittent**	Short-acting bronchodilator	No daily medication needed

(a) For children, bronchodilators are used as needed, but only up to
3 times a day
(b) Children generally start with a mast cell stabilizer (*e.g.,* cromolyn
or nedocromil)

References

1. Bone RC. Bronchial asthma: Diagnostic and treatment issues. *Hospital Practice.* 1993: 45-47.

2. Williams PV. Management of asthma. *Clinical Symposia.* 1997; 49(3): 1-27.

3. National Asthma Education Program. Expert Panel Report : *Guidelines for the diagnosis and management of asthma.* 1997. Bethesda, MD: National Institutes of Health, 1997.

4. Cydulka RK, Reilly M. Reactive airway disease. *Foresight: Risk Management For Emergency Physicians.* 1999; 45: 4-5.

5. Kaliner M. The late-phase reaction and its clinical implications. *Hosp Pract.* 1987; 22: 73.

6. Prendergast TJ , Ruoss SJ. Pulmonary disease. In McPhee SJ, Lingappa VR, Ganong WF, Lange JD. *Pathophysiology of Disease: An Introduction to Clinical Medicine.* 3rd Edition. New York: Lange Medical Books/McGraw-Hill, 2000. 202-203.

7. Light RW. Clinical pulmonary function testing, exercise testing, and disability evaluation. In George RB, Light RW, Matthay MA, Matthay RA (eds.). *Chest Medicine: Essentials of Pulmonary and Critical Care Medicine.* New York: Lippincott Williams & Wilkins, 2000. 93.

8. Heaf PJD, Gillam PMS. Peak flow rates in normal and asthmatic children. *Br Med J* 1962; 1: 1595-1596.

9. Darr, CD. Asthma and bronchiolitis. In Rosen P, Barkin R, *et al.* (eds.). *Emergency Medicine: Concepts and Clinical Practice.* New York: Mosby, 1997. 1137-1149.

10. Kerem E, Levison H, Schuh S, *et al.* Efficacy of albuterol administered by nebulizer vs. spacer device in children with acute asthma. *J Pediatr.* 1993; 123: 313.

11. Nelson HS. Adrenergic therapy of bronchial asthma. *J Allergy Clin Immunol.* 1986; 77: 771.

12. Rowe BH, Bretzlaff JA, Bourdon C, Bota GW, Cmargo CA. Intravenous magnesium sulfate treatment for acute asthma in the emergency department: A systematic review of the literature. *Ann Emerg Med.* 2000; 36(3): 181-190.

Review Questions

1. A 12-year-old male presents to the emergency department for treatment of asthma. Therapy to correct this patient's condition should be aimed at:
    A. Stimulating mast cells to clear the airways of inflammatory mediators.
    B. Administering intravenous steroids immediately, before nebulizer treatments can be started, to prevent a potential late response.
    C. Bronchodilators and anti-inflammatory agents to reverse the underlying disorder.
    D. Mast cell stabilizers and anticholinergic medications to bind IgE antibodies.
    E. Diuretics and anti-inflammatory medications to decrease edema and smooth muscle contraction.

Asthma is an inflammatory disorder; therefore, anti-inflammatory therapies such as inhaled or intravenous steroids are usually appropriate, but should not be administered until beta-2 agonists have been provided to improve air entry and reverse bronchoconstriction. The answer is C.

2. Which of the following is true regarding the use of peak expiratory flow (PEF) measurements in asthmatic patients?
    A. PEF determinations help make the diagnosis of asthma and guide therapy.
    B. PEF determinations provide an estimate of residual lung volume and inspiratory capacity.
    C. PEF determinations are useful in patients as young as 3-year-olds.
    D. PEF determinations are necessary before intravenous steroids can be considered for use.
    E. PEF determinations provide a relatively accurate prediction of the FEV1.

PEF measurements are meant to serve as a guide to the effectiveness of therapy and are not used to make a diagnosis of asthma. When multiplied by 9, PEF measurements provide a relatively accurate prediction of the FEV_1, a measurement otherwise only obtainable by pulmonary function testing. The answer is E.

3. Which of the following mechanisms is thought to be responsible for the secondary phase of asthma occurring 4 to 12 hours after the initial exacerbation?
   A. Allergen induction and IgE binding to mast cells.
   B. Release of inflammatory mediators by T-cells, eosinophils, and basophils.
   C. Parasympathetic inhibition and increased mucus secretions.
   D. Detachment of adhesion molecules and circulating immune complexes.
   E. Programmed cell death and leakage of lymph into the bronchioles.

IgE antibody stimulation of mast cells is thought to be responsible for the initial symptoms of an asthma attack. The late response occurs in up to 50% of adult and 30% to 40% of pediatric patients and is believed to be the result of cytokine stimulation and activation of inflammatory cells such as T-cells, eosinophils, and basophils. The answer is B.

4. A 9-year-old patient with no history of respiratory disease presents with acute dyspnea and wheezing after exposure to pollen. The patient has a positive family history of allergies and a mother with asthma. The physical exam is significant for moderate wheezing and pulsus paradoxus. After one treatment with nebulized albuterol, the patient reports significant relief and the lung sounds improve. What type of asthma would this patient have?
   A. Moderate persistent asthma
   B. Intrinsic asthma
   C. Extrinsic asthma
   D. Episodic asthma
   E. Anaphylactic asthma

Extrinsic asthma is believed to be caused by IgE activation of inflammatory cells after exposure to an allergen. It is also referred to as allergic asthma. Intrinsic asthma is more common in adults than in children and is usually only controlled by steroids. There is not enough information to classify this patient under the 1997 Expert Panel Report's scheme. The answer is C.

5-10. Match the agent with the correct mechanism of action.
   A. Beta-2 agonist
   B. Phospholipid A_2 inhibitor
   C. Calcium channel blocker and smooth muscle relaxant
   D. Mast cell stabilizer
   E. Leukotriene inhibitor

   5. Albuterol
   6. Zafirlukast
   7. Cromolyn
   8. Methylprednisolone
   9. Magnesium sulfate
   10. Terbutaline

5. A.

6. E.

7. D.

8. B.

9. C.

10. A.

11. A 34-year-old woman with a history of severe persistent asthma is intubated en route to the hospital for respiratory failure. The patient's lung sounds were decreased bilaterally upon initial assessment. The silent chest in severe asthma exacerbations is due to:
   A. Lung hyperinflation and compression of the left ventricle
   B. Severe bronchoconstriction as the result of inflammation
   C. Air leakage in the distal airways
   D. Mucus hyposecretion and increased cardiac output
   E. Airflow obstruction due to interstitial fluid shifts and lung edema

The answer is B.

Chronic Obstructive Pulmonary Disease

Chronic obstructive pulmonary disease (COPD) is a term used to represent a spectrum of disease states characterized by the presence of airflow obstruction due to emphysema or bronchitis.[1] COPD is also referred to as chronic obstructive lung disease (COLD) and chronic airway obstruction (CAO). At least 15 million Americans are estimated to suffer from COPD, making it the fifth most common leading cause of death in the United States.[2] Since the early 1980s, both the prevalence and mortality have continued to increase.

Risk Factors

Several risk factors for COPD have been identified, but by far, **the primary cause is almost invariably related to tobacco smoke exposure.**[1] Both passive and active smoking substantially increase the risk for COPD. Tobacco smoke impairs ciliary movement, inhibits the function of macrophages in alveoli, and leads to overstimulation of mucus glands.[1] Stimulation of sensitive irritant receptors in the airways can induce smooth muscle contraction and bronchoconstriction.

Other risk factors for COPD include air pollution, genetic factors, infections, occupational exposure to noxious gases or dusts, and alpha$_1$-antitrypsin deficiency.[1] Exposure to sulfur dioxide and nitrogen dioxide have been proposed to cause bronchitis, although the role of these pollutants appears to be small compared to tobacco smoke exposure. Infections with viruses and bacteria have also been thought to cause COPD exacerbations, and there is some evidence that severe viral pneumonia early during infancy may predispose patients to COPD. The genetic transmission of COPD has not been proven although studies involving twins have suggested a genetic link to the development of bronchitis despite a negative smoking history. The only known genetic abnormality that has been shown to cause COPD is alpha$_1$-antitrypsin deficiency.[1] Deficiency of the enzyme alpha$_1$-antitrypsin leads to autodigestion of lung tissue by other enzymes known as proteases. Emphysema may develop early in patients with this well-known genetic factor; smoking accelerates the progression to COPD in patients with a deficiency of this enzyme.

Clinical Manifestations

Emphysema and bronchitis are the disease entities that represent the two ends of the clinical and pathophysiologic spectrum of COPD. For this reason, each disease is discussed separately eventhough most patients with COPD have a combination of both components (Table 8-1).

Table 8-1
The clinical spectrums of chronic obstructive pulmonary disease.

Characteristics	Pink Puffers	Blue Bloaters
Age	>60	Young (50's)
Disease process	Emphysema	Chronic bronchitis
Cough?	Mild	Chronic cough
Weight changes?	Weight loss	Weight gain
Sputum?	Scant	Copious
Degree of hypoxia	Mild	Can be severe
Response to bronchodilators	Mild improvement	Increased
Cough type	"Dyspneic"	"Tussive"
Accessory muscle use?	Yes	No
Hyperventilation?	Yes	No

PINK PUFFERS

The first class of patients with COPD are commonly referred to as pink puffers because these patients have the ability to maintain near-normal oxygen levels by overventilating. Pink puffers have a predominantly **emphysematous** component to their disease. Usually diagnosed after the age of 60, dyspnea is severe, although PO_2 and PCO_2 levels are only slightly abnormal (mild hypoxia; mild hypocapnia) since equal portions of ventilated and perfused lung segments are lost. Cough and production of sputum are not as pronounced as in patients with a bronchitic component. Examination of the chest frequently reveals a prolonged expiratory component with wheezing on forced expiration. These patients often lean forward, bracing themselves on their forearms in the tripod position, to maximize the efficiency of the accessory muscles for expiration and diaphragmatic excursions. Over time, patients with emphysema become progressively dyspneic and more often than not endure a slowly declining course.

Pathogenesis of Emphysema

Permanent destruction of the elastic segments of alveoli by mechanical, chemical, or other factors is the pathologic hallmark of emphysema. When the alveolar walls and supporting structures are lost, the airways become narrow and have a greater tendency to collapse during expiration and trap air in the distal alveoli. Permanent dilation of the pulmonary air spaces occurs beyond the terminal bronchioles with destruction of the airway walls. For this reason, patients with emphysema develop what is known as the barrel chest. Both the residual and functional residual volumes are almost always increased in emphysema due to the greater lung compliance that results from the formation of large air spaces and free-floating segments of damaged pulmonary tissue. The vital capacity is typically decreased considerably.

BLUE BLOATERS

The second class of COPD patients have predominant chronic bronchitis and are referred to as blue bloaters. These patients commonly have a history of chronic cough and sputum production for many years. For patients to be diagnosed with chronic bronchitis, they must have a history of increased mucus production and chronic cough for at least 3 months of the year for 2 consecutive years.[1,2] Unlike the patient with emphysema, the patient with bronchitis is generally younger, overweight, and cyanotic. Despite chronic cough and significant sputum production, the respiratory rate is frequently normal or slightly increased without accessory muscle use. PCO_2 is higher and PO_2 is lower in patients with chronic bronchitis. On auscultation, coarse rhonchi and wheezes can usually be heard.

Pathogenesis of Chronic Bronchitis

Irritation of the mucosa by smoke, chemicals, fumes, pollutants, and other irritants leads to hyperplasia of mucus glands and disruption of the normal function of cilia in the respiratory tissue lining the airways. Airway passages become narrower from mucosal inflammation, edema, and mucus plugging; the smaller bronchi and bronchioles are particularly affected. Alterations in the respiratory lining may lead to secondary infection with a variety of bacterial organisms including *streptococci* species and *haemophilus influenza*. Viruses commonly implicated include the rhinovirus and adenovirus.

Management

The goals of pharmacologic intervention in cases of acute COPD exacerbations are to induce bronchodilation, decrease inflammation, and promote expectoration.[4] Several classes of medications can be used to achieve these goals.

BETA-2 AGONISTS

As with the treatment for acute exacerbations of asthma, beta-2 agonist aerosols represent the first-line class of agents to be used in the management of acute, severe COPD.[1,4,5] Beta-2 agonists increase airflow and reduce dyspnea in patients with COPD.[6] Albuterol, pirbuterol, metaproterenol, terbutaline, and isoetharine are more selective than other beta agonists such as epinephrine and ephedrine. These medications have a diminished half-life in acute exacerbations of COPD and may be administered under shorter intervals (every 30-60 minutes) as tolerated.[1]

ANTICHOLINERGIC AGENTS

In patients with a history of inadequate response to beta-2 agonists, anticholinergic aerosols (*e.g.*, ipratropium) can be considered for use.[7] As opposed to beta-2 agonists, these agents have a prolonged half-life in patients with COPD and usually should be administered every 4 to 8 hours during acute, severe exacerbations. Anticholinergic aerosols can also be combined with beta-2 agonists although combination therapy is not more effective than increased doses of individual agents.[8]

OXYGEN

Patients with acute, severe COPD have the potential to become hypoxic. Oxygen therapy is often initiated with the aim of keeping the oxygen saturation (SpO_2) above 90%.[1] The standard dual-prong nasal cannula is the most common and effective route of oxygen delivery for COPD patients. The percentage of delivered oxygen (FIO_2) can be estimated by adding 20% to the oxygen liter flow rate multiplied by 4 (20% + 4 x O_2 flow rate). Face masks can be used in patients who are strictly mouth breathers or in patients with nasal congestion or obstruction. Venturi masks allow for the administration of a constant FIO_2. In patients who are severely hypoxic (*e.g.*, SpO_2 <80%), oxygen can be administered via a nonrebreathing mask with a reservoir. This method of oxygen delivery can provide an FIO_2 greater than 90%. For purposes of prehospital management, and since transport times are relatively short, suppression of ventilation due to the hypoxic drive is unlikely during the administration of oxygen. A general rule of thumb to follow with COPD patients is **if the patient is hypoxic and needs oxygen, provide it.**

METHYLATED XANTHINES

If appropriate administration of aerosol therapy cannot be initiated, methylated xanthines can be used. Theophylline is well-known for its toxicity and numerous drug-drug interactions; nevertheless, it remains a viable alternative for patients who cannot use aerosol therapy reliably. In some patients, theophylline has anti-inflammatory properties.[9]

STEROIDS

Corticosteroids have a limited utility in treating acute exacerbations of COPD.[1,4,10,11] A study of over 1800 patients determined that treatment with systemic glucocorticoids resulted in moderate clinical improvement during the first 2 weeks of therapy in hospitalized patients, but conferred no benefit in terms of long-term mortality.[11] Many experts agree that corticosteroids are only useful if patients have an asthma-like component to their disease.[10] The inhaled route of delivery is preferred in these cases.[10]

References

1. American Thoracic Society Statement. Standards for the diagnosis and care of patients with chronic obstructive pulmonary disease. *Resp Crit Care Med* (Supplement) 1995; 152 (5): S78-S100.

2. Honig EG, Ingram RH. Chronic bronchitis, emphysema, and airways obstruction. *In* Fauci AS, Braunwald E, Isselbacher KJ, *et al.* (editors). *Harrison's Principles of Internal Medicine.* 14th Ed. New York: McGraw-Hill, 1998. 1451-1457.

3. Kobzik L, Schoen FJ. The Lung. *In* Cotran RS, Kumar V, Robbins SL. *Robbins Pathologic Basis of Disease* 2nd Ed. Philadelphia: W.B. Saunders Co., 1994. 683-689.

4. Ferguson GT, Cherniack RM. Management of chronic obstructive pulmonary disease. *N Eng J Med* 1993; 328: 1017-1022.

5. Postma DS. Inhaled therapy in COPD: What are the benefits? *Respir Med* 1991; 85: 447-449.

6. Nisar M, Earis JE, Pearson MG, *et al.* Acute bronchodilator trials in chronic obstructive pulmonary disease. *Am Rev Respir Dis* 1992; 146: 555-559.

7. Karpel JP. Bronchodilator responses to anticholinergic and beta-adrenergic agents in acute and stable COPD. *Chest* 1991; 99: 871-876.

8. Karpel JP, Kotch A, Zinny J, *et al.* A comparison of inhaled ipratropium, oral theophylline plus inhaled beta-agonist, and the combination of all three in patients with COPD. *Chest* 1994; 105: 1089-1094.

9. Sullivan P, Bekir S, Jaffar Z, *et al.* Anti-inflammatory effects of low-dose oral theophylline in atopic asthma. *Lancet* 1994; 343: 1006-1008.

10. Hudson LD, Monti CM. Rationale and use of corticosteroids in chronic obstructive pulmonary disease. *Med Clin N Am* 1990; 74: 661-690.

11. Niewoehner DE, Erbland ML, Deupree RH, *et al.* for the Department of Veterans Affairs Cooperative Study Group. Effect of systemic glucocorticoids on exacerbations of chronic obstructive pulmonary disease. *N Eng J Med* 1999; 340: 1941-1947.

Review Questions

1. What pathologic changes are thought to be responsible for the development of the barrel chest of emphysema?
   A. Permanent dilatation of the pulmonary air spaces with destruction of the airway walls
   B. Stretching of bronchi with air trapping in the pleural space
   C. Formation of small air spaces in segments of lung with air leakage into the pleura
   D. Alveolar expansion during expiration due to decreased surfactant formation
   E. Increased vital capacity due to air trapping in the distal alveoli

The vital capacity is decreased considerably in emphysema, not increased. Permanent destruction of the elastic segments of alveoli is the pathologic hallmark of emphysema. The answer is A.

2. All of the following classes of medications can be used in acute COPD exacerbations EXCEPT:
   A. Beta-2 adrenergic receptor agonists
   B. Systemic corticosteroids
   C. Methylated xanthines
   D. Cholinergic agonists
   E. Anticholinergic agents

Cholinergic agents such as physostigmine increase secretions in the lung and are absolutely contraindicated. The answer is D.

3. You are on the scene with an elderly male patient in moderate respiratory distress. Vital signs are: BP 132/88 RR 26 HR 100. Auscultation of the lungs reveals coarse rhonchi and wheezes. What is the single greatest risk factor for COPD?
   A. Previous exposure to sulfur dioxide and nitrogen dioxide
   B. A history of Alpha1-antitrypsin deficiency
   C. Exposure to significant air pollution
   D. A history of severe viral pneumonia during infancy
   E. Tobacco smoke exposure

All of the above are risk factors for developing COPD, but tobacco smoke exposure is by far the most important. The answer is E.

4-8. Match the following clinical characteristics to the most appropriate type of COPD patient.
   A. Blue bloaters (chronic bronchitis)
   B. Pink puffers (emphysema)
   C. Neither of the above

   4. A 66-year-old woman with dyspnea, mild hypoxia, and a history of weight loss.
   5. A 55-year-old morbidly obese smoker with dyspnea who improves significantly after two treatments with nebulized albuterol
   6. A 72-year-old male smoker with accessory muscle use, hyperventilation, and a barrel chest on physical examination.
   7. A 50-year-old female with a history of chronic occupational smoke exposure who presents with copious sputum, chronic cough, and severe hypoxia.
   8. An 8-year-old female with a history of wheezing and rhonchi after exposure to a new pet cat.

4. B.

5. A.

6. B.

7. A.

8. COPD is an adult disease. Other causes of dyspnea and wheezing must be considered in pediatric patients. The answer is C.

Pulmonary Embolism

Despite new technologies for recognition and management, deaths attributable to pulmonary thromboembolic disease continue to be substantial. Of patients with pulmonary emboli (PE) presenting to the emergency room, approximately **1 in 10 die within the first 60 minutes.**[1] Each year an estimated 500,000 patients suffer from a pulmonary embolic event and about 50,000 of these patients die.[2-4] Considering the prevalence of this disease, every emergency care provider is likely to encounter this potentially lethal disorder.

Risk Factors

All known clinical risk factors for deep vein thrombosis (DVT) and pulmonary embolism have in common one or more predisposing factors from **Virchow's triad**: venostasis, vessel wall inflammation and/or endothelial injury, and hypercoagulability.[5] A variety of inherited and acquired hypercoagulable states are known and listed in Table 9-1. **The strongest risk factor for PE is a history of a previous DVT or PE.**[3-6] Recent surgery, pregnancy, prolonged immobilization, or the presence of an underlying malignancy should raise the index of suspicion in patients with suspected PE.

Table 9-1
Inherited and Acquired Hypercoagulable States

Inherited Hypercoagulable States	Acquired Hypercoagulable States
Antithrombin III deficiency	Pregnancy
Protein C deficiency	Chronic disseminated intravascular Coagulation (Trousseau's syndrome)
Protein S deficiency	Oral birth control pills
Protein C substrate deficiency	Nephrotic syndrome
Abnormal fibrinogens	Lupus anticoagulant (anticardiolipin antibodies)
Excessive t-PA inhibitor production	Heparin-induced thrombocytopenia

Pathogenesis

Pulmonary thromboembolism should not be regarded as a pulmonary disease; rather, it is a complication of underlying blood clots that were already formed in the venous system. With few exceptions, almost all **emboli arise within the large deep veins of the pelvis and lower extremities** (*i.e.*. popliteal, femoral, or iliac veins,[5] Figure 9-1). Thrombus almost always starts in the veins of the calf and propagates to veins above the knee in 87% of the cases of DVT.[5-7] Over 90% of pulmonary emboli arise from thrombi within popliteal, femoral, and iliac veins.[5-7] This pathologic process creates a dilemma for clinicians and prehospital providers because most DVTs are clinically silent (*i.e.*, remain undetectable on physical exam). DVTs and pulmonary emboli can only be detected with specific radiological tests.

Once thrombi are dislodged from the venous circulation in the lower extremities, emboli are sent to the pulmonary circulation, commonly settling in the blood vessels of the lung. In some cases, a saddle embolus forms when a clot impacts against the bifurcation of the pulmonary arteries.[5] Emboli can occlude the main pulmonary artery or break off into segments and pass into the progressively branching pulmonary vessels as multiple small emboli. Occlusion of circulation to lung segments creates a ventilation-perfusion (V/Q) mismatch (Figure 9-2).

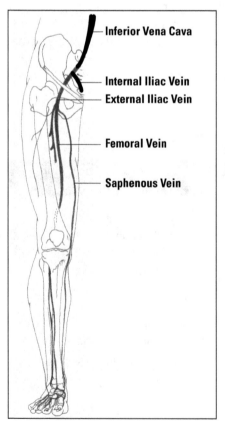

Inferior Vena Cava

Internal Iliac Vein

External Iliac Vein

Femoral Vein

Saphenous Vein

Figure 9-1 The anatomy of the lower extremity venous system.

Alveoli, deprived of circulation, continue to be ventilated despite an inability to exchange oxygen and carbon dioxide. Without blood flow, these air spaces become alveolar dead space. Since the blood content is devoid of oxygen as a result of poor oxygenation at the alveolar level, hypoxemia can ensue. Despite this fact, some patients avoid hypoxemia by hyperventilating, allowing remaining functional alveoli to compensate for the existing areas of V/Q mismatch.

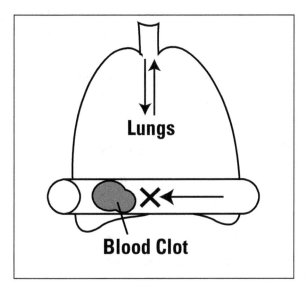

Figure 9-2
Ventilation-Perfusion (V/Q) mismatching. See text for explanation.

Clinical Manifestations

Even though PE is a fairly common complication of thrombotic disease, its clinical manifestations are elusive and can easily be confused with other disease processes. The classic triad of hemoptysis, dyspnea, and chest pain is present in less than 20% of cases of PE (Table 9-2).[6] The most common symptoms and signs of PE include: dyspnea, pleuritic chest pain, apprehension, cough, tachypnea (rate>16), rales, and tachycardia.[10] Other signs and symptoms ranging from fever, sweating, syncope, and cyanosis may also be present; however, no set of signs and symptoms is specific for PE.[11] Therefore, **clinical diagnosis of PE is unreliable and should never be attempted.**

Taking a thorough and directed history can frequently provide more useful information than physical exam alone. Indeed, in the management of PE, **the prehospital provider's history may provide the most important clue to the underlying disease process for patients who deteriorate before interrogation by emergency department staff.** Since several signs and symptoms of pneumonia and asthma overlap with PE, PE is often confused with these diseases. In fact, confusing PE with pneumonia is the single most common discrepancy for pulmonary causes of death in patients with PE.[12] Patients with PE who are misdiagnosed with asthma show little or no response to the administration of bronchodilators.

Table 9-2

Clinical Manifestations of Pulmonary Embolism

Symptoms	Percent	Signs	Percent
Dyspnea	84	Tachypnea (<16/min.)	92
Pleuritic chest pain	74	Crackles	
Apprehension	59		58
Cough	53	Loud S2 Heart Sound	53
Hemoptysis	30	Tachycardia (>100/min.)	44
Sweating	27		
		Fever	43
		S3 or S4 Gallop	34
		Lower Extremity Edema	24

Complications

Serious potential complications of PE include pulmonary infarction (death of lung tissue) or heart failure due to increased back-pressure secondary to occluded circulatory segments. Complete infarction of lung tissue is uncommon because the lung has three sources of oxygen supply: the pulmonary artery, the airways, and collateral arterial circulation. Although the lung has an extensive cross-sectional area of circulation, if the embolic occlusion is large enough, pulmonary vascular resistance can increase to the point of inducing right heart failure.[13] The risk of right heart failure, therefore, is in direct proportion to the size of the embolic obstruction.

Definitive Diagnosis and Treatment

Once in the emergency department, an extensive diagnostic work-up should take place. Laboratory tests such as the D-dimer and A-a gradient are frequently determined to find evidence of blood clot degradation and possible V/Q discrepancies.[14] Duplex Doppler exams, V-Q scans, and helical (spiral) computed tomography scanning provide additional functional and structural information that can help rule in or rule out PE.[4] The gold standard for diagnosis is angiography, although even with this technique small emboli can occasionally be missed.[4]

During transport, oxygen can be administered to maintain an adequate SPO_2 and to treat hypoxemia. Barring any contraindications, anticoagulation with unfractionated heparin or low molecular weight heparin (enoxaparin) can be initiated as soon as the diagnosis of PE is entertained, even before diagnostic confirmation.[15] This treatment is frequently initiated upon arrival in the emergency department. Patients may be started on warfarin, but only after heparin is initiated to avoid the potential complications of clot extension and hypercoagulability.[4,15] Thrombolysis is an option for severely hemodynamically unstable patients and for patients expected to have multiple recurrences of PE. Compression stockings, surgical embolectomies, and vena cava filters (*e.g.*, Greenfield filter) represent additional treatment modalities.

Other Types of Emboli

FAT EMBOLI

There are other conditions that can lead to embolization to the pulmonary circulation. Fat emboli, occasionally occurring after fractures of the long bones (*i.e.*, tibia, femur), can cause pulmonary damage in spite of the fact that most fat emboli pass **through** the pulmonary circulation, affecting various other end-organs (*e.g.*, brain). In instances of severe skeletal trauma, fat embolism can be detected in up to 90% of patients, but only 1% become symptomatic.[5] It is thought that small particles of fat cause occlusion of pulmonary and cerebral blood vessels while free fatty acids released from fat globules result in toxic injury.[8] The occlusion of pulmonary and cerebral blood vessels explains the neurologic and pulmonary symptoms that manifest 24 to 72 hours after injury.[5,8] A skin rash is also common; the fat globules decrease the platelets by binding to them, leading to a petechial skin rash.[8]

AIR EMBOLI AND AMNIOTIC FLUID EMBOLI

Air emboli and amniotic fluid emboli are other causes of pulmonary emboli. Amniotic fluid emboli are most common at the end of the first stage of labor.[9] Air emboli are typically iatrogenically induced (resulting from the action of the provider; *e.g.*, during placement of central lines, etc.).

References

1. Carson JL, Kelley MA, Duff A, *et al*. The clinical course of pulmonary embolism. *N Engl J Med* 1992; 326: 1240.

2. Rubenstein I, Murray D, Hoffsten V. Fatal pulmonary emboli in hospitalized patients. *Arch Int Med* 1988; 148: 1425-1426.

3. Bell WR, Smith TL. Current status of pulmonary thromboembolic disease: pathophysiology, diagnosis, prevention and treatment. *Am Heart J* 1982; 103: 239-262.

4. Moser KM. Venous thromboembolism. *Amer Rev Resp Dis* 1990; 141(1): 235-238.

5. Kobzik L, Schoen FJ. The Lung. *In* Cotran RS, Kumar V, Robbins SL. *Robbins Pathologic Basis of Disease*, 2nd Ed. Philadelphia: W.B. Saunders Co., 1994.

6. Feied C. Pulmonary embolism. *In*: Rosen P, Barkin R, *et al*. *Emergency Medicine: Concepts and Clinical Practice*. New York: Mosby, 1997. 1770-1800.

7. Huet Y, Brun-Buisson C, Lemaire F, *et al*. Cardiopulmonary effects of ketanserin infusion in human pulmonary embolism. *Am J Resp Dis* 1987; 135: 114-117.

8. Van Besouw JP, Hinds CJ. Fat embolism syndrome. *Br J Hosp Med* 1989; 42: 304.

9. Price TM *et al*. Amniotic fluid embolism: Three case reports with a review of the literature. *Obstet Gynecol Surv* 1985; 40: 462.

10. UPET: The urokinase pulmonary embolism trial: A national cooperative study. *Circulation* 1973; 47(Suppl).

11. USPET: Urokinase streptokinase pulmonary embolism trial: Phase III results. *JAMA* 1974; 229: 1606.

12. Thulbeck WB. Accuracy of clinical diagnosis in a Canadian teaching hospital. *Can Med Assoc J* 1981; 443: 125.

13. Vlahakes GJ, Turley K, Hoffman JIE. The pathophysiology of failure in acute right ventricular hypertension: Hemodynamic and biochemical correlations. *Circulation*. 1981; 63: 87-95.

14. Kline JA, Johns KL, Colucciello SA, Israel EG. New diagnostic tests for pulmonary embolism. *Ann Emerg Med* 2000; 35(2): 168-180.

15. Tapson VF. Management of the critically ill patient with pulmonary embolism. *J Crit Illness* 2000; 15(7 Supplement): S18-S23.

Review Questions

1. A patient transported to the emergency department for acute dyspnea and tachycardia is found to have a large pulmonary embolism detected by spiral computed tomography. All of the following are risk factors for developing a pulmonary embolism EXCEPT:
A. Venostasis, vessel wall inflammation
B. Known hypercoagulable state
C. Pregnancy
D. Prolonged strenuous physical activity
E. Recent surgery

Prolonged immobilization, not physical activity, is a strong risk factor for pulmonary embolism. The most important risk factor is a history of a previous DVT or PE. The answer is D.

2. What are the two leading signs and symptoms most sensitive for pulmonary embolism?
A. Tachypnea and dyspnea
B. Diaphoresis and tachycardia
C. Fever and syncope
D. Pleuritic chest pain and apprehension
E. Crackles on lung exam and cyanosis

All of the other choices are common signs and symptoms of PE too, but no set of signs and symptoms is sensitive enough to rule in PE on clinical grounds. Confusing PE with pneumonia is the single most common cause of misdiagnosis. The answer is A.

3. All of the following are acceptable actions during prehospital transport of a patient with suspected pulmonary embolism EXCEPT:
A. Supplemental oxygen to maintain SPO_2 above 95%
B. Prehospital 12-lead ECG
C. Heparin or low molecular weight heparin if approved by medical control during a prolonged transport
D. Intravenous thrombolytics if approved by medical control during a prolonged transport
E. Application of compression stockings and intravenous fluids titrated to keep the cannulated vein open

Anticoagulation may be considered even before the formal diagnosis of PE is made, but should be done with caution and only in special situations. Thrombolytics should never be administered in the prehospital arena for PE. Supportive measures and attention to the ABCs remain are the fundamental aspects of care rendered by prehospital providers for suspected PE. The answer is D.

Section III

Cardiovascular Pathophysiology

Basic Cardiac Physiology

In the chapters that follow, the pathophysiology of common cardiac emergencies is presented. To fully understand the pathogenesis of these diseases, one must first attain an appreciation for basic cardiac physiology. ECG interpretation should be studied and mastered independently after the processes in basic cardiac physiology are learned. Several excellent references for learning the essentials of 12-lead ECG interpretation are listed at the end of this chapter. Appendix II in this text provides a systematic approach for analyzing the 12-lead ECG.

Cardiac Action Potentials and Myocardial Contraction

ACTION POTENTIALS

The action potential is the central event that initiates cardiac muscle contraction. The word **potential** is a confusing term. Potential refers to the state of electrical tension in an electrical source that enables the source to do work under suitable conditions.[1] Electrical potential is analogous to temperature in relation to heat, and is measured in volts (millivolts). The change in cell membrane potential, which occurs as the result of the movement of sodium, potassium, and calcium, produces electrical signals that alter cellular activities. This change in membrane potential is known as an **action potential**. An action potential represents the electrical activity of the cardiac cell membrane during the exchange of electrolytes throughout the process of muscle contraction. The voltage changes during an action potential can be measured and graphed in the laboratory by placing a microelectrode in a cardiac cell.

DEPOLARIZATION

For an action potential to occur, the cell membrane of cardiac muscle must first lose its negative charge. This process is known as **depolarization**. Under normal conditions, an electrical gradient is maintained by sodium/potassium ATPase pumps embedded in the cell membrane. These pumps move potassium in and sodium out of cells. Although potassium carries a positive charge like sodium and potassium, the negatively charged organic acids and other molecules inside the cell are more numerous, thus imparting an overall negative charge to the cell under resting conditions. When depolarization occurs, this balance is temporarily upset. Sodium is allowed to move into the cells and is followed by calcium along an osmotic gradient (*i.e.*, high to low). Potassium moves out of the cell when sodium and calcium move into the cell. This series of events is schematically described in Figure 10-1.

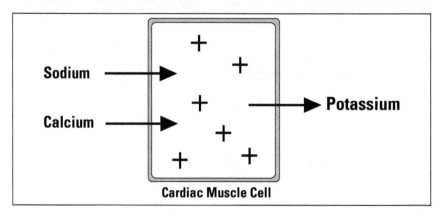

Figure 10-1 Electrolyte exchange during cardiac depolarization.

PHASES OF THE ACTION POTENTIAL

The phases of the cardiac action potential are numbered and correspond to intracellular changes in sodium, calcium, and potassium concentrations[2] (Figure 10-2). The example provided demonstrates the stages of an action potential for ventricular muscle. During **phase 4**, the ventricular cells are in **diastole**, a period of cardiac inactivity between beats. Channels in the cell membrane are predominantly permeable to potassium at this stage. **Phase 0** represents **depolarization** of the cell membrane secondary to increased sodium influx through a voltage-sensitive channel. A slight overshoot (+20 millivolts) occurs during this rapid upstroke of electrical activity. The next phase, **phase 1**, is the **termination of depolarization** and the beginning of a period of **partial repolarization**. The overshoot is corrected as some sodium leaves the cell membrane due to closure of the sodium channels. **Phase 2** is **systole**, or the period when the heart is actively contracting. The action potential is a plateau at this phase due to a slow inward flux of calcium through slow voltage-dependent channels. During this phase, coupling of the cardiac muscle myofibrils occurs causing contraction. **Phase 3** represents **rapid repolarization** or restoration of the resting membrane potential. The slow calcium channels are deactivated, the sodium channels are reset, and potassium continues to leave the cell until the ATP pump exchanges enough sodium and potassium to restore the phase 4 resting membrane potential.

PACEMAKER ACTION POTENTIALS

The action potentials for the sinoatrial (S-A) and atrioventricular (A-V) nodes are slightly different though the stages are comparable and correspond to similar events.[3] The S-A node is the primary pacemaker of the heart, dispatching depolarizations at a faster rate (60-100 beats/minute in adults) than the A-V node (40-60 beats/minute) and the ventricular cells in the myocardium (<40 beats/minute). Despite having a faster overall rate, action potentials of the S-A and A-V nodes are referred to as slow response action potentials because phase 0 is a gradual rather than rapid upstroke of electrical activity. A slow response action potential is compared with a ventricular action potential in Figure 10-3.

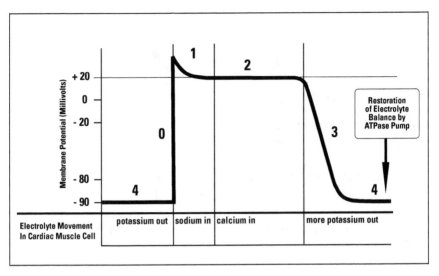

Figure 10-2 Action potential for ventricular muscle cell. See text for details.

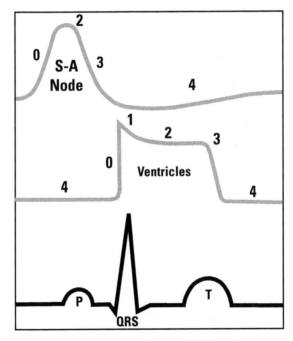

Figure 10-3 Correlation of cardiac action potentials in the S-A node and ventricles with the electrocardiogram.

REFRACTORY PERIODS

A period of time exists between depolarizations when a normal stimulation does not activate a cell. These periods are known as **refractory periods** and can be **absolute** (*i.e.*, no action potential can be generated) or **relative** (*i.e.*, if the stimulus is strong enough, an action potential can be generated). Refractory periods allow the contractile cells of the heart time to relax between contractions, permitting time for the ventricles to fill with adequate amounts of blood before systole.

Biochemical Correlation

Action potentials provide the means for the biochemical activation of contractile fibers in the myocardium, the muscular layer of the heart. Either voltage-dependent membrane channels or beta receptors allow cyclic AMP (cAMP) to be formed within the muscle cells. Cyclic AMP changes the surface configuration of proteins to allow more calcium to enter the cardiac cells. Increased calcium influx causes the storage sites for calcium within the cells (*e.g.*, sarcoplasmic reticulum) to release additional amounts of calcium. The release and influx of calcium is important because it allows the actin and myosin in muscle fibers to bind together in a series of what are known as crossbridge cycles. During these cycles, calcium and ATP facilitate these reactions, causing muscle fiber complexes to shorten (contract) and relax.

Electrophysiologic Correlation

The sequence of electrophysiologic events that occur after action potentials are generated at the S-A node and elsewhere can be recorded on an electrocardiogram (ECG). **P waves** represent the depolarization of atrial muscles but do not represent the repolarization of these tissues because this process occurs during the QRS complex. The **QRS complex** represents depolarization of ventricular muscle tissue. The **T wave** is the final segment (sometimes followed by a U wave) and represents ventricular repolarization.

Pressures, Forces, and Volumes During Myocardial Contraction

PRESSURES

A variety of terms are used to describe the events of cardiac contractility. As mentioned previously, systole is the period where the heart is contracting and diastole is the period of cardiac inactivity between beats. The systolic pressure is the highest arterial pressure during a cardiac cycle; the diastolic pressure is the lowest. The mean arterial pressure (MAP) is the average blood pressure between systole and diastole. It can be calculated by multiplying the difference between systolic and diastolic pressures by 1/3 and adding this value to the diastolic pressure (**MAP= Diastolic + 1/3 x [Systolic-Diastolic]**).

PRELOAD AND AFTERLOAD

Before blood can be pumped through the vessels during these periods, two forces must be overcome. The first force, **preload**, is the force exerted on the myocardial contractile cells by the end-diastolic volume: the volume of blood contained in the ventricle immediately prior to contraction. Preload is related to the amount of stretch exerted on the heart muscles at the end of diastole. **Afterload** is the force against which the ventricle must contract. When the force of afterload is overcome and blood is ejected from the ventricle, the remaining volume is known as the **end-systolic volume**. The **stroke volume** is the amount of blood ejected from the heart during each heartbeat. When this value is known (measured by invasive techniques in an intensive care unit), it can be multiplied by the heart rate to give the total **cardiac output**.

Cardiac Output = Stroke Volume x Heart Rate

THE FRANK-STARLING CURVE

The Frank-Starling relationship describes the effect of ventricular cell length on the strength of contraction. This relationship states that as the end-diastolic volume (preload) increases, the greater the tension of the muscle fibers, contractility, and quantity of blood pumped out of the heart during systole. **In other words, the more the heart fills with blood, the more forceful the contractions; up to a certain point.** According to this relationship, contractility can then be estimated by determining the **ejection fraction** (Figure 10-4). The ejection fraction is the percent of the end-diastolic volume ejected from the heart during systole. Many patients know their ejection fraction values; the value is given as a percentage and a normal ejection fraction is at or near 55%.[2]

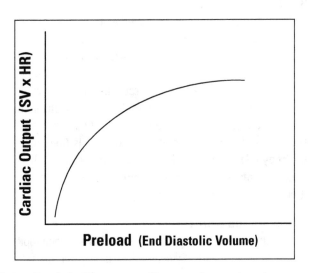

Figure 10-4 The Frank-Starling curve. See text for explanation.

PRESSURE DIFFERENCES AND BLOOD FLOW

Several factors influence the physical flow of blood through peripheral blood vessels after systole. The Hagen-Poiseuille equation mathematically describes the variables responsible for flow.[4]

$$\text{Blood Flow} = (\text{Change in Pressure}) \times \left(\frac{\pi r^4}{8\mu L}\right)$$

πr^4 Radius of Blood Vessel
μ Viscosity of Blood
L Length of Blood Vessel

This equation relates the force for flow, the pressure difference, with the forces of resistance (*i.e.* blood vessel radius, length, etc.). The first part of the equation states the driving force for blood flow: the change in pressure in the blood vessels. The second part of the equation takes into consideration the factors that increase resistance to flow (*i.e.*, viscosity, radius and length of blood vessel, etc.). The important point to remember about the Hagen-Poiseuille equation is that **the pressure gradient drives blood flow**. This concept has important clinical implications and will be addressed again in later sections.

Control of Cardiac Contractility

DEFINITIONS

The autonomic nervous system affects both cardiac conduction (*i.e.*, heart rate) and contractility. Three terms are used to describe the effects of sympathetic and parasympathetic control of the heart.[5] **Chronotropic** effects relate to changes in heart rate. A positive chronotropic effect increases the heart rate by increasing the firing of the S-A node whereas the opposite occurs as a negative chronotropic effect. **Dromotropic** effects relate to the conduction velocity, principally in the A-V node. A positive dromotropic effect increases conduction velocity through the A-V node while a negative effect slows the conduction of action potentials from the S-A node to the ventricles. **Inotropy** relates to the ability of the heart to contract; hence, this term is synonymous with contractility. A positive inotropic effect increases contractility; a negative inotropic effect decreases contractility.

Sympathetic Nervous Control

The sympathetic nervous system generally has **positive** chronotropic, dromotropic, and inotropic effects on the heart. Sympathetic neurons from the thoracic segments at the levels of T_{1-6} utilize norepinephrine as the principal neurotransmitter to stimulate beta-1 receptors in the heart.[1-3] When these neurons and receptors are activated, more action potentials occur during phase 4 of the cardiac action potential and the heart rate increases. The P-R interval on the ECG **decreases** as action potentials are conducted faster through the A-V node. Positive inotropic effects result from sympathetic stimulation when the heart rate is increased because more action potentials are generated during a given period of time. Contractility increases due to greater calcium utilization via increased entry of calcium into the contractile cells as well as greater release of calcium from the intracellular sarcoplasmic reticulum.

Parasympathetic Nervous Control

As opposed to the effects of the sympathetic nervous system, the parasympathetic division generally produces **negative** chronotropic, dromotropic, and inotropic effects. Muscarinic receptors in the heart are stimulated by acetylcholine, the principal neurotransmitter of the parasympathetic nervous system, via the vagus nerve (cranial nerve X).[3] Heart rate is decreased by a decreased rate of phase 4 depolarization during the cardiac action potential. Conduction velocity through the A-V node is decreased and can be assessed by measuring an **increased** P-R interval on the ECG as action potentials are conducted less frequently from the atria to ventricles. Calcium entry into cells is decreased during phase 2 of the action potential, thus inducing a negative inotropic effect.

The Cardiac Cycle: Summary

THE WIGGER'S DIAGRAM

The events of the cardiac cycle can be summarized with the Wigger's diagram.[1,2] This diagram shows the relationship between pressure changes in the various anatomical regions of the heart and electrophysiologic events taking place on the ECG (Figure 10-5).

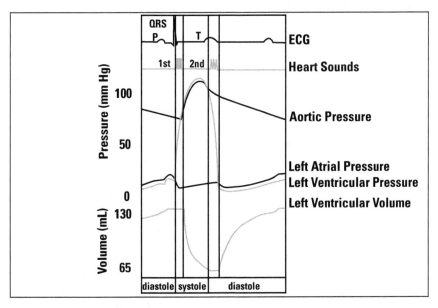

Figure 10-5 The Wigger's diagram.

References

1. Mohrman DE, Heller LJ. *Cardiovascular Physiology*, 3rd Ed. New York: McGraw-Hill, 1991.

2. Berne RM, Levy MN. *Cardiovascular Physiology*, 6th Ed. St. Louis: Mosby, 1992.

3. Netter FH. *The CIBA Collection of Medical Illustrations Volume 5: The Heart.* New York: CIBA-GEIGY, 1969.

4. Marino PL. *The ICU Book.* Philadelphia: Williams & Wilkins, 1998.

5. Yealy DM, Delbridge TR. Dysrhythmias. *In* Rosen P, Barkin R, *et al. Emergency Medicine: Concepts and Clinical Practice.* New York: Mosby, 1997.

Suggested Reading for ECG Interpretation

Brose JA, *et al. The Guide to EKG Interpretation* (White Coat Pocket Guide Series). 2000.

Dubin D. *Rapid Interpretation of EKGs*, 5th Ed. 1998.

Ehrat KS. *The Art of EKG Interpretation: A Self-Instructional Text*, 4th Ed. 1998.

Koenig DM, *et al. 12 Lead EKG Stat! A Lighthearted Approach: Essentials of 12 Lead EKG Interpretation.* 1995.

Seelig CB. *Simplified EKG Analysis: A Sequential Guide to Interpretation and Diagnosis.* 1992.

Summerall CP. *Lessons in EKG Interpretation: A Basic Self-Instructional Guide.* 2nd Ed. 1992.

Wagner GS. *Marriot's Practical Electrocardiography.* 9th Ed. 1994.

Zimmerman FH. *Clinical Electrocardiography.* 1994.

Review Questions

1. A 63-year-old patient is found to have the rhythm demonstrated below (Figure 10-1). Based on the available information, the rate would most likely be:

A. Less than 30 beats per minute
B. 90 to 100 beats per minute
C. 80 beats per minute
D. 40 to 60 beats per minute
E. Progressing rapidly to asystole

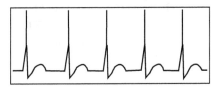

The rhythm is a junctional rhythm, and background ECG paper is omitted for the purpose of this question. Junctional rhythms depend on the A-V node for ventricular contraction. Although accelerated junctional rhythms are possible, the A-V node has an intrinsic pacemaker rate of 40 to 60 depolarizations per minute; hence, the heart rate is in the range of 40 to 60 beats per minute. The answer is D.

2. The mechanism of diuretics, morphine, and nitrates used to relieve symptoms related to congestive heart failure is:

A. Afterload reduction
B. Decreased release of atrial natriuretic peptide
C. Decreased ventricular remodeling
D. Decreased chronotropic effect on the heart
E. Preload reduction

While some afterload reduction also occurs, most of the symptoms of heart failure are relieved by the preload reduction offered by these agents. The answer is E.

3. Which of the following principles explains why, in a fluid-depleted patient with a normally functioning heart, the administration of intravenous fluids increases cardiac output?

A. Crystalloids provide added electrolytes for increased cardiac contraction
B. Ejection fraction decreases, lessening the workload of the heart
C. Decreased venous capacitance occurs in the vascular beds with hypotonic fluids
D. The Frank-Starling mechanism: the more the heart fills, the greater the force of contraction
E. Sequestered edema is removed as the osmotic pressure increases

The Frank-Starling mechanism for cardiac contraction explains how contractility increases as the heart chambers are stretched, up to a certain point. The analogy of a water-filled balloon can be made; as the balloon fills with water, the stream of water released from the opening is greater when the balloon if fully filled. The answer is D.

4. A 23-year-old involved in a serious motor vehicle accident presents with the following vital signs: HR 140, BP 80/P RR 28. The patient's abdomen is distended and rigid. Two large bore intravenous lines are placed in the upper extremities. What physiologic principle explains the rationale for proper catheter selection in trauma patients requiring fluid resuscitation?

    A. Laplace's Law: The catheter size is not important because smaller veins have greater surface tension than larger veins

    B. The Hagen-Poiseuille equation: The shorter the length and greater the radius, the greater the blood flow through the catheter

    C. Bernoulli's Law: Long, narrow catheters provide higher fluid velocities and allow for greater infusions of fluid to be delivered rapidly

    D. Boyle's Law: The size of the catheter radius and length is not important because the pressure of fluid in the catheter decreases as the amount of volume infused increases

    E. Newton's Law: The kinetics of fluid flow are related to the velocity of the fluid, not the radius or length of the catheter

The numerator in the Hagen-Poiseuille equation includes the radius of the tube (*i.e.*, blood vessel) to the fourth power, and the denominator includes length of the tube; thus, an increase in radius (smaller gauge) and decrease in length of the catheter allows for the greatest rate of fluid administration. The answer is B.

5-9. Match the appropriate physiologic effect with the appropriate sympathetic or parasympathetic response.

    A. Positive chronotropic

    B. Positive inotropic

    C. Positive dromotropic

    D. Negative chronotropic

    E. Negative dromotropic

    5. Increased heart rate

    6. Decreased heart rate

    7. Increased conduction at the A-V node

    8. Decreased conduction at the A-V node

    9. Increased heart contractility

5. A.

6. D.

7. C.

8. E.

9. B.

10. The finding of persistent tachycardia in a patient with heart failure should be considered:
   A. Ominous since the heart rate is increasing to compensate for a low stroke volume
   B. Reassuring because the increased heart rate is a well-tolerated compensatory mechanism to sustain cardiac output over time
   C. An indication for immediate cardioversion to restore the normal contractile properties of the ventricles
   D. Reassuring because an increased heart rate is related to a depletion of atrial natriuretic peptide
   E. Of no significance in heart failure patients since cardiac output is related to stroke volume and contractility, not heart rate

Cardiac output equals stroke volume multiplied by heart rate. When stroke volume decreases due to the failing ventricles, the heart rate is increased as a temporary measure to sustain cardiac output. Persistent tachycardia in heart failure patients can lead to ischemia, injury, and infarction secondary to greater oxygen consumption, as well as rapid depletion of available energy substrates and circulating neurohumoral molecules. The answer is A.

Conduction Pathways

The pathways for nervous conduction in the heart are reviewed in Figure 11-1. Impulses originate at the S-A node in the right atrium of the heart and are propagated through several intranodal tracts to the A-V node. These pathways above the A-V node are termed **supraventricular** for their location above the ventricular conducting pathways. Impulses leave the A-V node and enter the common A-V bundle, known as the Bundle of His, and divide into the right and left bundle branches. The nervous pathway from the A-V node to the Bundle of His is classified as the **junctional** conducting zone, representing the junction between supraventricular and ventricular pathways. The bundle branches are further divided into an anterior and posterior branch (fascicles) on the left and one branch on the right; all electrical activity below the Bundle of His is referred to as ventricular. Each bundle branch gives rise to Purkinje fibers embedded in the ventricles, innervating the myocardium.

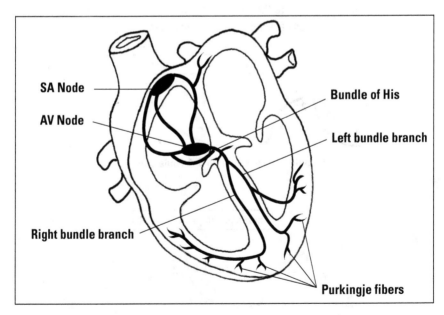

Figure 11-1 The cardiac conduction pathways.

Mechanisms of Dysrhythmia Formation

The three principle mechanisms for the formation of dysrhythmias are: altered automaticity, reentry, and triggered activation.[2-4] These mechanisms can be applied to the three divisions of the conducting system (supraventricular, junctional, and ventricular) to explain the cause of various dysrhythmias.

ALTERED AUTOMATICITY

The consequence of alterations during phase 4 of the cardiac action potential is known as altered automaticity. Nonpacemaker cells in the atria, ventricles or elsewhere outside of the S-A node can undergo spontaneous depolarization, triggering extra beats. Automaticity can also be enhanced when the slope of phase 4 is increased, causing the generation of multiple abnormal extra electrical impulses (Figure 11-2). If the sites of altered automaticity are not suppressed, sustained dysrhythmias ensue. Ischemia, myocardial infarction, electrolyte disturbances, and medications such as digitalis are common causes of increased automaticity. The ventricular tachycardia that occurs after myocardial infarction is usually the result of altered automaticity. In instances where catecholamine release is increased, the slope of phase 4 can be increased. Conversely, automaticity can occur when parasympathetic input to the S-A node is decreased, permitting unopposed sympathetic discharge.

Altered automaticity can generate rhythms from any site outside of the S-A node.[2] Other examples of dysrhythmias caused by altered automaticity include idioventricular rhythms, atrial tachycardia, and junctional tachycardia. These dysrhythmias often require a warm-up period before they are sustained. They also tend to take longer to terminate than dysrhythmias caused by other mechanisms.

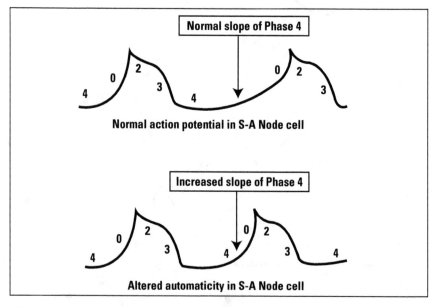

Figure 11-2 The mechanism of altered automaticity on S-A node action potentials. See text for explanation.

REENTRY

The mechanism of reentry occurs when a cardiac impulse travels in a circular course, creating abnormal impulses that lead to premature beats and tachydysrhythmias. In contrast to the aberrant impulse development that occurs with altered automaticity, reentry is caused by defects in the conduction pathways in the heart. Reentry develops when two different limbs of a conduction circuit in the heart have a difference in refractory (electrical recovery time of the cardiac cells) periods.[2] Reentrant rhythms occur when an electrical impulse propagates through the two unequally conducting limbs, one refractory, one nonrefractory. The end result of this conduction pattern is the formation of a circus rhythm as impulses travel in a retrograde (reverse) direction when the initial refractory limb becomes nonrefractory. This confusing concept is best explained schematically (Figure 11-3). When the initial refractory limb recovers, the impulse can travel in a reverse direction up the limb rather than down it, resulting in a self-perpetuating circular rhythm.

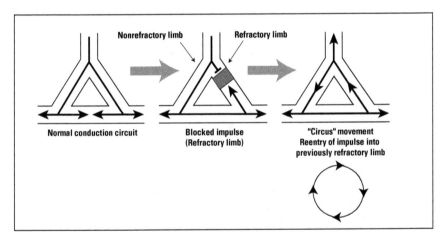

Figure 11-3 The mechanism of reentry.

Wolff-Parkinson-White Syndrome

A good example of the reentry phenomenon is the Wolff-Parkinson-White (WPW) syndrome. Impulses originate normally in the S-A node and pass through the intranodal fibers to the A-V node. In WPW, an accessory conduction pathway called the bundle of Kent provides a shortcut from the atria to the ventricles, allowing impulses to rapidly pass through the accessory bundle directly to the ventricle[2,3] (Figure 11-4). A delta wave forms on the ECG when both impulses arrive at the ventricles via an abnormal route; the widened delta wave reflects the sum of the two different ventricular depolarizations. In this condition, the P-R interval is shortened because the accessory bundle provides a quicker route to ventricular depolarization than the normal, slower passage through the A-V node. Eventually, retrograde conduction can occur in this condition, leading to circus movements, excessive reactivation of the ventricles, and paroxysmal tachycardia. With reentry, the normal 1:1 conduction from the S-A node to the ventricles is disrupted by the circus rhythm.

Reentry is the most common mechanism for narrow-complex tachydysrhythmias such as ventricular tachycardia, supraventricular (atrial) tachycardia, and various atrial and ventricular bigeminal and trigeminal rhythms.[2,5] Unlike dysrhythmias that result from altered automaticity, reentrant dysrhythmias can occur without an associated warm-up period and can terminate abruptly.[5]

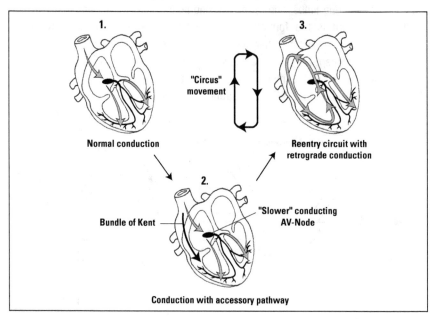

Figure 11-4 The Wolff-Parkinson-White Syndrome: An example of reentry.

TRIGGERED ACTIVATION

Triggered activation is another cause of dysrhythmias and is caused by a small rebound depolarization that occurs prematurely following the period of repolarization.[2] This rebound depolarization, or early afterpolarization, may have enough potential to trigger a cardiac action potential. This mechanism of dysrhythmia formation becomes clinically significant when the heart rate is slower in contrast to the mechanisms of altered automaticity and reentry. An example of a triggered dysrhythmia is polymorphic ventricular tachycardia (torsades de pointes).

Treatment of Dysrhythmias

DEFIBRILLATION

External cardioversion and defibrillation are techniques used to terminate dysrhythmia such as atrial fibrillation, ventricular tachycardia, and ventricular fibrillation.[6]

These techniques, introduced in the 1950s, are an important part of the prehospital provider's armamentarium and can be lifesaving when applied in emergencies.[7]

Investigators have proposed different hypotheses regarding the mechanism of action; however, the exact mechanism of effective defibrillation is unknown.[7] Defibrillating shocks may cause transient depolarization of myocardial tissue or prolong the refractory period of the cardiac action potential.[8,9] The ability of an electrical shock to defibrillate the heart depends on it waveform and energy.[10] Cardioversion, as opposed to defibrillation, involves delivery of a shock synchronized with the QRS complex. Regardless of the timing, a defibrillation waveform describes the energy, or current, mathematically as a factor of time.[11] A monophasic waveform has a single positive phase that either rapidly or gradually returns to zero voltage with current flowing in the direction between defibrillation electrodes.[11] Biphasic waveforms have a positive and negative phase reflecting a reversal of current flow between the defibrillation electrodes.[11]

Recent clinical trials have compared the use of monophasic and biphasic shocks for external defibrillation.[10,6,12,13] In general, biphasic waveforms are superior to monophasic shocks and are being incorporated into modern defibrillators.[6]

ANTIDYSRHYTHMIC PHARMACOLOGY

The Vaughan-Williams Classification

Antidysrhythmic medications are classified according to mechanism of action and effect on the cardiac action potential. The Vaughan-Williams classification has four categories with an additional category reserved for miscellaneous agents.[5] Table 11-1 lists each class, major mechanism of action, and phase of the cardiac action potential affected for the common antidysrhythmics used in emergency care. Although considered to be the standard of care according to current advanced cardiac life support algorithms, the benefit of many of these agents has not been established in well-controlled clinical trials.[14,15]

Class I Antidysrhythmics

Class I antidysrhythmics have different effects during phase 0 of the cardiac action potential. These agents slow depolarization to various degrees and have different effects on repolarization. Class Ia and Ib are commonly used in emergency situations with class Ic agents generally reserved for treatment failure.

Pro-arrhythmic side effects are typically greatest with class Ic agents, especially with orally administered preparations.[5] These agents have the potential to stretch the intervals of the ECG, prolonging the P-R interval, QRS complex, and QT duration. The ECG should always be monitored closely when using class Ic antidysrhythmics.

Table 11-1

The Vaughan-Williams Classification for Antidysrhythmic Medications

Class	Representative Agents	Mechanisms of Action	Phase of Action Potential Affected
IA	**Procainamide** **Quinidine**	Slowed depolarization Slowed conduction Prolonged repolarization Prolonged action potential duration	Phase 0
IB	**Lidocaine** **Phenytoin**	Slowed depolarization Shortened repolarization Shortened action potential duration	Phase 0
IC	**Flecainide** **Encainide** **Lorcainide**	Slowed depolarization Prolonged repolarization Prolonged action potential duration	Phase 0
II	**Propranolol** **Esmolol** **Acebutolol** **Metoprolol**	Beta-blockers	Slow S-A and A-V node conduction, decreasing *frequency* of action potentials
III	**Amiodarone** **Bretylium** **Sotalol** **Ibutilide**	Prolonged action potential Antifibrillatory Prolonged refractory period	Phase 4 (all phases affected)
IV	**Verapamil** **Diltiazem**	Calcium channel blockers	Phase 2

Class II Antidysrhythmics

Class II agents are beta-blockers: agents that decrease heart rate, contractility, and cardiac oxygen consumption. These medications do not have a specific effect on the cardiac action potential; however, the frequency of action potentials generated is decreased as the sympathetic input to the conducting system is blocked at the beta-1 receptor level. Unlike class I agents, only the P-R interval is affected by beta-blockers.[5] Even though many beta-blockers are relatively specific for the beta-1 receptor, they should be used with caution in patients with COPD, asthma, and pregnancy.

Class III Antidysrhythmics

Three of the class III antidysrhythmics exclusively prolong the refractory period (phase 4 of the cardiac action potential) and prevent fibrillation of cardiac muscle tissue. The fourth class III drug, sotalol, is also a beta-blocker. These medications have potentially serious side effects and are usually reserved as second-line alternatives to class I agents.

Class IV Antidysrhythmics

The calcium channel blockers verapamil and diltiazem constitute class IV. In addition to blocking the slow calcium channels in the myocardium (phase 2 of the cardiac action potential), this class also slows A-V conduction and vascular smooth muscle relaxation. Of the two approved antidysrhythmic calcium channel blockers, verapamil has a greater effect on delaying A-V conduction and a lesser effect on the peripheral vasculature.[5] Verapamil is contraindicated in patients with A-V blocks because of the potent A-V conduction delay induced by this agent. An additional caveat to the use of verapamil is **its absolute contraindication in patients with the Wolf-Parkinson-White syndrome**. Use of verapamil, as well as beta-blockers, can accelerate the underlying tachycardia by allowing the accessory pathway to conduct impulses without opposition, thereby creating an increased ventricular response rate.

Miscellaneous Antidysrhythmics

Adenosine, a naturally occurring purine nucleoside, is **one of the most highly effective medications used to terminate narrow-complex tachycardias.**[5] This drug shortens the action potential duration without affecting ventricular contractility as soon as 5 seconds after administration. The action potential is shortened as a result of adenosine's ability to hyperpolarize atrial myocardial cells, decreasing atrial contractions. Due to the short half-life of adenosine (less than 40 seconds), it is a favorable agent for use in the emergency management of supraventricular tachycardias.

Magnesium, a naturally occurring calcium channel blocker, is another miscellaneous antidysrhythmic used to terminate reentrant rhythms, ventricular tachycardia, and polymorphic ventricular tachycardia (torsades de pointes).[5] It is generally a second-line agent for these conditions.

Digitalis, a cardiac glycoside, has a host of effects on cardiac muscle tissue. The main mechanism of action is inhibition of the sodium-potassium-ATPase pump embedded in the cardiac cell membranes. Inhibition of this pump alters the action potential and indirectly raises intracellular calcium levels, increasing the force of heart muscle contraction and slowing electrical transmission through the heart. Because of the numerous side effects and longer duration to onset of action of this agent, **digitalis is not a drug of first choice in the emergency management of dysrhythmias such as atrial fibrillation with a rapid ventricular response.** Digitalis has the potential for many drug-drug interactions.

Amiodarone

Of the previously described antidysrhythmic medications, one deserves special mention. In ventricular tachycardia or pulseless ventricular tachycardia that persists after attempts to defibrillate electrically, treatment with the antidysrhythmic amiodarone (Cordarone, Cordarone X) confers a higher rate of survival to hospital admission.[14] A number of other studies found significant improvement in patients surviving to the emergency department from out-of-hospital cardiac arrests.[16,17] Amiodarone is a powerful, effective antidysrhythmic that can terminate both supraventricular and ventricular dysrhythmias as well as dysrhythmias due to accessory pathways such as the Wolff-Parkinson-White syndrome. Amiodarone has actions in classes I, II, III, and IV of the Vaughn-Williams Classification, but is predominantly a membrane stabilizer (class III). Its class III action is mediated by inhibition of the rapid component of the delayed potassium channels. The automaticity is decreased in the S-A and A-V nodes and Purkinje system and mild negative inotropy occurs as a result of down-regulation of beta adrenergic receptors and alpha receptor blockade. The defibrillation threshold may also be decreased by amiodarone. Acute side effects are rare, but when used in the long term, significant pulmonary toxicity, neurotoxicity, thyroid abnormalities, and liver dysfunction may occur.

References

1. Netter FH. *The Ciba Collection of Medical Illustrations: Volume 5 Heart.* West Caldwell, NJ: CIBA-GEIGY Corp., 1978.

2. Wagner GS. *Marriott's Practical Electrocardiography.* 9th Ed. Philadelphia: Williams and Wilkins, 1994.

3. Gilmour RF, Zipes DP. Basic electrophysiologic mechanisms for the development of arrhythmias: clinical application. *Med Clin North Am* 68:795. 1984.

4. Ward DE, Camm AJ. *Clinical Electrophysiology of the Heart.* London: Edward Arnold, 1987.

5. Yealy DM, Delbridge TR. Dysrhythmias. *In:* Rosen P, Barkin R, *et al. Emergency Medicine: Concepts and Clinical Practice.* New York: Mosby, 1997.

6. Dell'Orfano JT. Update on external cardioversion and defibrillation. *Curr Opin Cardiol* 2001; 16(1): 54-57.

7. Trohman RG, Parrillo JE. Direct current cardioversion: Indications, techniques, and recent advances. *Crit Care Med* 2000; 28(10): 170-173.

8. Zipes DP, Fisher J, King RM, *et al.* Termination of ventricular fibrillation by depolarizing a critical amount of myocardium. *Am J Cardiol* 1975; 36: 37-44.

9. Jones JL. Waveforms for implantable cardioverter defibrillators (ICDs) and transchest defibrillation. In: *Defibrillation of the Heart: ICDs, AEDs, and Manual.* Tacker WA (Ed.). St. Louis, Mosby-Year Book, 1994, 46-81.

10. Higgins SL. A comparison of biphasic and monophasic shocks for external defibrillation. Physio-Control biphasic investigators. *Prehosp Emerg Care* 2000; 4(4): 305-313.

11. Niemann JT. Defibrillation waveforms. *Ann Emerg Med* 2001; 37(1): 59-60.

12. Schneider T, Martens P, Paschen H, *et al.* Multicenter, randomized, controlled trial of 150J biphasic shocks compared with 200-360J monophasic shocks in resuscitation of out-of-hospital cardiac arrest victims. *Circulation* 2000; 102: 1780-1787.

13. Bain AC, Swerdlow CD, Love CJ, *et al.* Multicenter study of principles-based waveforms for external defibrillation. *Ann Emerg Med* 2001; 37: 5-12.

14. Kudenchuk PJ, Cobb LA, Copass MK, *et al.* Amiodarone for resuscitation after out-of-hospital cardiac arrest due to ventricular fibrillation. *N Eng J Med* 1999; 341: 871-878.

15. Advanced Life Support Working Party of the European Resuscitation Council. Guidelines for advanced life support: a statement by the Advanced Life Support working Party of the European Resuscitation Council, 1992. *Resuscitation* 1992; 24: 111-121.

16. Gonzales ER, Kannewurf BS, Ornato JP. Intravenous amiodarone for ventricular arrhythmias: overview and clinical use. *Resuscitation* 1998; 39(1-2): 33-42.

17. Pfisterer M, Kiowski W, Burckhardt D, Follath F, Burkart F. Beneficial effect of amiodarone on cardiac mortality in patients with asymptomatic complex ventricular arrhythmias after acute myocardial infarction and preserved but not impaired left ventricular function. *Amer J Cardiol* 1992; 69(17): 1399-1402.

Review Questions

1. What is the most common mechanism of action for the dysrhythmia shown below in Figure 11-1?

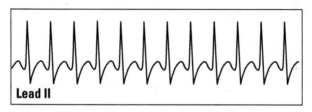

Lead II

  A. Altered automaticity
  B. Triggered mechanisms
  C. Ectopic ventricular pacemaker
  D. Reentry
  E. Loss of functioning S-A node

This dysrhythmia is SVT. The most common pathophysiologic mechanism for SVT is reentry. The answer is D.

2. The drug of choice for the dysrhythmia in Question 1 is classified under the Vaughn-Williams scheme as:
  A. Class II (beta blocker)
  B. Ia (Sodium channel blocker)
  C. Ib (sodium channel blocker)
  D. III (antifibrillatory)
  E. Miscellaneous

The drug of choice for SVT is adenosine. Adenosine is classified as a miscellaneous agent under the Vaughn-Williams classification scheme for antidysrhythmic medications. The answer is E.

3. The most common mechanism of action for this dysrhythmia (Figure 11-2) is:

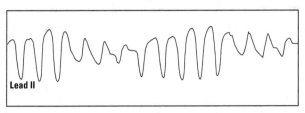

A. Triggered activation
B. Altered automaticity
C. Reentry
D. A-V nodal block
E. Hypermagnesemia

Polymorphic ventricular tachycardia, known also as torsades des pointes, is commonly caused by triggered activation. This condition can be associated with hypomagnesemia, not hypermagnesemia; hence, treatment with magnesium may terminate the dysrhythmia in some cases. The answer is A.

4. Which of the following agents (Figure 11-3) is contraindicated in a patient with this dysrhythmia?

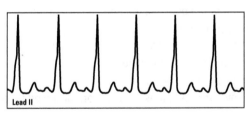

A. Amiodarone
B. Verapamil
C. Procainamide
D. Ablation surgery
E. Sotalol

For the purposes of prehospital care, undifferentiated tachycardia associated with Wolff-Parkinson-White Syndrome (WPW) should not be treated with calcium channel blockers nor beta-blockers. The other agents are drugs of choice for WPW. Surgical techniques can be used to ablate the accessory pathway. The answer is B.

5. The patient with this dysrhythmia has normal heart function and has had this dysrhythmia for less than 48 hours. All of the following (Figure 11-4) are acceptable agents for treating the accelerated heart rate associated with this dysrhythmia EXCEPT:

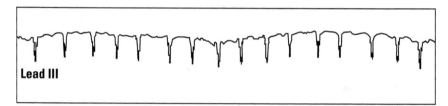

Lead III

    A. Verapamil
    B. Diltiazem
    C. Esmolol
    D. Digoxin
    E. Atenolol

Because of the delayed onset of action, digitalis glycosides should not be used for rate control in patients with atrial fibrillation associated with a rapid ventricular response. The answer is D.

6. The mechanism(s) of amiodarone includes all of the following EXCEPT:
    A. Antifibrillatory properties
    B. Potassium channel blockade
    C. Beta-adrenergic receptor blockade
    D. Calcium channel blockade
    E. All of the above are mechanisms of action for amiodarone

Amiodarone is classified as a class III antidysrhythmic, and prolongs both the cardiac action potential duration and refractory period via the mechanisms listed above. The answer is E.

Acute Coronary Syndromes I:
Pathophysiology of Coronary Artery Disease

Coronary heart disease (CHD) is the leading cause of death in the United States with more than 1.5 million cases of acute myocardial infarction and over 500,000 deaths annually.[1,2] Unstable angina, stable angina, and myocardial infarction are conceptually grouped together as a continuum of diseases known as the **acute coronary syndromes** (Figure 12-1).[1,4]   Acute coronary syndromes represent a spectrum of disease entities that share the same underlying pathophysiology.   Dependence on intact circulation and the consequences of ischemia are central concepts defining the pathophysiology of these disorders.

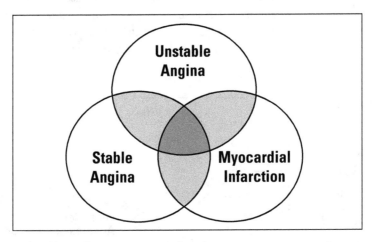

Figure 12-1 Venn diagram representing the acute coronary syndromes.

Plaque Formation

THE CULPRIT PLAQUE

The formation of vulnerable or culprit plaques in the coronary arteries is the initial event in the pathogenesis of acute coronary syndromes.[3-5] The process of plaque formation and coronary artery calcification is an organized, regulated, and dynamic process rather than a passive accumulation of calcium crystals and cholesterol as was once thought.[4,5] These plaques, designated by the American Heart Association as developed **human fibrolipid plaques**, form when low density lipoproteins (e.g., cholesterol) are oxidized and consumed by macrophages (immune cells derived from monocytes).[6]   Macrophages are transformed into foam cells, actively consuming oxidized lipoproteins by the process of phagocytosis; the accumulation of these cells within the smooth muscle cell layer of coronary arteries forms a plaque. Foam cells release different tissue growth factors that stimulate proliferation of smooth muscle and induce calcification of the surrounding tissue. The end result is the formation of a fibrolipid plaque with a core of lipid-containing cholesterol and its breakdown products surrounded by a capsule of connective tissue. The core of the plaque is further surrounded by more highly activated foam cells that continue to release growth factors as well as inflammatory cell mediators. A fibrous cap forms during this process, and separates the lipid core of the plaque from the arterial lumen.

THROMBOSIS

The consequence of fibrolipid plaque formation in the coronary arteries is thrombosis: a condition leading to decreased oxygen supply to the myocardium. Excluding the rare exceptions of spontaneous coronary artery dissection, vasospasm, and arteritis, nearly all thromboses occur as the result of a ruptured fibrolipid plaque.[5] The core of a fibrolipid plaque contains many foam cells, which are extremely thrombogenic. Tissue factor, fragments of collagen, and the crystalline surfaces of cholesterol accelerate the process of coagulation.[4,5] In addition, foam cells cause the plaque to weaken, making it more likely to rupture with the release of thrombogenic material and formation of a local blood clot. Figure 12-2 outlines the processes preceding plaque formation and rupture.

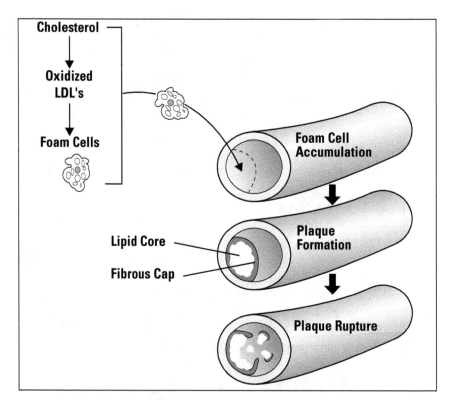

Figure 12-2 The pathogenesis of plaque formation and rupture.

INFLAMMATION

Inflammation within the plaque reduces collagen synthesis within the plaque, making the structure weaker and more prone to rupture.[4,5] The fibrous cap that forms on top of the plaque is a dynamic structure comprised of disorganized collagen and sparseness of smooth muscles cells. Inflammation causes the smooth muscle cells to die through the process of apoptosis (programmed cell death). A ruptured plaque typically results in formation of a local blood clot (thrombus) that later becomes organized and leads to the development of atherosclerosis (narrowing of the arteries due to lipid accumulation) or total occlusion of the coronary arteries.

PLAQUE RUPTURE

A rapid disruption or complete rupture of the fibrolipid plaque may result in acute occlusion with clinical manifestations ranging from unstable angina to myocardial infarction.[3] In most instances, episodes of plaque formation do not result in major acute coronary syndromes such as infarction or death; stable lesions can form over the course of several weeks.[4]

In episodes of eventful plaque disruption, intermittent attacks of myocardial ischemia or even total myocardial cell death can occur as the result of thrombus formation. Platelets expressing the IIbIIIa receptor migrate to the thrombogenic collagen and tissue factors when the plaque ruptures, and initiate the formation of a clot.[4] Intense local vasoconstriction can occur in response to the presence of increased platelet deposition, causing clumps of blood clots to embolize into the myocardial vascular bed. In some instances, vascular occlusion may last only 10 to 20 minutes.[7] **In instances of non-Q wave and Q wave myocardial infarction, coronary blood flow is reduced abruptly and completely in sections of myocardial tissue.**[7]

VASOCONSTRICTION

Although rupture of fibrolipid plaques is the usual cause of acute coronary syndromes, other mechanisms with the potential to alter myocardial oxygen supply and demand must be also considered. Vasoconstriction can occur as a secondary response to local platelet aggregation, exposure to damaged vascular endothelium, cold stimuli, or excessive sympathetic nervous system stimulation. Drugs such as cocaine can induce vasoconstriction without thrombus formation.[4] Other factors contributing to reductions in coronary blood flow include coronary inflammation and progressive coronary obstruction[4] (Figure 12-3).

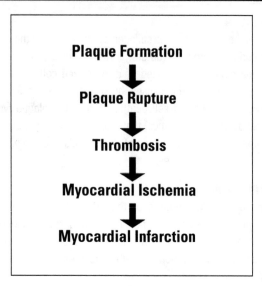

Figure 12-3 A summary of the pathologic processes involved in the acute coronary syndromes.

References

1. Jones EB, Robinson DJ. Unstable angina: Year 2000 update. Multi-modal strategies for reducing mortality, urgent revascularization, and adverse cardiovascular events. *Emergency Medicine Reports.* 2000; 21(10): 105-120.

2. Braunwald E, Jones RH, Mark DB, et al. Diagnosing and managing unstable angina. *Circulation.* 1995; 90: 613-622.

3. Theroux P, Fuster V. Acute coronary syndromes: Unstable angina and non-Q wave myocardial infarction. *Circulation.* 1998; 97(12): 1195-1206.

4. Davies MJ. The pathophysiology of acute coronary syndromes. *Heart.* 2000; 83(3): 361-366.

5. Stary H, Chandler A, Dinsmore R, et al. A definition of advanced types of atherosclerotic lesions and a histological classification of atherosclerosis. A report from the committee on vascular lesions of the council on atherosclerosis, American Heart Association. *Circulation.* 1995; 92: 1355-1374.

6. Champe PC, Harvey RA. *Biochemistry.* 2nd ed. Philadelphia: J.B. Lippincott Co., 1994

7. Diver DJ, Bier JD, Ferreira PE, *et al.* Clinical and arteriographic characterization of patients with unstable angina without crucial coronary artery narrowing. *Am J Cardiol.* 1994; 74: 531-537.

Review Questions

1. All of the following are acute coronary syndromes EXCEPT:
   A. Unstable angina
   B. Acute myocardial infarction
   C. Stable angina
   D. Malignant hypertension
   E. All of the above are acute coronary syndromes

Hypertension, while an independent risk factor for heart disease, is not an acute coronary syndrome. The answer is D.

2. Glycoprotein IIbIIIa receptor antagonists are of benefit for a patient with myocardial ischemia because these agents:
   A. Prevent the direct formation of thrombin
   B. Increase plasmin, dissolving existing clots
   C. Make collagen more thrombogenic
   D. Interfere with thromboxane A2, preventing platelet activation
   E. Prevent platelet aggregation and clot formation

The glycoprotein IIbIIIa receptors are expressed on platelets. Drugs that antagonize these receptors prevent the progression of clot formation by blocking the final common pathway for platelet aggregation. The answer is E.

Acute Coronary Syndromes II: Angina

Angina is the clinical manifestation of an imbalance between myocardial blood supply and oxygen demand. Although the clinical presentations vary, angina shares the same pathophysiology as the other acute coronary syndromes.[1] Since **unstable** angina is frequently the forerunner to myocardial infarction, and given that some instances of infarction are occasionally classified under the heading of unstable angina, this clinical entity is the primary focus of this chapter.

Clinical Classifications

GENERAL DEFINITIONS
The term angina pectoris coarsely translated from Latin means breast pain. Angina is classified into three distinct categories based on pathophysiology and clinical presentation. **Stable** or **typical** angina is commonly caused by atherosclerosis and can be precipitated by stress, cold, exercise, emotion, or eating. Stable angina typically progresses to **unstable** angina, which is also known as **pre-infarction** or **crescendo** angina. Both coronary vessel spasm and atherosclerotic occlusion may be present. **The patient with unstable angina requires no stress to provoke episodes of chest pain**. The essentials of diagnosis for unstable angina are discussed below. Prinzmetal's angina, also known as **variant** or **vasospastic** angina, is caused by vasospasm of the coronary arteries and may or may not be associated with severe atherosclerosis. As in unstable angina, chest pain may develop at rest. The diagnosis is made when the ECG and other ancillary data are considered when differentiating this disorder from true unstable angina.

DEFINITION OF UNSTABLE ANGINA
Defining unstable angina can be difficult as this syndrome occupies a wide spectrum of clinical presentations and often overlaps with noncardiac causes of chest pain. In 1994, the Agency for Health Care Policy and Research (AHCPR) of the National Heart, Lung, and Blood Institute published a practice guideline defining unstable angina.[2] Three possible presentations are defined in the guideline: new onset exertional chest pain, chest pain at rest, or recent acceleration of angina[3,4] (Table 13-1).

Variant or Prinzmetal's angina, non-Q wave myocardial infarction, and post-myocardial infarction angina are additional components within the realm of unstable angina.

Table 13-1

Clinical Criteria for Diagnosing Unstable Angina

I. **Angina at Rest** (usually greater than 20 minutes)
II. **Angina with Exertion-New Onset** (less than 2 months)
III. **Recent Increase in Severity of Angina** (less than 2 months)

Pathogenic Mechanisms

ENERGY DEFICIENCY

The development of myocardial cell ischemia is the result of an energy deficiency. In normal myocardial cells, arterial blood supplies the essential nutrients for **aerobic** metabolism: oxygen and glucose. When the blood supply is reduced or completely cut off, cardiac cells rely on glycogen molecules as reserve stores for glucose. This process of **anaerobic** metabolism does not require oxygen, but is only capable of sustaining myocardial cells for a limited time since glycogen stores are rapidly depleted. During a period of ischemia, myocardial cells may become electrically inactive and incapable of contracting.

OXYGEN SUPPLY AND DEMAND

Ischemia is ordinarily the result of **increased demand** or **decreased supply** of the oxygen and glucose carried by the blood to the myocardial cells. Cells that are overworked become ischemic when the ability of the coronary arteries to supply the cells with nutrients is outstripped by the demands of an increased workload. Stressors that can lead to increased myocardial demand include fever, exercise, surgery, or any exertion poorly tolerated as a consequence of other disease processes. The cardiac cell electrical **recovery phase** is most affected by increased oxygen and glucose demand; accordingly, ST-segment and T-wave changes are common during these circumstances.[5] Ischemia of increased demand is generally tolerated better than ischemia of decreased supply. Decreased blood supply is the result of the chronic process of atherosclerosis: the development of fibrolipid plaques in the coronary arteries. Instances of decreased blood supply can cause significant ischemia. Arterial vasospasm and inflammation are additional contributory mechanisms of decreased supply (Figure 13-1).

MYOCARDIAL ISCHEMIA

The outcome of ischemia differs according to the various anatomical areas of the heart affected. The ventricles are the thickest sections of cardiac muscle and sustain the greatest workload throughout systole and diastole. The effects of preload (the force distending the ventricular wall during diastole) and afterload (the force distributed in the ventricular wall during the ejection of blood) are greatest in the left ventricle; hence, **the left ventricle is the area of myocardium most susceptible to ischemia.**[1,5] The right ventricle has an intermediate susceptibility, and the left and right atria are least affected by reductions in blood flow, as the forces of preload and afterload on the walls of these chambers are comparably less than that exerted on the left ventricle. Coronary arteries, arising from the aorta, coarse through the layers of myocardium from the outside to the inside. **The subendocardial layer is the furthest from the coronary arteries and therefore the most vulnerable to injury during episodes of ischemia due to decreased blood supply or increased demand** (Figure 13-2).[5]

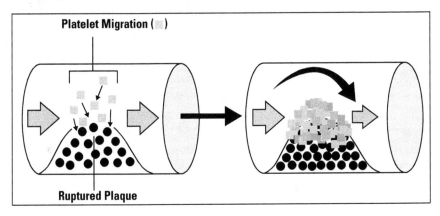

Figure 13-1 Plaque rupture leads to platelet aggregation and resultant reduction in the blood vessel diameter. Further thrombosis and vasoconstriction severely limit blood flow, leading to decreased blood supply.

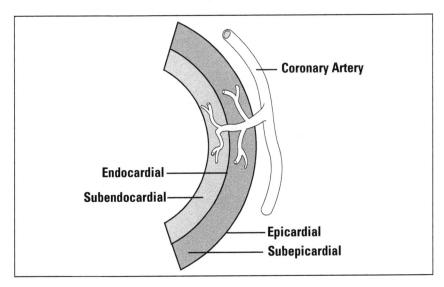

Figure 13-2 Diagram of the blood flow to the myocardial layers. The innermost layer, the subendocardium, is the most distant from the coronary arteries and therefore the most susceptible to ischemia.

ECG CHANGES

The ST-segments and T-waves represent periods of the recovery or repolarization phase of the cardiac action potential. Ischemia disables myocardial fibers from maintaining prolonged activation. As a result, transient ST-segment depression, T-wave inversion, or ST-elevation during acute episodes of ischemic pain are typical ECG findings in patients with unstable angina.[1,3-5] The above findings, including ST-segment depression greater than 1 mm or marked symmetrical T-wave inversion in multiple precordial leads, are predictors of complications in unstable angina.[3-5]

NON-Q WAVE MYOCARDIAL INFARCTION

As a rule, non-Q wave myocardial infarctions are classified under the broad heading of unstable angina. In non-Q wave myocardial infarction, plaque rupture and thrombus formation bring about complete occlusion of coronary blood vessels, but collateral blood vessels maintain perfusion, sparing myocardial tissue. **Non-Q wave myocardial infarctions represent unfinished ischemic events that leave anatomical distributions of myocardium in jeopardy of eventual infarction as the result of diminished blood flow.**[6] Findings on the ECG suggestive of non-Q wave myocardial infarction include ST-segment depression and biphasic or inverted T-waves (Figure 13-3).

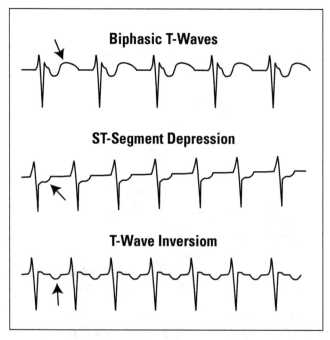

Figure 13-3 ECG changes in non-Q wave myocardial infarction.

Management

ANTICOAGULANT/ANTIPLATELET AGENTS

The goals of treatment for unstable angina are aimed at preventing thrombus formation and preventing ischemia. Aspirin irreversibly blocks cyclo oxygenase, the enzyme necessary for the eventual formation of thromboxane A2, a powerful platelet modulator, and is the most widely used antiplatelet agent.[7,8] Several studies have shown aspirin reduce the risk of acute myocardial infarction by over 50%.[7-9] Heparin, in both unfractionated and low molecular weight formulations, also prevents further thrombus formation. Due to the improved safety profile, low molecular weight heparin has emerged as the new anti-thrombotic drug of choice for unstable angina and myocardial infarction.[10,11] A new class of antiplatelet medications known as the glycoprotein IIb/IIIa receptor antagonists are also effective at decreasing mortality in patients with unstable angina.[12,13] These agents block the IIb/IIIa receptor on platelet surfaces, preventing the progression of thrombosis by blocking the final common pathway for platelet aggregation.

ANTIANGINAL AGENTS

Antianginal agents, with the exception of beta-blockers, alleviate the clinical symptoms of angina, but have not been conclusively shown to reduce mortality from myocardial infarction.[13] Although used in nearly all chest pain patients, there is no evidence that oxygen improves outcomes when used routinely.[9,13] Likewise, calcium channel blockers have not been shown to confer any benefit with regards to reducing mortality in patients with unstable angina.[9,13,14] Some studies show that the calcium channel blocker nifedipine, once a commonly used antianginal agent, may increase mortality rates when used alone.[14] Morphine, although an effective analgesic, anxiety-reducing agent, and probable preload reducer, has yet to be adequately evaluated in terms of the long-term benefit in patients with angina.[9,13] Beta-blockers such as propranolol, metoprolol, and atenolol decrease the incidence of acute myocardial infarction in patients with unstable angina, reducing myocardial oxygen demand by decreasing heart rate and myocardial contractility.[2,3,13] Nitrates have been used for years with known clinical success for relieving the pain associated with unstable angina, but have not been shown to definitively improve the prognosis.[15] Some studies have shown a reduction in mortality from acute myocardial infarction in unstable angina patients treated with nitrates.[15]

OTHER INTERVENTIONS

Ongoing studies continue to assess the merit of new medications and procedural interventions. New adjunctive agents on the horizon include direct thrombin inhibitors and newer formulations of glycoprotein IIb/IIIa receptor antagonists.[16] In patients with significant documented coronary artery disease, coronary artery bypass grafting remains an option for patients with unstable angina. The role of infectious agents and inflammation as possible etiological factors continues to be appraised, and may eventually contribute to a better understanding and correction of the underlying pathophysiology of angina (Figure 13-4).

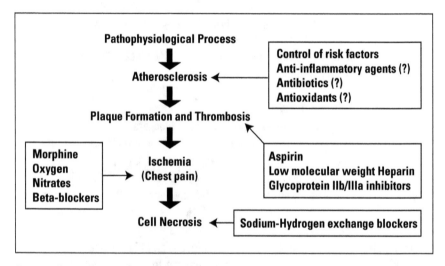

Figure 13-4 A summary of the pathologic processes leading to ischemia and cell death. Pharmacologic interventions are possible at each stage and are noted.

References

1. Fuster V, Badimon L, Badimon JJ, *et al.* The pathogenesis of coronary artery disease and the acute coronary syndromes. *N Eng J Med* 1992; 326, 242-250.

2. Braunwald E, Jones RH, Mark DB. Diagnosing and managing unstable angina. *Circulation* 1994; 90: 613-2548.

3. Jones EB, Robinson DJ. Unstable angina: Year 2000 update. Multi-modal strategies for reducing mortality, urgent revascularization, and adverse cardiovascular events. *Emergency Medicine Reports* 2000; 21(10): 105-120.

4. Ambrose JA, Dangas G. Unstable angina: Current concepts of pathogenesis and treatment. *Arch Intern Med* 2000; 160: 25-37.

5. Wagner GS. *Marriot's Practical Electrocardiography.* 9th ed. Philadelphia: Williams & Wilkins, 1994.

6. Theroux P, Fuster V. Acute coronary syndromes: Unstable angina and non-Q wave myocardial infarction. *Circulation* 1998; 97(12): 1195-1206.

7. Cairnes JA, Gent M, Singer J, *et al.* Aspirin, sulfinpyrazone, or both in unstable angina. *N Eng J Med* 1985; 313: 1369-2375.

8. Lewis HD, Davis JW, Archibald DG, *et al.* Protective effects of aspirin against acute myocardial infarction and death among men with unstable angina. *N Eng J Med* 1983; 309: 396-403.

9. Yusef S, Wittes J, Friedman L. Overview of the results of randomized clinical trials in heart failure II: Unstable angina, heart failure, primary prevention with aspirin and risk modification. *JAMA* 1988; 260: 2259-2263.

10. Cohen M, Demers C, Gurfinkel EP, *et al.* A comparison of low molecular weight heparin with unfractionated heparin for unstable coronary disease. *N Eng J Med* 1997; 37: 447-452.

11. Hirsh J. Low molecular weight heparin: A review of the results of recent studies of the treatment of venous thromboembolism and unstable angina. *Circulation* 1998; 98: 1575-1582.

12. Chong PH. Glycoprotein IIb/IIIa receptor antagonists in the management of cardiovascular diseases. *Am J Health-System Pharm* 1998; 55: 2363-2386.

13. Braunwald, E. Unstable angina: An etiologic approach to management. *Circulation* 1998: 2219-2222.

14. Muller JE, Morrison J, Stone PH, *et al.* Nifedipine therapy for patients with threatened and acute myocardial infarction: A randomized, double-blind, placebo-controlled comparison. *Circulation* 1984; 69: 740-747.

15. Yusef S, Collins R, MacMahon S, *et al.* Effect of intravenous nitrates on mortality in acute myocardial infarction: An overview of the randomized trials. *Lancet* 1989; 1: 1088-1092.

16. Fonarow, GC. Management of acute coronary syndromes. *Family Practice Recertification* 2000; 22(12): 35-50.

Review Questions

1. A 63-year-old with a past medical history significant for diabetes, hypertension, and a one-pack-per-day smoking habit for 25 years presents with substernal chest pain. The chest pain occurred at rest. What anterior coronary syndrome is this patient most likely to have?
   A. Stable angina
   B. Unstable angina
   C. Typical angina
   D. Variable angina
   E. Definite anterior wall myocardial infarction

The patient with unstable angina requires no stress to provoke episodes of chest pain. New onset angina with exertion or a recent increase in severity of angina are the other two possible presentations according to the guideline established by the AHCPR in 1994. The answer is B.

2. What is the most likely pathogenic mechanism for the disease process in unstable angina?
   A. Energy deficiency as a result of an oxygen supply-demand imbalance
   B. Increased aerobic metabolism
   C. Complete thrombosis of human fibrolipid plaques
   D. A complete ischemic event with complete cessation of blood flow to myocardial tissue
   E. Increased glucose metabolism and uptake by myocardial cells

Unstable angina usually represents an unfinished ischemic event as the result of an oxygen supply-demand imbalance. The answer is A.

3. A 74-year-old female with hypertension and known left ventricular hypertrophy is diagnosed with unstable angina. Her ECG shows evidence of myocardial ischemia. Which of the following would explain the physiologic status of her heart?
   A. The left ventricle is the most susceptible to ischemia
   B. The left and right atria is the least affected by reductions in blood flow
   C. The subendocardial layer is the most vulnerable to injury during ischemia
   D. All of the above statements are true
   E. All of the above statements are false

The answer is D.

4. A 53-year-old with a strong family history of MI (both mother and father died of MI at early age) and a history of heavy smoking is diagnosed with unstable angina. Which of the following ECG changes would be LEAST likely?
   A. ST-segment depression
   B. ST-segment elevation
   C. Absence of Q waves
   D. T-wave inversions
   E. Q waves

Q waves indicate myocardial infarction. This topic is discussed in the next chapter. Non-Q wave MI should always be suspected in patients with unstable angina because ECG findings often overlap with those found in angina (e.g., biphasic T-waves, ST-segment depression). The answer is E.

5. Which antianginal class reduces the mortality associated with unstable angina?
   A. Beta-blockers
   B. Oxygen
   C. Calcium channel blockers
   D. Morphine sulfate
   E. Nitrates

As of this writing, the only agents of those listed above shown to decrease mortality associated with unstable angina are the beta-blockers. Anticoagulants, aspirin, and angiotensin converting enzyme inhibitors (ACE-I) also reduce the risk of death in patients with coronary syndromes. The answer is A.

14

Acute Coronary Syndromes III:
Acute Myocardial Infarction

Acute myocardial infarction (AMI) remains the leading cause of death in most Western industrialized nations.[4] AMI is the leading cause of death in the United States and is responsible for a 40% mortality in European nations in patients under the age of 75.[1-3] Of the 4 to 6 million patients with chest pain seen in emergency departments in the United States, more than 1 million experience an AMI and **approximately 25% die before reaching the hospital.**[2] Due to the widespread prevalence and high attendant mortality of AMI, this disease remains one of the greatest challenges for prehospital care providers. Despite recent advances in early diagnosis, improved drug therapy, and understanding of the pathophysiology of AMI, the expected reduction in adverse clinical outcomes has yet to be fully realized.[5]

Pathogenesis

As part of the continuum of acute coronary syndromes, AMI shares the same pathophysiology as angina. The integral event in AMI is an abrupt decrease in blood flow secondary to a previously narrowed coronary artery.[6] Virtually all myocardial infarcts are caused by the development of a thrombus at the site of a ruptured fibrolipid (atherosclerotic) plaque.[7] Platelet aggregation, stimulated by the release of epinephrine, serotonin, ADP, and exposed collagen, induces the increased formation of thromboxane A2 and a change in the glycoprotein IIbIIIa receptor on platelets. Factors VII and X of the blood coagulation cascade are also activated.[6] The thrombus, in addition to waxing and waning in size, can cause intense local vasoconstriction, inflammation, and further platelet deposition. The end result is thrombosis and cessation of blood flow to myocardial tissue with ischemia, injury, and ultimately, infarction.[7]

Transmural infarcts involve simultaneous death of all myocardial muscle layers and develop over a time frame of a few hours.[7] Alternatively, nontransmural infarcts (non-Q wave) are caused by many small areas of tissue death of different ages and commonly follow episodes of unstable angina.[7]

Risk Factors

Studies have shown several factors play an important role in the process of atherosclerosis (*i.e.*, the formation of fibrolipid plaques; Table 14-1).

Of the known cardiac risk factors, hypercholesterolemia, low HDL levels, tobacco use, and (possibly) diabetes are modifiable. Other risk factors include the post-menopausal state, physical inactivity, obesity, homocystinemia, and hyperfibrinogenemia.[6]

Table 14-1

Independent Risk Factors for Myocardial Infarction
Hypertension
Smoking
Diabetes
Family History of CAD
Low HDL level
Hypercholesterolemia
High Lipoprotein (a) level
Male Gender

HYPERCHOLESTEROLEMIA

High levels of cholesterol are thought to contribute to the formation of the initial lesion of atherosclerosis: the fatty streak.[8] Deposition of cholesterol-rich low-density lipoproteins (LDL) in the intimal layer of the coronary arteries undergo chemical modifications and lead to the formation of a fibrolipid plaque.[8] Removal of lipid material such as LDL particles is facilitated by the "good" cholesterol, high-density lipoproteins (HDL). Low levels of HDL cholesterol are associated with an increased risk of cardiac events.[6]

SMOKING

Tobacco users have an increased chance for developing AMI. The role between the toxins in cigarette smoke and atherogenesis remains poorly understood, even though smoking is known to induce inflammatory states, increase fibrinogen levels, and conceivably promote thrombosis.[6]

DIABETES

Diabetes mellitus is known to stimulate atherosclerosis in humans.[9] Diabetes is associated with high levels of triglycerides and low HDL and is connected with increased conversion of LDL cholesterol to atherosclerotic precursors. Diabetics may also have higher levels of lipoprotein (a) (known as lipoprotein 'little a'), a molecule that inhibits the body's ability to break down blood clots (fibrinolysis).[6]

HYPERTENSION

High blood pressure has been shown in multiple prospective epidemiological studies to be a strong independent risk factor for the development of atherosclerosis and AMI.[10] Hypertension increases the risk of AMI in men two-fold and increases the risk in women two- to three-fold.[10] Left ventricular hypertrophy, an ominous ECG finding associated with poorly controlled hypertension, can cause confusion with the diagnosis of anterior wall infarcts and is associated with an increased risk of developing coronary atherosclerotic disease.

OTHER PREDISPOSING CONDITIONS

Unalterable risk factors for atherosclerosis and AMI include age, sex, and genetic predisposition. Although men are at increased risk at an earlier age than women, coronary heart disease and AMI is the leading cause of death for women over the age of 50.[6] The genetic mechanisms behind the development of coronary heart disease remain an important focus of cardiovascular research.

Clinical Manifestations

PATHOPHYSIOLOGY OF CHEST PAIN

Various pain pathways are involved in angina and chest pain associated with AMI. Painful stimuli travel through the middle and inferior cervical cardiac and thoracic cardiac nerves to the sympathetic chain ganglia of the neck and upper thorax.[11] From these ganglia, the nerve fibers continue to spinal nerves T_1 to T_5 via white rami communicans. While difficult to explain on an anatomical basis, referred pain is likely to travel through cardiac sensory fibers located from C_8 to T_5.[11]

Silent AMI

In up to 30% of all patients presenting with AMI, symptoms are **atypical**.[12] The incidence of painless MI drastically increases with age and can be seen in up to 70% of patients over age 85.[13] Silent MI is thought to occur in 40% of all patients with diabetes mellitus.[14] In both of these instances, an altered perception of cardiac pain, perhaps due to damaged sympathetic neurons innervating the heart, is felt to be responsible for atypical symptoms.

PHYSICAL EXAM

Anterior infarctions tend to cause overstimulation of the sympathetic nervous system, leading to tachycardia. Parasympathetic overstimulation frequently occurs in response to posterior infarctions and is associated with bradycardia.

An S_4 heart sound, a sign of increased resistance to ventricular filling, may be audible in patients with AMI. In some instances, an S_3 or ventricular gallop may be auscultated. This extra heart sound results from decreased myocardial contractility and volume overloading of a ventricle. If a transmural infarct has taken place, a pericardial friction rub may be heard. Friction rubs are caused by inflammation of the fibrous sac that envelops the heart (pericardium).

ECG Findings

ELECTROPATHOPHYSIOLOGY

From an electrophysiologic standpoint, myocardium deprived of oxygen can be classified by three zones: the zone of infarction, the zone of injury, and the zone of ischemia.[12] Ischemia results in repolarization impairment in myocardial tissue. Therefore, **the recovery phase of the ECG (S-T segment, T waves) is initially affected.** Figure 14-1 illustrates the zones of infarcted muscle and the expected ECG changes.

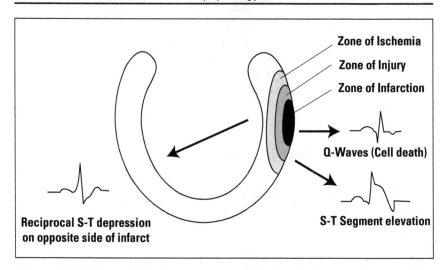

Figure 14-1 Myocardial infarction: zones of ischemia, injury, infarction with associated ECG changes. Adapted from Netter FH. *The CIBA Collection of Medical Illustrations. Volume 5: Heart.* Eighth printing. West Caldwell, NJ: CIBA-GEIGY Corp., 1992.

DIAGNOSTIC CRITERIA

Table 14-2 summarizes the ECG findings suggestive of AMI and the positive predictive values associated with these findings.

Infarction produces Q waves due to the inability of dead myocardial tissue to depolarize. The opposing currents from other areas of the heart cause the formation of Q waves on the ECG. **For Q waves to be clinically significant, they must have a duration of greater than 0.03 seconds or a height of greater than 1/3 of the amplitude of the QRS complex.**[13] The S-T segment changes that occur during myocardial ischemia may disappear when the tissue either infarcts or recovers when blood supply is reestablished.[13] S-T segment elevation or depression greater than or equal to 1 mm in any limb lead (I-III, aVR, aVF, aVL) or S-T elevation greater than 2 mm in any precordial lead (V_{1-6}) is considered 94% specific for AMI.[14] The specificity for detecting AMI on ECG increases when at least 1 mm of S-T depression in at least two leads exists or when greater than 1 mm of S-T elevation or abnormal Q waves are present in greater than two leads.[4]

Table 14-2

Positive Predictive Values for ECG Findings in AMI	
ECG Finding	**Positive Predictive Value**
>1 mm ST elevation or Q waves in > 2 leads	76%
ST depression in > 2 leads	38%
New ischemia, or strain >1 mm	21-38%
Old infarction, ischemia, or strain	8%
Nonspecific ST-T changes only	5%
Normal	2%

ANATOMICAL LOCALIZATION

The normal heart receives its blood supply from two coronary arteries (Figure 14-2). The left and right coronary arteries originate at the sinus of Valsalva at the base of the ascending aorta, giving rise to several branches that supply segments of myocardial tissue.

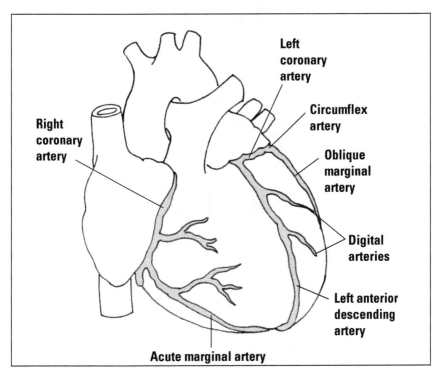

Figure 14-2 The anatomy of the blood supply to the heart.

Although immense variation exists in the pattern of coronary arteries, knowledge of the normal distribution is necessary to recognize regional patterns of ischemia and infarction on the ECG. Table 14-3 lists the ECG criteria for localization of anatomical areas of ischemia, injury, and infarction due to coronary artery occlusion.[13]

CONFOUNDING ECG PATTERNS

The initial ECG is interpreted as normal or with nonspecific changes **in up to 10%** of all patients presenting with documented AMI in the emergency department.[15] Confounding ECG patterns include left bundle branch block (LBBB), left ventricular hypertrophy, and non-Q wave MI.[16] In addition, infarctions in evolution may only show nonspecific ST-segment or T-wave changes on the initial ECG. Patients with acute, isolated posterior MI or ventricular-paced rhythms may also have misleading ECG findings.[16]

Table 14-3
Anatomical Localization of Infarct by ECG Findings

Anatomical Location	Inferior Wall	Anterior Wall	Lateral Wall	Right Ventricle	Posterior Wall
Leads	II,III,aVF	V_{1-4}	I, aVL, V_5, V_6	V_4 R (<1 mm)	V_{1-3} (ST-depression)
Blood Supply	Right Coronary (90%) Left Circumflex (10%)	Left Anterior Descending (LAD)	Left Circumflex, LAD, Right Coronary	Right Coronary	Left Circumflex, Right Coronary

LBBB and Ventricular Paced Rhythms

Table 14-4 lists ECG characteristics of AMI in patients with LBBB and ventricular-paced rhythms. In both conditions criteria are not based on the QRS complex or T wave changes.[17,18]

Table 14-4

Diagnosis of AMI with LBBB or Ventricular-Paced Rhythm
1. Concordant ST elevation > 1 mm
2. Discordant ST elevation > 5 mm
3. ST depression 1 mm in leads V_1, V_2, V_3

Non-Q Wave MI

Of all patients with AMI, 25% to 40% have a nontransmural infarct (*i.e.*, incomplete infarction of myocardial layers) without pathologic ST-segment elevation or abnormal Q waves.[16] Diagnosis is confirmed when a patient with chest pain demonstrates positive serum enzymes for AMI. The non-Q wave MI results from incomplete coronary artery occlusion that leads to death of myocardial cells. These infarcts are typically smaller than conventional infarctions and have a better prognosis for recovery.

Posterior Wall MI

Coronary arterial disease affecting either the left circumflex or right coronary artery with its posterior descending branch may lead to infarction of the posterior wall of the heart. The ECG usually shows a large R wave with increased voltage in V_1-V_3.[16] **Posterior MI most often occurs in conjunction with an inferior or lateral wall MI.** ST-segment elevation greater than 1 mm in posterior leads V_8 and V_9 confirm the presence of posterior MI.

Cocaine

ECG findings in cocaine abusers who present with chest pain and suspected AMI can be misleading. Significant false negative and false positive readings commonly occur. Cocaine binds and blocks the action of the amine reuptake pump in presynaptic neurons, leading to substantial elevations in epinephrine and norepinephrine as well as serotonin.[19] Elevations of these neurotransmitters leads to excessive beta- and alpha-adrenergic tone, increasing myocardial oxygen demands by increasing heart rate and shortening diastole, while also decreasing the diameter of coronary arteries and increasing coronary vascular resistance. Cocaine also has the potential to increase platelet aggregation and atherogenesis.[19] It is likely that most patients with cocaine-related MI suffer from diffuse small-vessel injury rather than occlusion of a large central coronary artery.[19] Taking into account the unique pathophysiology, the ECG alone is inadequate when evaluating patients with suspected cocaine-related MI.

Serum Markers of Cardiac Injury

When cardiac tissue is damaged, enzymes are released from the cytoplasm of cardiac cells and the contractile apparatus of the myocardial cell. Enzyme markers, when combined with information from the ECG, serve as valuable diagnostic adjuncts by enhancing the sensitivity for early detection of myocardial injury. Of the available enzymes, creatinine kinase (CK-MB), troponin-I, troponin-T, and CK (creatinine kinase) are commonly used. Most hospitals exclusively use troponin-I and CK-MB; hence, the discussion below is limited to these two serum markers. Each of these enzymes have unique release patterns, half-lives, and sustained elevations in plasma (Figure 14-3).[4]

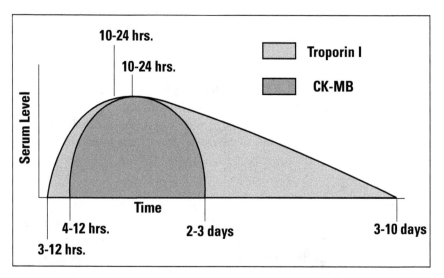

Figure 14-3 Comparison between serum levels of troponin-I and CK-MB enzymes over time in AMI.

CK AND CK-MB

The CK and CK-MB enzymes help diagnose myocardial infarction, especially when the ECG is difficult to interpret. CK is an enzyme found in nearly all tissues.[4] It is elevated not only in myocardial infarction, but also with trauma, muscle breakdown (rhabdomyolysis), vigorous physical activity (*e.g.*, marathon running), infections, and various other systemic diseases.[4,15] CK-MB is a specific isoenzyme located within the cytoplasm of cardiac cells. An isoenzyme, also known as an **isozyme**, is an enzyme that catalyzes the same reaction as other enzymes, differing only by amino acid sequence. This marker becomes detectable between 4 to 12 hours after AMI and remains elevated in the serum for 2 to 3 days.[4] Conditions such as rhabdomyolysis, renal failure, and hypothyroidism can cause false elevations of CK-MB.[15,16,26]

TROPONINS

Cardiac troponin I and T are regulatory proteins found in cardiac muscle. These enzymes are found both within the cytoplasm of cardiac cells as well as the actual contractile apparatus of the cardiac cells.[17] Of the two proteins, troponin I is commonly used in emergency departments. Troponin I rises in 3 to 12 hours after AMI and returns to baseline in 5 to 14 days.[18] It has replaced former markers of cardiac injury such as lactate dehydrogenase (LDH) as a more specific marker of myocardial infarction. Unlike CK-MB, it has a greater concentration in cardiac muscle and is not reported to increase in renal failure, hypothyroidism, after physical exercise, or in other acute or chronic muscle diseases.[19,27]

Additional Diagnostic Modalities

A 2-D echocardiogram should be performed to detect myocardial wall motion abnormalities in cases of suspected AMI without ECG changes. Echocardiography can also be used to diagnose right ventricular infarcts and pericardial effusions. The ejection fraction can be determined if heart failure is suspected. With the addition of Doppler studies, complications of AMI such as mitral insufficiency and ventricular septal defect can be diagnosed.

Other diagnostic modalities used for the evaluation of patients presenting to the emergency department with chest pain include radionuclide scanning, graded exercise testing, and cardiac catheterization.

Treatment

The goals for treatment for AMI are to limit the progression of infarction, prevent ischemic tissue from becoming infarcted, and to protect the remaining normal myocardial tissue from injury or ischemia (Table 14-4).

Effective drug therapy for myocardial infarction involves administering agents that rapidly restore perfusion. As discussed below, the use of additional agents may be used to reduce pain, decrease myocardial workload, and facilitate healing of damaged cardiac tissue.

EARLY INTERVENTIONS

Oxygen

Oxygen in commonly administered for patients with AMI although no studies to date have shown a mortality reduction associated with its use.[28,29] If a patient has an oximetry reading greater than 95%, no more than 2 liters per minute of oxygen should be administered. In other words, **if a patient is oxygenating well, the use of additional oxygen cannot be justified.** As the understanding of the pathophysiology of AMI becomes more clear, the role for oxygen therapy may become more defined. Oxygen may contribute to inflammation and oxidative damage, although this risk has not been confirmed in recent studies. Moreover, oxygen is hypothesized to cause vasoconstriction, an action that could have deleterious consequences in the coronary arterial system.

Nitroglycerin

Nitroglycerin and isosorbide dinitrate are powerful venodilators that decrease venous return to the heart. These medications are also reported to redistribute blood to the ischemia-prone endocardium, reduce afterload, and dilate the coronary arteries.[20] Although a mortality reduction was suggested with a meta-analysis of early trials on the use of nitrates in AMI, recent mega-trials have not shown any long term mortality reduction with the use of these agents.[20,21] Nitrates have not been shown to reduce the recurrence rate of AMI. Despite these findings, some clinicians maintain that nitrates are useful for relieving ischemic pain and improving left ventricular function.[20]

Morphine

Morphine sulfate is a potent opioid analgesic with anxiolytic effects. Even though relief of pain and anxiety decreases myocardial oxygen consumption and workload, no studies have shown a mortality reduction with the use of morphine.[6,17] Large doses of morphine (over 20 mg) are occasionally necessary to relieve pain in patients with AMI. The uncommon side effect of hypotension arises only in volume-depleted patients.[4]

Aspirin

Aspirin exhibits a powerful antiplatelet effect by inhibiting the production of thromboxane A2. In early trials with aspirin, a 50% mortality reduction was seen at 3 months.[20] Larger recent studies continue to show a substantial mortality reduction, especially when aspirin is combined with thrombolytics.[20] Early administration of aspirin is safe, inexpensive, and potentially life-saving.

REPERFUSION STRATEGIES

Thrombolytics

In instances of AMI with ST-segment elevation, the use of thrombolytics improves survival. The indications for thrombolytics are based solely on ECG data and are listed in Table 14-5.

Table 14-5

Indications for Thrombolytics in Acute Myocardial Infarction
ST-segment elevation greater than 1 mm in two or more contiguous leads
New onset Left Bundle Branch Block

These agents activate plasminogen that in turn activates plasmin, the complex that leads to dissolution of blood clots (Figure 14-4). Plasminogen binds to fibrin, a constituent of a formed thrombus. As the clot is dissolved, active thrombin is generated and platelet aggregation is secondarily activated. Hence, **thrombolytics should always be combined with antiplatelet medications such as aspirin.**[4] Contraindications to thrombolytic therapy are numerous; generally, any patient with active internal bleeding, a history of a bleeding disorder or recent surgery, severe hypertension (>180 systolic or >120 diastolic), or recent stroke should not receive thrombolytics.[4] Agents currently approved for use are listed in Table 14-6.

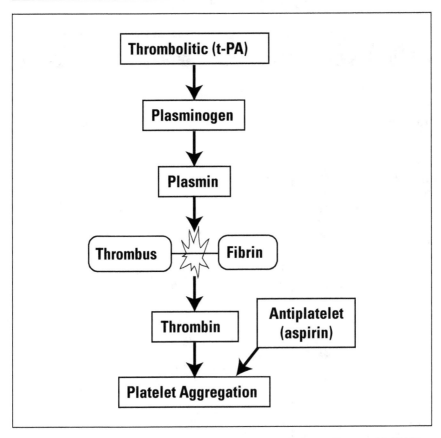

Figure 14-4 The mechanism of action of thrombolytic agents used in AMI.

Percutaneous Transluminal Coronary Angioplasty

Percutaneous transluminal coronary angioplasty (PTCA) is a surgical procedure that involves passage of a balloon-tipped catheter into the coronary arteries. It effectively restores blood flow to coronary arteries in more than 90% of all cases.[22,30] Several major clinical trials have shown a slight advantage of PTCA over thrombolysis. When performed by highly skilled practitioners (*e.g.*, interventional cardiologists) within 60 minutes of the onset of AMI, mortality is reduced to a greater extent than with thrombolytics.[22,30] Downfalls of PTCA are increased cost, availability of skilled operators, and the possibility of reocclusion several months after the procedure.

CARDIOPROTECTIVE PHARMACOLOGIC THERAPY

In addition to thrombolytics, PTCA, and other therapeutic options, cardioprotective drugs constitute an important measure that should be instituted in most patients with AMI. Two classes of drugs, the beta-blockers and angiotensin converting enzyme inhibitors (ACE-I) reduce mortality for patients having sustained an AMI.

Table 14-6
Pharmacologic Interventions and Mortality Reduction for AMI

Treatment	Mechanism of Action	Mortality Reduction
Aspirin	antiplatelet; decreases thromboxane A2	Yes
Thienopyridine Derivatives (ticlopidine, clopidogrel)	antiplatelet; affects ADP-mediated platelet activation	Yes
Glycoprotein IIb/IIIa Inhibitors (tirobifan, eptifibatide, abciximab)	prevent platelet aggregation	Yes
Heparin	activates antithrombin III; blocks coagulation cascade	Yes*
Low Molecular Weight Heparin (enonxiparin, daltaparin)	activates antithrombin III more specific blockade of factor Xa of coagulation cascade	Yes*
Thrombolytics (streptokinase, TPA, TNK-TPA, reteplase)	dissolve clot; restore perfusion to cardiac tissue	Yes**
Beta Blockers (metoprolol, atenolol)	decreased myocardial oxygen demand, control pain	Yes
Angiotensin Converting Enzyme Inhibitors (lisinopril, enalapril)	prevent ventricular remodeling	Yes
Nitrates (isosorbide dinitrate, nitroglycerin)	decreased preload, dilatation of coronary arteries(?), prevent ventricular remodeling(?)	No
Morphine	decreases sympathetic stimulation, decreases heart rate	No
Oxygen	increase SpO_2; prevent further ischemia(?)	No

* Synergistic with aspirin
** Synergistic with heparin

Beta-Blockers

Beta-blockers slow the heart rate, decrease systemic arterial pressure, and decrease myocardial contractility; through these actions, myocardial oxygen demand is reduced. The excitatory effects of catecholamines on the heart are also reduced.[20] Studies show a reduction for the risk of heart failure, arrhythmias, sudden death, and recurrent MI in AMI patients treated with beta-blockers.[21] Cardioselective beta-blockers provide a more specific blockade of adrenergic beta-1 receptors. Representative cardioselective agents include metoprolol (Lopressor®), esmolol (Brevibloc®), and atenolol (Tenormin®). These drugs have numerous contraindications and are used with caution in patients with asthma and COPD. When used in appropriately selected patients, beta-blockers represent an excellent class of first-line agents to be used in not only AMI, but also in angina and hypertension.[21]

ACE-Inhibitors

ACE-inhibitors block the conversion of angiotensin I to angiotensin II: a powerful vasoconstrictor. In addition to these affects, it is presumed that ACE-inhibitors also prevent ventricular remodeling after infarction, induce an anti-ischemic effect, and increase plasma levels of plasminogen-activator inhibitor.[20] ACE-inhibitors are clearly of long-term benefit in patients who have suffered an AMI. Unlike beta-blockers, ACE-inhibitors are not useful in cases of angina; however, virtually any patient with a history of cardiovascular disease, heart failure, or hypertension, is likely to derive a positive benefit from long-term therapy with these agents.[21] ACE-inhibitors should not be used in patients with renal artery stenosis, renal failure, symptomatic hypotension, or cardiogenic shock. ACE-inhibitors commonly used include captopril (Capoten®), enalapril (Vasotec®), lisinopril (Prinivil®, Zestril®), and ramipril (Altace®).

Landmark AMI Studies

Over the course of the past 20 years, several large multicenter studies have been performed to assess the impact of various interventions on the mortality associated with AMI. Tremendous strides have been made during this time. These landmark studies are summarized in Table 14-7.

Table 14-7
Landmark Clinical Trials for AMI

Trial Acronym	Year	Finding
GISSI-1	1986	Streptokinase associated with better survival if given < 3hrs
ISIS-2	1988	Streptokinase & aspirin had additive effect for survival
TIMI-1	1989	tPA better than streptokinase
GUSTO	1993	tPA & heparin used together showed best survival
PAMI	1993	PTCA reduced mortality more than tPA
MIAMI	1985	Improved survival with metoprolol (beta blocker) after AMI
SAVE	1992	Improved survival with captopril (ACE-I) after AMI
PRISM, PURSUIT, CAPTURE	1997-1998	Glycoprotein IIb/IIIa inhibitors show improved survival after AMI/ non-Q-wave MI

Data compiled from sources 31-40.

References

1. Gillum RF. Trends in acute myocardial infarction and coronary heart disease in the United States. *J Am Coll Cardiol* 1994; 23: 1273-1277.

2. American Heart Association. *2000 Heart and Stroke Statistical Update.* Dallas, TX: American Heart Association; 1999.

3. The Task Force of the European Society of Cardiology and the European Resuscitation Council. The prehospital management of acute heart attacks: Recommendations of a Task Force of the European Society of Cardiology and the European Resuscitation Council. *Eur Heart J* 1998; 19: 1140-1164.

4. Robinson DJ, Jerrard DA, Kuo DC. Acute myocardial infarction: Clinical guidelines for patient evaluation and mortality reduction. *Emergency Medicine Reports* 1998; 19(6): 53-67.

5. Bahr RD, Welch R for Third National Congress of Chest Pain Centers in Emergency Departments Focusing on Acute Myocardial Ischemia. A report on the proceedings of the third national congress of chest pain centers in the emergency department: Putting the pieces together. *Clinician* 1999; 17(3): 1-23.

6. Antman EM, Barunwald E. Acute myocardial infarction. *In:* Fauci AS, Braunwald E, Isselbacher KJ, *et al* (eds.). *Harrison's Principles of Internal Medicine: Volume I.* 14th ed. New York: McGraw-Hill, 1998.

7. Davies MJ. The pathophysiology of acute coronary syndromes. *Heart.* 2000; 83(3): 361-366.

8. Ross R. The pathogenesis of atherosclerosis: A perspective for the 1990s. *Nature* 1993; 362: 801.

9. Berliner J, et al. Atherosclerosis: Basic mechanisms—oxidation, inflammation, and genetics. *Circulation* 1995; 91: 2488-2496.

10. Kannel WB. Coronary atherosclerotic sequelae of hypertension. *In:* Oparil S, Weber MA (eds.). *Hypertension: A Companion to Brenner and Rector's The Kidney.* Philadelphia: W.B. Saunders Co., 2000.

11. Cahill DR. *Lachman's Case Studies In Anatomy.* New York: Oxford University Press, 1997.

12. Lusiani L, Perrone A, Pesavento R, *et al.* Prevalence, clinical features, and acute course of atypical myocardial infarction. *Angiology* 1994; 45: 49-55.

13. Aronow WS. Prevalence of presenting symptoms of recognized acute myocardial infarction and of unrecognized healed myocardial infarction in elderly patients. *Am J Cardiol* 1987; 60: 1182-1187.

14. Jacoby RM, Nesto RW. Acute myocardial infarction in the diabetic patient: Pathophysiology, clinical course, and prognosis. *J Am Coll Cardiol* 1992; 20: 736-744.

15. Netter FH. *The CIBA Collection of Medical Illustrations. Volume 5: Heart.* Eighth printing. West Caldwell, NJ: CIBA-GEIGY Corp., 1992.

16. Wagner GS. *Marriot's Practical Electrocardiography.* 9th ed. Baltimore: Williams & Wilkins, 1994.

17. Gruppo Italiano per lo Studio della Sopravivenza nell'Infarcto Miocardico. Comparison of frequency, diagnosis, and prognostic significance of pericardial involvement in acute myocardial infarction treated with and without thrombolytics. *Am J Cardiol* 1993; 71: 1377-1381.

18. Bertolet BD, Hill JA. Unrecognized myocardial infarction. *Cardiovasc Clin* 1989; 20: 173-182.

19. Brady WJ. Missing the diagnosis of acute MI: Challenging presentations, electrocardiographic pearls, and outcome-effective management strategies. *Emerg Med Reports* 1997; 18(10): 92-102.

20. Sgarbossa EB, Pinski SL, Barbagelata A, et al. Electrocardiographic diagnosis of evolving acute myocardial infarction in the presence of left bundle branch block. *N Engl J Med* 1996; 334: 481-487.

21. Sgarbossa EB, Pinski SL, Gates KB, et al. Early electrocardiographic diagnosis of acute myocardial infarction in the presence of ventricular paced rhythm. *Am J Cardiol* 1996; 77: 423-424.

22. Hoffman RS, Hollander JE. Evaluation of patients with chest pain after cocaine use. *Crit Care Clin* 1997; 13(4): 809-828.

23. Bhayana V, Henderson AR. Biochemical markers of myocardial damage. *Clin Biochem* 1995; 28: 1-29.

24. LeMar HJ, West SG, Garrett CR, et al. Covert hypothyroidism presenting as a cardiovascular event. *Am J Med* 1991; 91: 549-552.

25. Aufderheide TP, Gibler WB. Acute Ischemic Coronary Syndromes. In: Rosen P, Barkin R, *et al. Emergency Medicine: Concepts and Clinical Practice.* New York: Mosby, 1997. 1692-1695.

26. Adams JE, Abendschein DR, Jaffee S. Biochemical markers of myocardial injury: Is MB creatinine kinase the choice for the 1990s? *Circulation* 1993; 88: 750-763.

27. Ross G, Bever F, Zi U, Hockman EM. Troponin I sensitivity and specificity for the diagnosis of acute myocardial infarction. *JAOA* 2000; 100(1): 29-32.

28. Rapaport E. Pharmacological therapy for acute myocardial infarction. *Postgraduate Med* 1997; 102(5).

29. Fonarow GC. Management of acute coronary syndromes. *Family Practice Recertification* 2000; 22(12): 35-50.

30. Faxon DP. Thrombolytic therapy versus primary angioplasty. *Postgraduate Med* 1997; 102(5).

References for Table 14-7

31. Gruppo Italiano per lo Studio della Streptochinasi nell'Infacto Miocardico (GISSI). Effectiveness of intravenous thrombolytic treatment in acute myocardial infarction. *Lancet* 1986; 1 (8478): 397-402.

32. ISIS-2 (Second International Study of Infarct Survival) Collaborative Group. Randomized trial of intravenous streptokinase, oral aspirin, both, or neither among 17,187 cases of suspected acute myocardial infarction: ISIS-2. *Lancet* 1988; 2: 349-360.

33. TIMI Study Group. Comparison of invasive and conservative strategies after treatment with intravenous tissue plasminogen activator in acute myocardial infarction: results of the Thrombolysis in Myocardial Infarction (TIMI) Phase II Trial. *N Engl J Med* 1989; 320: 618-627.

34. GUSTO. An international randomized trial comparing four thrombolytic strategies for acute myocardial infarction. The GUSTO investigators. *N Engl J Med* 1993; 329 (10): 723-725.

35. Primary Angioplasty in Myocardial Infarction (PAMI) Study Group. A comparison of immediate angioplasty with thrombolytic therapy for acute myocardial infarction. *N Engl J Med* 1993; 328(10): 673-679.

36. MIAMI Trial Research Group. Metoprolol in acute myocardial infarction (MIAMI): A randomized placebo-controlled international trial. *Eur Heart J* 1985; 6: 199-226.

37. Pfeffer MA, Braunwald E, Moye LA, *et al.* for the SAVE Investigators. Effect of captopril on mortality and morbidity in patients with left ventricular dysfunction after myocardial infarction. Results of the survival and ventricular enlargement trial. *N Engl J Med* 1992; 327: 669-677.

38. Platelet Receptor Inhibition in Ischemic Syndrome Management (PRISM) Study Investigators. A comparison of aspirin plus tirofiban with aspirin plus heparin for unstable angina. *N Engl J Med* 1998; 338: 1498-1505.

39. The PURSUIT Trial Investigators. Platelet Glycoprotein IIb/IIIa in Unstable Angina: Receptor Suppression Using Integrilin Therapy. Inhibition of platelet glycoprotein IIb/IIIa with eptifibatide in patients with acute coronary syndromes. *N Engl J Med* 1998; 339: 436-443.

40. The CAPTURE Investigators. Randomized placebo-controlled trial of abciximab before and during coronary intervention in refractory unstable angina: The CAPTURE Study. *Lancet* 1997; 349: 1429-1435.

Review Questions

1. Your unit is called to the scene for a 66-year-old male with substernal chest pain, that started 15 minutes ago while shoveling snow. Which of the following is NOT an appropriate question to ask this patient regarding independent risk factors for myocardial infarction?
    A. History of hypertension?
    B. History of diabetes mellitus?
    C. Smoking history?
    D. Caffeine intake?
    E. LDL cholesterol level?

There is currently no evidence to support an association of caffeine with myocardial infarction. The answer is D.

2. ST elevation in leads II, III, and aVF is noted for the patient in the above scenario. Which of the following is NOT a known pathogenic mechanism for these changes?
    A. Abrupt cessation of blood flow to the right coronary artery
    B. Activation of the coagulation cascade
    C. Ruptured fibrolipid plaque in right coronary artery or left coronary artery
    D. Platelet inhibition by circulating plasmin
    E. Vasoconstriction and inflammation in the right coronary artery

Platelets are activated, not inhibited, during the pathogenesis of myocardial infarction. The answer is D.

3. For the patient in the above scenario, if the ECG was normal, what percentage of patients with documented myocardial infarction have an initial ECG that is normal or nonspecific?
    A. 1%
    B. 40%
    C. 50%
    D. 10%
    E. 4%

The answer is D.

4. A 55-year-old male with multiple cardiac risk factors (diabetes, smoking history, positive family history) has chest pain radiating to the left upper extremity. What must the ECG show for this patient to qualify for prehospital thrombolytic therapy?

A. ST-segment elevation in V_1, aVL only
B. ST-segment elevation in V_{1-3}
C. New onset left anterior fascicular block
D. Q wave over 1 mm in leads II, III, aVF
E. U-waves in leads I, aVL, V_{5-6}

Indications for thrombolytics in AMI depend on the following ECG findings: ST-segment elevation greater than 1 mm in two or more contiguous leads or new onset left bundle branch block. The answer is B.

5. Initial treatment in the field for the patient in Question 4 should include all of the following EXCEPT:

A. Oxygen if the Sp_{O2} is less than 95%
B. Nitroglycerin spray to control pain
C. One baby aspirin by mouth
D. Intravenous morphine sulfate for pain
E. Intravenous beta-blocker to slow heart rate

Beta-blockers are usually administered only after an evaluation by a physician in the emergency department. The answer is E.

6. Of the correct field measures in Question 5, which of the following decreases mortality in patients with AMI?

A. Oxygen
B. Nitroglycerin
C. Aspirin
D. Morphine sulfate
E. Beta-blockers

Aspirin has been shown to decrease mortality associated with AMI by as much as 50% in some studies. Beta-blockers also decrease mortality in patients with AMI, but are not usually administered until a complete evaluation by a physician in the emergency department. The answer is C.

7. Which portion of the electrocardiograph is most likely to show changes during an AMI?
   A. Recovery phase
   B. Ventricular depolarization phase
   C. Atrial depolarization phase
   D. Atrial repolarization phase
   E. Isoelectric phase

The recovery phase is represented on the ECG by the ST- and T-segments. The answer is A.

8. Which of the following statements is correct with regards to posterior wall myocardial infarction?
   A. A decreased R-wave in V1 is highly suggestive of posterior wall MI
   B. Posterior leads on the ECG are not needed for diagnosis
   C. Posterior wall MI is most likely to be associated with an anterior wall MI
   D. Posterior wall MI is most likely to be associated with an inferior-lateral wall MI
   E. V1-3 usually shows ST-segment elevation

Posterior MI, like inferior or inferior-lateral wall MI, is usually due to blockage of the right coronary or left circumflex artery. The answer is D.

Heart Failure

Heart failure has been compared to the mythical multi-headed beast Hydra because of its many causes and numerous clinical presentations.[1] Heart failure is a complex syndrome defined by an inability of the heart to pump a sufficient supply of blood to meet the metabolic requirements of the body.[2,4] As opposed to other cardiac diseases, the incidence of heart failure is increasing; each year over 400,000 new cases are diagnosed.[2,3] Overall, approximately 4.7 million people in the United States have heart failure and the incidence in patients 65 years and older has doubled each decade.[1,5] The risk of death for patients with mild heart failure is 5% to 10% annually, increasing to 30% to 40% in patients with advanced disease.[3,6] **Approximately one half of all patients with heart failure do not live beyond 5 years once diagnosed.**[5]

For the purposes of this chapter, the term congestive heart failure (CHF) is avoided. This term, while descriptive for most patients, implies congestion as the cause rather than the result of the failing heart.

Pathogenesis

ETIOLOGY

The major causes of heart failure can be classified according to anatomical disorders, systemic disease, and pulmonary dysfunction. **The most common causes of heart failure are coronary artery disease and hypertension.**[4] Virtually any disease that affects the coronary arteries, heart tissue (pericardium, myocardium, endocardium), peripheral blood vessels, or lungs can cause heart failure. Table 15-1 lists the most common causes of heart failure; the three leading causes are listed in order.

MECHANISMS

As the heart fails, cardiac output decreases and filling pressures (preload) increase. Multiple mechanisms are activated to compensate for depressed ventricular ejection of blood. Since 80% to 90% of patients with heart failure have symptoms due to impairment of **left ventricular function**, the mechanisms discussed below pertain mostly to this dysfunction.[3] Isolated right ventricular heart failure is rare but may occur in lung diseases such as COPD and cor pulmonale (primary pulmonary hypertension); **the most common cause of right ventricular failure is left ventricular failure.**[2]

Table 15-1

Causes of Heart Failure
(#1) Coronary Arterial Disease
(#2) Hypertension
(#3) Valvular Heart Disease (aortic stenosis, mitral insufficiency)
Cardiomyopathies (dilated, restrictive, hypertrophic)
Pericarditis, Myocarditis **Pulmonary Disease** (emphysema, pulmonary fibrosis)
Systemic Diseases (thiamine deficiency, amyloidosis, sarcoidosis, thyroid disease)

Renin-Angiotensin-Aldosterone System

The renin-angiotensin-aldosterone system is activated when an insufficient amount of blood is pumped to the kidneys. Renin is released from the juxtaglomerular apparatus of the kidney in response to this low-flow state (Figure 15-1). Renin converts the biological precursor angiotensinogen to angiotensin I in the liver. Angiotensin I is then converted to the potent vasoconstrictor angiotensin II by angiotensin-converting-enzyme (ACE) in the lungs. Release of this substance causes an increase in afterload (*i.e.*, the force against which the ventricle must contract). In addition to its vasoconstricting properties, angiotensin II stimulates production of aldosterone, a hormone that promotes salt and water retention by activating the sodium-potassium-ATPase pumps of the principal cells in the cortical-collecting duct of the nephron (the functional unit of the human kidney).[8]

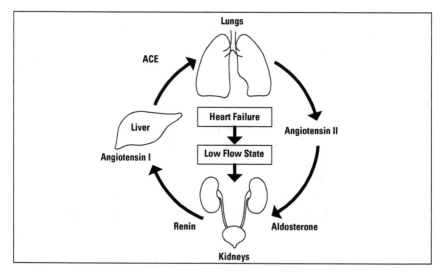

Figure 15-1 The renin-angiotensin-aldosterone system.

The overall effect of the renin-angiotensin-aldosterone mechanism is to increase water and salt retention, increasing both preload and afterload through the action of angiotensin II. By increasing preload, myocardial work is temporarily made more efficient by improved optimization of the Frank-Starling curve.[2] As reviewed in Chapter 10, the Frank-Starling mechanism states that as the cells in the myocardium (myocytes) are stretched, the number of actin-myosin filament interactions are increased, thereby increasing the force of ventricular contraction. While the myocytes contract more forcefully, this is only a temporary solution to the problem of left ventricular dysfunction. Stretched myocytes eventually becomes energy-depleted and die, leading to dilation and fibrosis of the myocardial wall.[9]

Myocardial Hypertrophy

Structural remodeling of the myocardium in response to increased filling pressures (preload) results in increased size (hypertrophy) of the remaining active myocytes due to the inability of myocytes to divide in adult life. Remodeling is a process wherein the hypertrophied ventricle becomes more spherical and dilated.[3] This process has a negative impact on cardiac performance because the mechanical stresses on the myocardial walls and the extent of regurgitant flow through the valves of the heart are increased[3] (Figure 15-2). In conditions where the ventricle is dysfunctional and **volume** overloaded (*i.e.*, myocardial infarction, valvular insufficiency), the myocardium responds by remodeling and becomes **dilated**. In cases where **pressure** is increased (*i.e.*, hypertension, aortic stenosis), **concentric** hypertrophy of ventricular tissue occurs.[2] As a result of the sustained exposure of the myocardial wall to abnormal volume and pressure, the Frank-Starling mechanism fails and cardiac output decreases[9] (Figure 15-3).

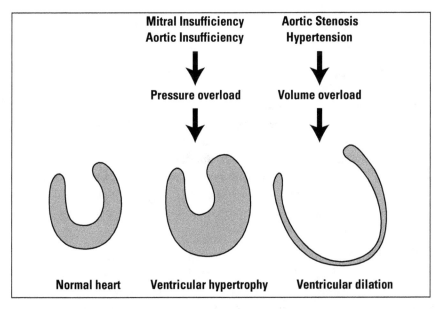

Figure 15-2 The Starling curve. See text for explanation.

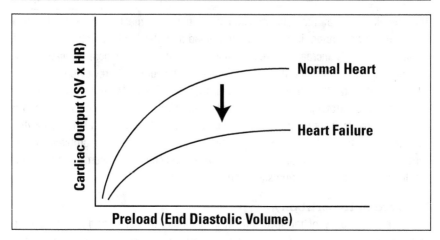

Figure 15-3 The effects of increased pressure and volume in heart failure: concentric and dilational hypertrophy.

Atrial Natriuretic Peptide

Atrial natriuretic peptide is a hormone secreted by atrial cardiac cells in response to atrial distension.[10] The increased afterload in heart failure and the deleterious effects of the renin-angiotensin-aldosterone system are counteracted by this peptide hormone. Atrial natriuretic peptide also works in the kidney to promote sodium excretion, reducing preload. As heart failure progresses, this hormone is gradually depleted.

Other Mechanisms

A variety of cell-signaling pathways and other neurohormonal substances play a central role in the pathogenesis of heart failure. Known mediators include endothelin, epinephrine, norepinephrine, vasopressin, prostaglandins, and substance P.[3,4] A toxic effect may be exerted by these substances. Apoptosis (programmed cell death) and fibrosis may be promoted by overstimulation of these pathways.[4]

SYSTOLIC VERSUS DIASTOLIC FAILURE

Many classification schemes exist to describe the pathophysiologic and clinical sequela of heart failure. For instance, heart failure can be classified as: forward versus backward, high output versus low output, right-sided versus left-sided, forward versus backward, and systolic versus diastolic.[7] **Of these schemes, the classification of systolic and diastolic dysfunction has the most utility because making the distinction between the two allows one to formulate appropriate treatment decisions**. Firm distinctions between any classification scheme are unrealistic and impractical. In clinical practice, considerable overlap exists between systolic and diastolic heart failure.

Systolic Failure

Systolic failure of the heart results from inadequate **contractility**. Common causes include diseases that directly injure or destroy the myocytes such as myocardial infarction or myocarditis.[7] Inadequate systemic perfusion results from decreased cardiac output and forward flow. The **ejection fraction is often significantly decreased** (<40%) in patients with systolic failure, accompanied by increased left ventricular end-diastolic and end-systolic volumes.[3]

Diastolic Failure

In up to 40% of patients with heart failure, the ejection fraction is normal.[11,12] Many of these patients have an impairment of ventricular relaxation and normal filling, otherwise known as diastolic failure. Diastolic failure results from inability of the myocytes to relax. Diseases culminating in diastolic failure include chronic hypertension, aortic stenosis, and cardiomyopathies.[7] The process of myocardial relaxation, in comparison to myocardial contraction, requires energy to relax; hence, **patients with diastolic failure have stiff hearts with supranormal filling pressures**.

ACUTE PULMONARY EDEMA

Pulmonary edema is one of the most serious manifestations of heart failure. Pulmonary edema refers to the accumulation of fluid in the interstitium of the lungs and has both cardiogenic and noncardiogenic etiologies. Noncardiogenic causes involve alterations in the permeability characteristics of the pulmonary capillary membranes and can result from septic shock, toxins, fat emboli, and high altitude.[7] Cardiogenic pulmonary edema is the result of abnormally high filling pressures in the heart and is frequently induced by the causes of heart failure (*i.e.*, AMI, valvular disease, hypertension, etc.).

In Chapter 2, Starling's law of the capillary was discussed in detail.

Starling's Law of the Capillary

$$\text{Flow} = K_f \left[(P_c - P_i) - \sigma(\pi_c - \pi_i) \right]$$

$(P_c - P_i)$ Difference in Hydrostatic Pressure
(Driving Force for Filtration)

$(\pi_c - \pi_i)$ Difference in Osmotic Pressure
(Driving Force for Reabsorption)

K_f **Filtration Coefficient** *(Permeability of Membrane)*

σ **Protein Permeability Coefficient**

This law explains the forces governing fluid shifts across membranes and is especially applicable to the capillary membranes in the lung. The net **hydrostatic** pressure is the driving force to send fluid out of the capillaries into the pulmonary interstitium as opposed to the net **osmotic** pressure (*i.e.*, the colloid osmotic pressure) which is the driving force for the retention of fluid within the vascular space (reabsorption).

Imbalances in these pressures can lead to the accumulation of fluid in the pulmonary interstitium. Likewise, abnormalities in the permeability of the capillary membranes (filtration and reflection coefficients) can precede the formation of pulmonary edema (Figure 15-4).

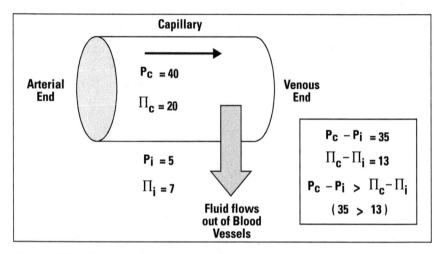

Figure 15-4 Starlings forces at the level of the pulmonary capillary membrane. Backed-up blood and fluid cause an increase in the capillary hydrostatic pressure, causing a net outward flow of fluid into the pulmonary interstitium.

Unlike the circulatory flow in other areas of the body, blood vessels within the lungs are arranged as a low-pressure circuit.[7] This low-pressure circuit leads to higher concentrations of proteins in the pulmonary interstitium (higher osmotic interstitial pressure). When the left ventricle fails, fluid is backed-up into the lungs, an area of higher osmotic interstitial pressures. The high pressures caused by the failing ventricular chambers are reflected backwards into the pulmonary blood vessels.[7] The hydrostatic pressure is also greater; this pressure differential favors movement of fluid **out** of the pulmonary capillaries **into** the interstitium when the ventricles fail. The lymphatic drainage of the lung is unable to fully compensate for this fluid overload.

Patients with heart failure and pulmonary edema may have decreased **intravascular** plasma volume compared to normal subjects.[7] This concept is of great importance because **patients with pulmonary edema and hypotension may be in need of fluid resuscitation to restore blood pressure, even though the pulmonary interstitium is overwhelmed by excess fluid.**[7] In other words, patients in florid pulmonary edema may be hypotensive as a result of a decreased intravascular volume.

The downward spiral of heart failure is represented in Figure 15-5.

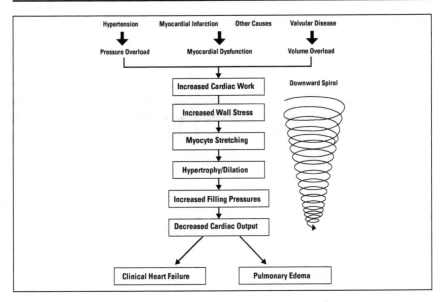

Figure 15-5 The downward spiral of heart failure. Adapted from Nagendran T. The syndrome of heart failure. *Hospital Physician* 2001: 48

Clinical Manifestations

The first step in evaluating a patient with suspected heart failure is a thorough history and physical examination. With an understanding of the pathophysiology, one can use the physical examination as an important tool to distinguish heart failure from the many other entities that mimic this syndrome. **This is especially important in acutely dyspneic patients for whom the cause of the dyspnea is unknown**. A host of symptoms and signs are associated with heart failure. The following section is limited to a discussion of symptoms and signs with plausible pathophysiologic explanations.

CLINICAL SYMPTOMS

Dyspnea is the most common symptom in patients with heart failure.[2,7] This symptom results from vascular congestion (*i.e.*, pulmonary edema), hypoxia, and decreased cardiac output to the peripheral tissues. Paroxysmal nocturnal dyspnea (PND) and orthopnea are caused by pooling of blood in the central blood vessels (*i.e.*, vena cava), which leads to increased filling pressures and pulmonary congestion. Both of these conditions tend to occur when the patient is in the supine position. PND refers to the acute onset of dyspnea. This condition occurs mostly at night, when the patient is recumbent. Nocturia (urination at night) and anorexia are other symptoms of heart failure that are presumed to result from abnormal activation of the renin-angiotensin-aldosterone system and hepatic congestion. Heart failure patients with cough generally have dyspnea first, as opposed to patients with COPD who have coughing and production of sputum **before** dyspnea.[2]

The New York Heart Association's classification is the most commonly used clinical scoring system to determine the degree of heart failure[3] (Table 15-3).

This classification is based entirely upon symptoms. Efforts to develop more quantitative measures exist but have only been adapted by clinical researchers.[3]

Table 15-3

New York Heart Association Classification of Heart Failure

Class I: Symptoms at levels that would be found in normal patients

Class II: Symptoms with ordinary exertion

Class III: Symptoms with less than ordinary exertion

Class IV: Symptoms at rest

CLINICAL SIGNS

Jugular Venous Distension

Systolic failure of the left ventricle causes increased filling pressures and a backing-up of blood in the major vessels supplying blood to the heart. Both the internal and external jugular veins drain into the superior vena cava; hence, in the failing heart, blood backs up into the right atrium, superior vena cava, and jugular veins. To assess the pulsations of the internal jugular, the examiner stands on the right side of the patient with the patient lying at an angle of approximately 30 degrees. The pulsations should be seen between the suprasternal notch and the attachments of the sternocleidomastoid muscle to the sternum and clavicle. The height of the pulsating venous column is recorded by measuring between the distance from the sternal angle (at the level of the second intercostal space) to the highest point of internal jugular pulsations. A distance greater than 3 to 4 centimeters is considered abnormal and is indicative of elevated filling pressure.[13]

Peripheral Edema

Peripheral edema in heart failure is usually bilateral and symmetrical, and occurs late in the course of the disease.[2] Up to 7 to 10 liters of fluid can be retained before edema is noted.[2] In chronically bedridden patients, the sacral area is commonly affected more than the extremities. Anasarca (severe generalized edema) may occur with severe heart failure.[2]

Kussmaul's Sign and Pulsus Paradoxus

In patients with failure of the right ventricle (e.g., constrictive pericarditis), tests can be used to check for increased venous pressure. Venous pressure normally **decreases** during deep inhalation. This pressure change occurs as a result of the negative intrathoracic pressure associated with inspiration, causing the lungs to expand with air, compressing the vena cavae and decreasing preload. In patients with right ventricular failure, venous pressure **increases** due to the inability of the excessively stiff ventricles to fill with blood. This diastolic dysfunction is known as **Kussmaul's sign** and is defined as jugular venous distension when a patient takes a deep inspiration. Kussmaul's sign can be found in patients with right ventricular heart failure by asking a patient to take a deep inspiration while observing the neck veins for distention. The neck veins may already be increased due to increased filling pressures; a positive sign is elicited when the neck veins become more distended with inspiration.

Pulsus paradoxus is often a difficult sign to evoke in patients with right ventricular failure. This sign can be found by inflating the blood pressure cuff 15 mm Hg over the patient's last known systolic pressure (determined immediately before looking for pulsus paradoxus) and asking the patient to take a deep breath while the cuff is deflated. If the systolic pressure decreases by more than 10 mm Hg during inspiration, pulsus paradoxus is present.[14] The systolic drop is produced when the stiffened heart collapses in on itself as a result of the reduction in venous return to the heart that occurs during inspiration.

Proportional Pulse Pressure

A useful clinical indicator of decreased ejection fraction and left ventricular systolic dysfunction is the proportional pulse pressure.

$$\frac{\text{Systolic-Diastolic}}{\text{Systolic}} \times 100 = \text{Proportional Pulse Pressure}$$

This pressure is determined by taking the difference between the systolic and diastolic pressures and dividing by the systolic pressure, converting the decimal value to a percentage. A decrease in the systolic pressure decreases both the numerator and denominator in the equation, thus decreasing the final value. If the value obtained is less than **32%**, a decreased ejection fraction and left ventricular systolic dysfunction is likely.[15]

Apical Impulse

The apical impulse is a palpable beat typically found at the fourth or fifth intercostal space and is described as a brief tap.[2,13,15] The apical impulse can best be palpated when the patient lies in the left lateral decubitus position while sitting upright at 45 degrees. A laterally shifted, downward, or sustained impulse is suggestive of left ventricular systolic function.[2] In cases of right ventricular failure, the apical impulse can be found more medially, closer to the sternum.[2,15]

S_3 & S_4

A third heart sound is caused by increased atrial pressure and noncompliance of the left ventricle during **rapid ventricular filling**. This sign is an indication of left ventricular systolic dysfunction.[2] The patient should be placed in the left lateral recumbent position while sitting upright at 45 degrees, using the bell of the stethoscope for auscultation of the heart.[15] The cadence of three heart sounds has been described as a gallop and is usually louder with inspiration.[13] An S_3 is regarded by many clinicians to be one of the most reliable signs of left ventricular failure; however, it is only considered an abnormal finding in patients over the age of 40.[13]

An S_4 caused by the reverberation of blood during ejection from the left atrium into the left ventricle may also be present in heart failure patients. This sign is due to **noncompliance of the left ventricle** and may be present as a normal finding in elderly patients with stiffened left ventricles.

Valsalva's Maneuver

A method for detecting left ventricular failure involves the use of blood pressure and the Valsalva maneuver. **This 30-second test is perhaps the most practical and accurate clinical sign for a patient with suspected heart failure**. The Valsalva maneuver involves taking a deep breath, inducing glottic closure, and forcibly contracting the abdominal muscles. This causes an increase in both intra-abdominal and intrathoracic pressure. The end result in normal subjects is a decrease in blood return to the right atrium.

To determine an abnormal response in patients with suspected heart failure, the blood pressure is inflated **15 mm Hg above the systolic pressure** with the patient in a supine position.[15] The patient is then asked to perform the Valsalva maneuver. In healthy patients, the Korotkoff (blood pressure) sound should **not** be heard during the straining phase of the Valsalva maneuver.[2] In patients with left ventricular systolic dysfunction and increased filling pressures, an audible Korotkoff sound is produced during the maneuver.[2,15] This clinical sign has been shown in several studies to correlate with confirmed left ventricular failure.[16,17] Furthermore, the blood pressure response to the Valsalva maneuver is related to a variety of neurohumoral parameters of heart failure including release of atrial natriuretic peptide.[18]

Signs of Pulmonary Edema

The early sign of tachypnea in patients with heart failure is often caused by the presence of **interstitial** pulmonary edema. When crackles and rhonchi are heard, the **alveoli** are likely to be affected by edema; **both** lungs are commonly affected. Alterations in the Starling's forces at the capillary level cause a derangement in the organization of body fluids. Peripheral edema in heart failure results from increased capillary hydrostatic pressure as a result of the backing-up of fluid in the pulmonary blood vessels. This increases the outward movement of fluid across the pulmonary capillary membranes into the interstitium.

In some instances, fluid accumulation around the bronchi may induce bronchoconstriction. This circumstance is referred to as **cardiac asthma**, a befitting designation considering the potential for confusion with asthma. Peribronchial fluid accumulation and bronchoconstriction manifest as audible wheezing.

Definitive Diagnosis

The definitive diagnosis of heart failure is made when data obtained from the ECG, echocardiogram, and chest x-ray is evaluated. In addition, serum assays of neurohormonal mediators (*e.g.*, atrial natriuretic peptide), the pulmonary artery catheter, or other tests may help confirm the diagnosis. **Echocardiography is the most useful diagnostic tool for heart failure**. The finding of a low ejection fraction (less than 40%) strongly suggests left ventricular systolic dysfunction and is useful for making long-term management decisions.[2,3] Echocardiography can be combined with Doppler flow studies to determine the geometry, thickness, and regional motion of the ventricles as well as the function of the valves and status of the pericardium.[2]

Of particular importance in the prehospital environment is the 12-lead ECG. An abnormal ECG is strong evidence of left ventricular dysfunction.[17] ECG abnormalities include left ventricular hypertrophy and left atrial enlargement.[9] Myocardial ischemia and infarction, the most common cause of heart failure, must be assessed with ECG analysis. Other dysrhythmias known to cause heart failure may be present including atrial fibrillation and ventricular tachycardia.[9]

Management

The ultimate goal in the management of heart failure is to restore perfusion so that the metabolic requirements of the body are satisfied. In order to attain this goal, the cardiac output and preload must be fully optimized. The Starling curve for the both the normal and failing heart best illustrates how hemodynamic changes can be made with the use of pharmacotherapeutic agents (Figure 15-6).

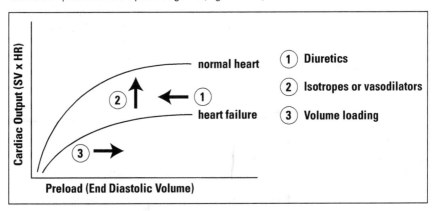

Figure 15-6 The effect of various pharmacotherapeutic agents on the Starling curve. Adapted from Marino PL *The ICU Book*. Philadelphia: Williams & Wilkins, 1998. 248.

STABILIZATION OF ACUTE PULMONARY EDEMA

The dyspneic patient with heart failure and suspected pulmonary edema must be evaluated and stabilized promptly. The pharmacologic agents used for acute pulmonary edema are listed in Table 15-4.

For patients with persistent hypoxia despite a high percentage of delivered oxygen (FiO$_2$), positive airway pressure may be applied. The two most popular modes are continuous positive airway pressure (CPAP) and bi-level positive (Bi-PAP) airway pressure. CPAP improves oxygenation, reduces tachypnea, corrects respiratory acidosis, increases cardiac output, decreases afterload, and reduces the need for endotracheal intubation and mechanical ventilation; however, no impact on mortality has been shown.[9,20,21] Bi-PAP has the advantage of reducing the amount of expiratory positive airway pressure that a patient would be exposed to with CPAP, allowing patients to better adapt to the technique.[9] Bi-PAP was shown to improve ventilation and vital signs more rapidly than CPAP in one study, but has not shown a reduction in mortality when used in patients with cardiogenic pulmonary edema.[22].

Table 15-4
Agents Used for the Management of Acute Pulmonary Edema

Agent	Mechanism of Action	Precautions
Oxygen	Maintain saturation above 95% Prevent hypoxia	May reduce cardiac output; may increase systemic vascular resistance; may constrict the coronary arteries
Nitrates (sublingual or buccal spray nitroglycerin, nitroprusside)	Reduce systemic vasoconstriction Increase cardiac output Decrease preload Decrease afterload*	If hypotension develops, consider right ventricular infarction and give fluid challenge
Loop Diuretics (furosemide,Bumetinide, torsemide)	Reduce volume overload by causing sodium and water excretion at the ascending loop of Henle in the Kidney Increase peripheral vasoconstriction Increase renin release	Hypotension is likely with right ventricular infarction, cardiac tamponade, hypovolemia
Morphine	Anxiolytic: relieves sense of breathlessness	Nausea and vomiting common; hypotension and hypoventilation possible at high doses

* In patients with left ventricular dysfunction

TREATMENT OF CHRONIC HEART FAILURE

Diuretics

Loop diuretics such as furosemide (Lasix®) and bumetanide (Bumex®) inhibit the reabsorption of sodium at the thick ascending loop of Henle in the kidney[3] (Figure 15-7). These agents increase water excretion by increasing sodium excretion (*i.e.*, water follows sodium according to principles of diffusion). They can relieve both pulmonary and peripheral edema rapidly (within hours to days) and are the only class of drugs shown to adequately control the fluid retention associated with heart failure.[3] Diuretics are used exclusively to relieve symptoms of fluid retention in heart failure; no proven mortality benefit has been found.[4] The use of diuretics alone cannot maintain clinical stability in patients with heart failure.[3,4] Thiazide diuretics are a second-line class of diuretic agents with a different mechanism of action in the nephron. Hydrochlorothiazide (HCTZ) is the prototypical thiazide diuretic.

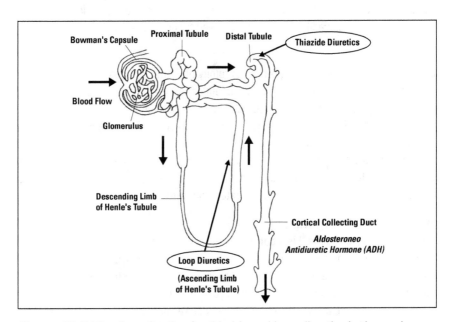

Figure 15-7 The sites of action for thiazide and loop diuretics in the nephron.

ACE-Inhibitors

Six ACE-inhibitors are approved for use in patients with heart failure.[3] ACE-inhibitors have several beneficial effects in patients with heart failure. These agents interfere with the renin-angiotensin-aldosterone system by inhibiting angiotensin-converting enzyme (ACE). Since ACE is identical to kininase II, the enzyme responsible for the degradation of kinins, inhibition of this enzyme allows more kinins to become active.[3] Kinins play an important role in the synthesis of prostaglandins, molecules that help protect the kidneys, and may be helpful for patients with heart failure. ACE-inhibitors also prevent cardiac remodeling, a process that contributes to the altered hemodynamics associated with heart failure.[3] ACE inhibitors have been evaluated in more than 7,000 patients in over 30 placebo-controlled clinical trials, and have been shown to confer a significant reduction in mortality for patients in heart failure.[3,4] ACE inhibitors are contraindicated in angioedema, renal insufficiency, renal artery stenosis, and pregnancy.[3,4] Common side effects include hypotension, dizziness, cough, and potassium retention.[3]

Beta-Blockers

Beta-blockers were previously thought to have detrimental effects in patients with heart failure and were contraindicated. Beta-blockers inhibit the negative effects of the sympathetic nervous system by attenuating the damaging effects of norepinephrine stimulation of beta-1, beta-2, and alpha-1 receptors on cardiac cells. Metoprolol (Lopressor®), bisoprolol fumarate (Zebeta®), and carvedilol (Coreg®, a combined alpha- and beta-blocker) improve both symptoms and ejection fraction in patients with moderate to severe symptoms of heart failure.[4] Beta-blockers have shown the greatest benefit in patients with documented reduced ejection fractions.[23] Despite the beneficial effects of beta-blockers, only carvedilol is currently approved for use (Table 15-5).[3]

Digoxin

Digoxin is the representative agent of the family of digitalis glycosides, and was first used more than 200 years ago for the treatment of heart failure.[23] Digitalis inhibits the sodium-potassium adenosine triphosphatase (ATPase) pumps in the cardiac cells, vagus nerve, and kidney.[3] This enzymatic inhibition serves to decrease sympathetic outflow to the heart while providing a modest increase in contractility. Renin is also suppressed, as well as other neurohormonal factors.[3] Although effective for relief of symptoms, better quality of life, increased functional capacity, and improved exercise tolerance, digoxin has failed to demonstrate a mortality benefit.[3,4]

Aldosterone Antagonists

Spironolactone (Aldactone®) is a potassium sparring diuretic that works at the cortical collecting duct in the kidney by antagonizing the action of the hormone aldosterone. This agent is used in patients with severe symptoms.[3,4,23] Long-term overstimulation of the heart and blood vessels with high levels of circulating aldosterone has been hypothesized to have adverse effects on the structure and function of the heart.[3] When used with loop diuretics for severe heart failure (NYHA class IV), a decrease in hospitalizations and mortality was observed.[3,4,23]

Nonrecommended Agents

Unapproved agents for the treatment of heart failure include angiotensin receptor blockers (losartan, candesartan), hydralazine, isosorbide dinitrate, Coumadin, and various antiarrhythmics.[4] The use of these agents has not been found to confer enough of a beneficial effect on mortality and symptom relief to recommend routine use. These unapproved agents should only used in carefully selected patients.

Vasodilators such as hydralazine and isosorbide dinitrate improve cardiac performance by dilating resistance vessels and reducing afterload.[3] As shown in Figure 15-6, afterload reduction helps shift the Starling curve upwards. These drugs are typically reserved for use in the intensive care unit setting, where hemodynamic variables can be closely monitored.

Dobutamine, milrinone, and amrinone are powerful inotropic agents that dramatically increase cardiac output in heart failure patients.[3,23] These drugs have a favorable effect on cardiac performance, as indicated by an upwards shift of the Starling curve (Figure 15-6), but are only used when well-defined goals are established (*e.g.*, stabilizing the patient before diuresis) and must be used under close hemodynamic surveillance (*i.e.*, ICU, CCU).[23]

Cardiogenic Shock

Cardiogenic shock is the end result of heart failure and serves as a paradigm for the progressive changes seen clinically in the development of shock. Progressive loss of functional myocardial tissue brings about a critical loss in stroke volume, and the heart rate increases to sustain cardiac output. The capacity of the failing heart to beat faster is limited and cardiac output falls to levels that are inadequate to support end-organ function. The signs of shock ensue and coronary perfusion decreases, in turn causing progressive myocardial ischemia with progression to further myocardial infarction. **Cardiogenic shock is associated with a grave prognosis**. Therapy is mainly supportive; the management of shock is discussed further in Chapters 17 to 19.

Table 15-5

Approved Agents for Treatment of Chronic Heart Failure

Loop Diuretics
furosemide (LASIX), torsemide (DEMADEX), bumetanide (BUMEX)

Thiazide Diuretics*
hydrochlorothiazide (MICROZIDE)

Digitalis Preparations
digoxin (LANOXIN)

ACE-Inhibitors*
captopril (CAPOTEN), enalapril (VASOTEC), lisinopril (PRINIVIL/ZESTRIL), quinapril (ACCUPRIL), fosinopril (MONOPRIL), ramapril (ALTACE)**

Beta-Blockers*
carvedilol (COREG)***, metoprolol (LOPRESSOR/TOPROL), atenolol (TENORMIN), bisoprolol (ZEBETA)

* Various combination preparations exist
** ramapril is approved for heart failure after MI
*** All these agents have beneficial effects on heart failure, but only carvedilol is approved for heart failure

References

1. Cleland JG. Heart failure: a medical Hydra. *Lancet* 1998; 352 (Suppl): SI 1-2.

2. Nagendran T. The syndrome of heart failure. *Hospital Physician* 2001: 46-57.

3. Packer MP, Cohn JN (eds.) for the Steering Committee and Membership of the Advisory Council to Improve Outcomes Nationwide in Heart Failure. Consensus recommendations for the management of chronic heart failure. *Amer J Cardio* 1999; 83(2A): 1A-79A.

4. Gomberg-Maitland M, Baran DA, Fuster V. Treatment of congestive heart failure: guidelines for the primary care physician and the heart failure specialist. *Arch Intern Med* 2001; 161: 342-352.

5. Guidelines for the evaluation and management of heart failure: Report of the American College of Cardiology / American Heart Association Task Force on Practice Guidelines (Committee of Evaluation and Management of Heart Failure). *Circulation* 1995; 92: 2764-2784.

6. Massie BM, Shah NB. Evolving trends in the epidemiologic factors of heart failure: rationale for preventive strategies and comprehensive disease management. *Am Heart J* 1997; 133: 703-712.

7. Falk JL, O'Brien JF, Shesser R. Heart failure. In: Rosen P, Barkin R, *et al. Emergency Medicine: Concepts and Clinical Practice.* New York: Mosby, 1997: 1631-1652.

8. Vander AJ. *Renal Physiology.* 5th ed. New York: McGraw-Hill, 1995.

9. Albrich JM. Congestive heart failure: A state-of-the-art review of clinical pitfalls, evaluation strategies, and recent advances in drug therapy (part I). *Emerg Med Reports* 1997; 18(16): 159-166.

10. Vander AJ, Sherman JH, and Luciano DS. *Human Physiology: The Mechanisms of Body Function.* 6th Ed. New York: McGraw-Hill, 1994.

11. Goldsmith S, Dick C. Differentiating systolic from diastolic heart failure: Pathophysiologic and therapeutic considerations. *Am J Med* 1993; 95: 645-655.

12. Gaasch WH. Diagnosis and treatment of heart failure based on left ventricular systolic or diastolic dysfunction. *JAMA* 1994; 271: 1276-1280.

13. Bates B, Bickley LS, Hoekelman RA. *A Guide to Physical Examination and History Taking.* 6th ed. Philadelphia: J.B. Lippincott Co., 1995.

14. Barach P. Pulsus paradoxus. *Hosp Phys* 2000; 36(1): 49-50.

15. Badgett RG, Lucey CR, Mulrow CD. Can the clinical examination diagnose left-sided heart failure in adults? *JAMA* 1997; 277: 1712-1719.

16. Zema MJ. Diagnosing heart failure by the Valsalva maneuver: Isn't it finally time? *Chest* 1199; 116(4): 851-852.

17. Marantz PR, Kaplan MC, Alderman MH. Clinical diagnosis of congestive heart failure in patients with acute dyspnea. *Chest* 1990; 97: 776-781.

18. Brunner-La Rocca HP, Weilenmann D, Rickli H, *et al.* Is blood pressure response to the Valsalva maneuver related to neurohormones, exercise capacity, and clinical findings in heart failure? *Chest* 1999; 116(4): 861-867.

19. Rihal CS, Davis KB, Kennedy JW, *et al.* The utility of clinical, electrocardiographic, and roentgenographic variables in the prediction of left ventricular dysfunction. *Am J Cardiol* 1995; 75: 220-223.

20. Bersten AD, Holt AW, Vedig AE, *et al.* Treatment of severe cardiogenic pulmonary edema with continuous positive airway pressure delivered by face mask. *N Engl J Med* 1991; 325: 1825-1830.

21. Lin M, Yang YF, Chiang HT, *et al.* Reappraisal of continuous positive airway pressure therapy in acute cardiogenic pulmonary edema: Short-term results and long-term follow-up. *Chest* 1995; 107: 1379-1386.

22. Mechta S, Jay GD, Woolard RH, *et al.* Randomized, prospective trial of bi-level vs. continuous positive airway pressure in acute pulmonary edema. *Crit Care Med* 1997; 25: 620-628.

23. Stevenson LW. Recent advances in the management of heart failure. *Fam Prac Recert* 2000; 22 (12): 51-58.

Review Questions

1. An 85-year-old female presents with crackles and a loud S3 gallop on physical exam. The patient has a history of previous MI in the past. A Valsalva's maneuver is positive and peripheral pitting edema is noted. Which of the following statement(s) is(are) true regarding this patient's condition?
   A. The patient's condition is associated with a 50% 5-year mortality
   B. The most common causes are coronary atherosclerotic heart disease and hypertension
   C. Left ventricular function is most likely significantly decreased
   D. Ejection fraction is likely to be below 55%
   E. All of the above are true statements

The answer is E.

2. Referring to the patient in Question 1, which of the following pathophysiologic characteristics would most likely be present?
   A. Increased ejection fraction
   B. Suppression of the renin-angiotensin-aldosterone system
   C. Supranormal elevation of atrial natriuretic peptide
   D. Inhibition of apoptosis
   E. Supranormal filling pressures in the heart

The renin-angiotensin-aldosterone system is stimulated in heart failure and atrial natriuretic peptide is depleted, not increased. Programmed cell death (apoptosis) occurs over time. The answer is E.

3. Which of the following statements is correct regarding the use of the Valsalva's maneuver for patients with presumed heart failure?
   A. The blood pressure is inflated to 15 mm Hg over the systolic pressure before the maneuver
   B. Glottic closure causes increased intrathoracic and intra-abdominal pressure
   C. Absence of Korotkoff sounds after the blood pressure cuff is deflated constitutes a positive test
   D. This 30-minute test is a valuable predictor of right ventricular dysfunction
   E. In normal patients, the maneuver increases preload, making the Korotkoff sounds audible after the cuff is deflated

The Valsalva's maneuver is a valuable bedside diagnostic test that takes no longer than 30 seconds to perform properly. The blood pressure is inflated to 15 mm Hg over the systolic pressure before the maneuver. The cuff is then deflated. In a normal patient,

Korotkoff sounds should not be heard immediately after cuff deflation. Auscultation of Korotkoff sounds during cuff inflation (above the patient's known systolic blood pressure) constitutes a positive test. When positive, this test is highly suggestive of left ventricular dysfunction. The answer is A.

4. In patients with heart failure, peripheral edema is caused by:
   A. Interstitial fluid depletion
   B. Accumulation of up to 700 mL of fluid in the interstitium
   C. Increased fibrosis of the capillary walls
   D. Increased capillary hydrostatic pressure
   E. Collapse of the right ventricle with expiration

According to Starling's law of the capillary, the hydrostatic pressure is the driving force for filtration. When this pressure is increased, fluid passes out of blood vessels into the interstitial (third) space. Seven to ten liters of fluid can accumulate before edema is noticed. The answer is D.

5. Signs of heart failure include all of the following EXCEPT:
   A. S3 heart sound due to rapid ventricular filling
   B. S4 heart sound due to noncompliance of the left ventricle
   C. Pulsus paradoxus: an increase of 20 mm Hg in the systolic blood pressure when the patient exhales as the cuff is deflated
   D. Proportional pulse pressure less than 30%
   E. Jugular venous distension secondary to systolic failure of the left ventricle

Pulsus paradoxus can be found by inflating the blood pressure cuff 15 mm Hg over the patient's last known systolic pressure and asking the patient to take a deep breath while the cuff is deflated. If the systolic pressure decreases by more than 10 mm Hg during inspiration, pulsus paradoxus is present. The answer is C.

6. Which of the following agents are used for stabilization of heart failure patients with acute pulmonary edema?
   A. Morphine, diuretics, BiPAP
   B. Morphine, diuretics, digoxin
   C. Morphine, diuretics, angiotensin II receptor antagonists
   D. Milrinone, ACE inhibitors, beta-blockers
   E. Hydralazine, ACE inhibitors, nitrates

Agents listed in the other answer choices are used for the chronic management of patients with heart failure. The answer is A.

7-8. Refer to Figure 15-1.
- A. Furosemide
- B. Dobutamine
- C. Lisinopril
- D. Oxygen
- E. Nitroglycerin

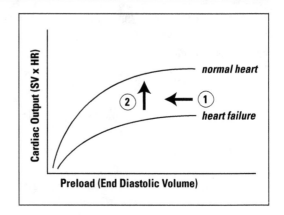

Preload (End Diastolic Volume)

7. Which agent causes a shift of the Starling curve as indicated by 1?
8. Which agent causes a shift of the Starling curve as indicated by 2?

7. Diuretics such as furosemide decrease preload. The answer is A.

8. Dobutamine is a potent inotrope that increases cardiac output. The answer is B.

9. A 68-year-old male presents to the emergency department with the chief complaint of dyspnea. A chest x-ray shows cardiomegaly and evidence of acute pulmonary edema. What is the most common cause of heart failure?
- A. Coronary artery disease
- B. Hypertension
- C. Valvular heart disease
- D. Alcoholic cardiomyopathy
- E. Chronic obstructive pulmonary disease

Coronary artery disease is the most common cause of heart failure. The answer is A.

10. The effect of diuretics for the patient in Question 9 includes all of the following EXCEPT:
- A. Reduction of systemic vasoconstriction
- B. Increased peripheral vasoconstriction
- C. Increased renin secretion by the juxtaglomerular apparatus of the kidney
- D. Decreased volume overload by increased excretion of sodium and water at the ascending loop of Henle in the kidney
- E. Induction of immediate vasodilation in the pulmonary vasculature

Diuretics are useful in the management of dyspnea secondary to acute pulmonary edema because of an immediate vasodilatory effect in the lungs. Over time, diuretics decrease preload. Nitrates, not diuretics, reduce systemic vasoconstriction. The answer is A.

16

Hypertensive Emergencies and Urgencies

Few disorders cause more confusion than hypertension when it comes to the management and disposition of patients. The decision to treat and what agents to use can only be made when the underlying pathophysiology and consequences of drug action are considered.

Epidemiology

Nearly one out of every four Americans has hypertension.[1,2] The disease is more prominent in African-Americans, and according to the most conservative estimates, affects at least 20 million patients in the United States.[2,3] Many patients with hypertension remain undiagnosed and untreated. Hypertensive emergencies are defined as acute, life-threatening increases in blood pressure that requires immediate blood pressure reduction to limit or prevent target-organ damage.

Definitions

It is important to distinguish between hypertensive **emergencies** and **urgencies** because management of the two differs drastically. A hypertensive urgency is defined as an acute, severe blood pressure elevation with a systolic blood pressure greater than 220 mm Hg and/or a diastolic blood pressure greater than 120 mm Hg.[4,5] Hypertensive emergencies are severe elevations in blood pressure complicated by severe end-organ damage, such as intracranial hemorrhage, encephalopathy, pulmonary edema, or acute renal insufficiency. Some authors use the term **malignant hypertension** to describe a hypertensive emergency. Malignant hypertension exists when one or more of the following signs of end-organ damage is seen with a diastolic blood pressure over 120 mm Hg: specific pathologic changes in the eye as detected by funduscopy, encephalopathy, renal insufficiency, and left ventricular failure and CHF with pulmonary edema.[8] Hypertensive urgencies are severe elevations of blood pressure **without evidence of end-organ damage.**[4] The most important consideration for patients with hypertensive emergencies or urgencies is the determination of the **rate of rise of the blood pressure** since a patient with chronic, poorly controlled blood pressure can tolerate a much higher blood pressure than a normotensive patient.[4] It is important to note that **differentiating between a true hypertensive emergency and a hypertensive urgency can only be accomplished when laboratory data, funduscopy, and the results of radiological studies are considered together**.[6] In the absence of conditions that

can be clinically diagnosed, such as heart failure, pulmonary edema, or encephalopathy, it is virtually impossible to clinically differentiate between the two in the field.

Pathogenesis

The cause of abrupt increases in systolic and diastolic blood pressure has yet to be associated with a specific etiology. Most cases of hypertension are the result of **essential** hypertension, the cause of which remains highly speculative. Major theories for the pathogenesis of hypertension include arterial wall damage because of alterations in the contractile properties of smooth muscle and arterial smooth muscle damage resulting from failure of autoregulatory systems.[6] Blood pressure elevation is likely to result from several pathologic processes occurring concomitantly.

SYMPATHETIC HYPERACTIVITY

The sympathetic nervous system occupies a central role in the regulation of blood pressure. Cardiac output and systemic vascular resistance are controlled by a variety of adrenergic receptor interactions.

Blood Pressure = Cardiac Output x Systemic Vascular Resistance
(Cardiac Output = Heart Rate x Stroke Volume)

Stimulation of adrenergic receptors stimulates the renin-angiotensin-aldosterone system, enhancing vasoconstriction, sodium retention, and volume expansion[7] (Figure 16-1). Overactivity of the sympathetic nervous system can occur as a result of disinhibition failure, which is the failure of inhibitory neurons to decrease sympathetic nervous activity in the brainstem.[7]

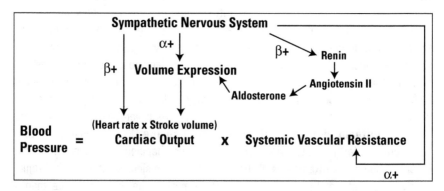

Figure 16-1 The effect of the sympathetic nervous system on the determinants of blood pressure: both cardiac output and systemic vascular resistance are affected by adrenergic receptor activation.

RENIN-ANGIOTENSIN-ALDOSTERONE OVERSTIMULATION

Overstimulation of the renin-angiotensin-aldosterone system leads to critically high levels of circulating vasoactive agents such as angiotensin II, norepinephrine, and vasopressin.[8] Circulation of these substances induces changes in the hemodynamics of the kidney, constricting blood vessels exiting the glomerular apparatus (Figure 16-2).

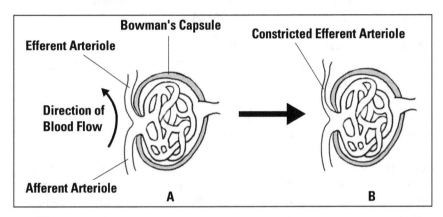

Figure 16-2 Efferent arteriolar constriction in the kidney: the mechanism leading to pressure diuresis in the kidney and the cycle of increased renin-angiotensin-aldosterone activity.

Narrowing of the efferent arteriole brings about a pressure diuresis by causing a pressure difference between the blood entering and exiting the circulation of the kidney, this leads to net elimination of free water. These events stimulate higher levels of renin to be released from the juxtaglomerular apparatus of the kidney, which in turn leads to the release of vasoactive substances in response to hypovolemia. This vicious cycle perpetuates itself as the body senses hypovolemia and reacts by releasing more vasoactive substances in an attempt to sustain a normal blood volume. The release of vasoactive substances causes endothelial damage, platelet aggregation, and release of other factors, causing progressive narrowing of blood vessels and vasoconstriction.

OTHER PATHOGENIC FACTORS

In addition to renin-angiotensin-aldosterone overstimulation and sympathetic hyperactivity, a host of other determinants are speculated to play a role in the pathogenesis of essential hypertension. Angiotensin II and the substance known as endotheilin-1 can act synergistically to stimulate the sympathetic nervous system and increase systemic vascular resistance. In patients with hypertension, vasodilatation by nitric oxide and other substances may be impaired. Obese patients are susceptible to hypertension because of low HDL cholesterol levels, high triglycerides, and increased insulin resistance, all leading to increased vascular damage. The pathophysiology of obesity-related hypertension is polyfactorial; both overactivity of the sympathetic nervous system and salt sensitivity play a role.[9] Insulin resistance, is a well-known risk factor for the development of any cardiovascular disease, including hypertension. Sensitivity of blood pressure to dietary salt intake varies from person to person, but in some patients can lead to high blood pressure.[9] Blood pressure is a trait that is polygenic (determined by many genes). Researchers continue to isolate specific genes postulated to play a role in regulating blood pressure and vasoactive substances.

SECONDARY HYPERTENSION

Sustained elevations in blood pressure can be caused by secondary factors or other primary disease processes that lead to hypertension. Reduced renal perfusion resulting from occlusion (*i.e.*, stenosis) of the renal blood vessels can lead to hypertension. This disorder elicits an abnormal response by various angiotensin-dependent mechanisms. Pheochromocytoma is a rare tumor that releases abnormal levels of catecholamines, invariably leading to increased blood pressure. Both hypothyroidism and hyperthyroidism can lead to elevations in blood pressure. Abnormalities in calcium metabolism, as occurs in hyperparathyroidism, can potentiate hypertension by causing changes in the renin-angiotensin-aldosterone system in addition to renal damage generated by this disorder. The most common cardiovascular cause of hypertension is coarctation of the aorta, a disorder that should be clinically suspected when blood pressure is higher in the arms than legs. Psychiatric illnesses such as anxiety disorders and depression tend to coexist in patients with hypertension but the association between these disorders is poorly understood from a purely physiologic standpoint.

Diagnosis

BLOOD PRESSURE MEASUREMENTS

The first step in evaluating a hypertensive emergency or urgency is to take an accurate blood pressure measurement. The technique used in prehospital care is an indirect measurement of blood pressure and is made with a sphygmomanometer, a device that enables the examiner to correlate the auscultated Korotkoff sounds with a pressure measurement in millimeters of mercury. This technique is notoriously unreliable and well recognized for its inaccuracy.[10-12] The Korotkoff sounds generated when an occluded artery is reopened are nearly inaudible to the human ear and wide intraobserver variations complicate interpretation of indirect measurements.[10-12] When the patient is brought to the emergency department or intensive care unit, more accurate determinations of blood pressure can be made with direct techniques involving the use of intra-arterial catheters. In the prehospital environment, indirect measurements are the only available means of estimating a patient's blood pressure.

Korotkoff Sounds

The Korotkoff sounds are divided into five phases, each one described by the ausculatory findings when the blood pressure cuff is inflated and then gradually deflated at the recommended rate of 2 to 3 mm Hg per second.[13] Table 16-1 lists the five phases of the Korotkoff sounds. Most trials use the fifth phase of the Korotkoff sounds for the diastolic blood pressure although there is still no universal agreement among clinicians, so differences of up to 25 mm Hg are possible if the fourth Korotkoff sound is used.[14]

Table 16-1
The Five Phases of the Korotkoff Sounds

Phase	Auscultatory Findings
Phase I	First appearance of faint, clear tapping sounds (the *systolic* blood pressure)
Phase II	Murmur or swishing sound
Phase III	Crisper sounds with increasing intensity
Phase IV	Abrupt muffling of sounds—sounds become soft and blowing
Phase V	Disappearance of sounds (generally used as the diastolic blood pressure)

Patient Positioning and Cuff Placement

The patient should be seated and made as comfortable as possible during blood pressure measurement. Cuff size is important and if not properly applied leads to falsely high or low measurements. The bladder of the cuff should be placed 2.0 to 2.5 cm above the antecubital space and should be 20% wider than the diameter of the extremity.[8] The bell of the stethoscope should always be used because it is better equipped to detect the low-frequency Korotkoff sounds. The arm should be positioned horizontally, at the level of the heart; vertical or diagonal positioning of the arm results in slightly higher measurements.

JNC-VI CLASSIFICATION

The 1997 Joint National Commission was composed of an executive committee of nine members and over 100 consultants who created recommendations for the management of chronic hypertension.[15] An understanding of this classification provides insight for prehospital providers when assessing patients with hypertension (Tables 16-2 and 16-3).

Table 16-2

The Three-Stage JNC-VI Classification for Hypertension and the Recommended Drug Classes for Specific Patient Populations

Blood Pressure (JNC-VI)

High Normal	<139 - <89
Stage I	<159 - <99
Stage II	<179 - <109
Stage III	>180 - >110

Essential Tremor
Nonselective beta-blockers

Diabetes Type I
low dose diuretics
ACE-inhibitors (if proteinuria)

Atrial Tachycardia/fibrilliation
Beta-blockers

Osteoporosis
Thiazides

Dyslipidemia
Alpha-blockers

Prostatism
Alpha-blockers

Migraine
Nonselective beta-blockers
Nondihydropyridine calcium channel blockers
(verapamil, diltiazem)

Table 16-3
Hypertension Risk Group Stratification as
Outlined in the JNC-VI Guidelines.

Hypertension Risk Groups

Group A: Uncomplicated HTN
No cardiovascular risk factors
No target organ damage
(Lifestyle modification & drug therapy if Stage II or III; can wait 12 months
if Stage I)

Group B: Comorbid Conditions
No target organ damage
At least one of below, excluding diabetes:
- Smoking
- Age > 60
- Men; menopausal women
- Family history of CV disease*
- Dyslipidemia

*(women under 65; men under 55)
(Lifestyle Modification & Drug Therapy if Stage II or III; can wait 6 months
if Stage I)

Group C: Complicated HTN
Target organ damage and one of below:
- Heart disease
- Left ventricular hypertrophy
- Diabetes
- Angina; prior myocardial infarction
- Prior CABG or revascularization
- Stroke or transient ischemic attack
- Nephropathy
- Retinopathy
- Aortic atherosclerosis
- Congestive heart failure

(Lifestyle Modification & Drug Therapy for all stages)

Management

AVAILABLE AGENTS

When a true hypertensive emergency is established, the following goals should be considered when deciding on an appropriate agent for immediate blood pressure reduction: reduction of systemic vascular resistance, preservation of cardiac output, improved arterial compliance, and maintenance of organ perfusion.[8] The above should be achieved within a 24-hour period, while avoiding compensatory neurohumoral reflexes such as reflex tachycardia, salt and water overload, and reflex vasoconstriction by vasoactive substances.[8] A wide variety of agents are available to accomplish these goals and are summarized in Table 16-4.

Table 16-4

Agents of Choice for the Management of Hypertensive Emergencies

Agent	Mechanism of Action	Specific Indications	Adverse Effects
Nitroprusside	Arteriolar and Venous Dilator	Hypertensive Emergencies	Risk of cyande toxicity, nausea, vomiting, fluid, retention, precipitous blood pressure drop, drug inactivated when exposed to light, may increase intracerbral pressure
Nitroglycerin	Venous Dilator	Hypertensive Emergencies associated with angina & myocardial infarction	Headache, nausea, metheemoglobinemia, tolerance for patients on nitrates for prolonged time
Labetalol	Alpha and Beta Blocker	Hypertensive Emergencies, especially aortic dissection, pheochromocytoma, preeclampsia	Heart failure, heart block, bronchospasm, bradycardia
Fenoldopam	Peripheral Dopamine-1 Agonist	Hypertensive Emergencies	Has diuretic effect which may exacerbate volume depletion
Hydralazine	Arteriolar Dilator	Preeclampsia & Ecclampsia	Tachycardia, flushing, worsening ofangina, local thrombophlebitis
Enalaprilat	Aniotensin Converting Enzyme Inhibitor	Hypertensive Emergencies associated with heart failure and pulmonary edema	May cause precipitous drop in blood pressure
Esmolol	Beta Blocker	Used in combination with Nitroprusside in aortic dissection	Nausea, bradycardia, heart block, heart failure, bronchospasm
Phentolamine	Alpha Blocker	Pheochromocytoma	Tachycardia, headache, angina

Most of these agents have an onset of action less than 5 minutes with a variable duration of action and all are administered parenterally. Nitroprusside is the most popular agent for the treatment of hypertensive emergencies, but other agents such as labetalol and fenoldopam can be equally effective and do not increase intracranial pressure.[16] Use of these agents requires close patient monitoring in a critical care setting.

Moratorium on Nifedipine

Over the past 20 years, nifedipine, an orally administered dihydropyridine calcium channel blocker, became immensely popular in the treatment of hypertensive emergencies.[17] Advantages of this agent included sublingual administration and administration in a noncritical care, nonmonitored setting. Despite several serious reports of adverse effects with sublingual or oral nifedipine in the medical literature, some systems still support the use of this agent.[18-21] Nifedipine is erratically absorbed via the oral or sublingual route and leads to an uncontrollable and unpredictable fall in blood pressure. Reflex catecholamine release and increased heart rate may occur, exacerbating underlying myocardial ischemia or infarction. Nifedipine can also lead to a steal phenomenon by causing peripheral vasodilatation with redirection of blood flow away from vital organs such as the heart and brain. Given the seriousness of the reported side effects and the variable absorption and unpredictable response, the use of nifedipine capsules for hypertensive emergencies should be abandoned.[17]

SPECIAL SITUATIONS

Hypertensive Encephalopathy

Hypertensive encephalopathy is a potentially lethal complication of hypertensive emergencies and typically occurs in patients with chronic, poorly-controlled hypertension.[5,7] In normal patients, perfusion of the cerebral tissue is equal to the mean arterial pressure minus the intracranial pressure.

> **Cerebral Perfusion Pressure (CPP) = MAP - Intracranial Pressure**
> **(MAP = Diastolic + 1/3x Systolic-Diastolic BP)**

The cerebral perfusion pressure (CPP) is controlled by the process known as autoregulation. When an increase in the blood pressure exceeds the autoregulatory ability of the brain, cerebral edema results and is manifested by progressive neurologic deterioration. Hypertensive encephalopathy presents with neurologic signs such as confusion, seizures, headache, nausea, and vomiting; the diagnosis is only apparent after other neurologic diseases such as stroke, subarachnoid hemorrhage, infections, or other disorders are ruled out.[5,7] Abrupt reductions in blood pressure must be avoided in patients with hypertensive encephalopathy as a decrease in the mean arterial pressure (MAP) may lead to cerebral hypoperfusion. A recommended blood pressure reduction of 25% within the first hour or treatment to a diastolic pressure of no less than 100 mm Hg is a legitimate treatment goal.[5]

Preeclampsia

Preeclampsia is a complex disorder that typically presents in the third trimester in greater than 3% of all pregnancies in the United States.[22] This disorder is characterized by a wide variety of proposed pathogenic factors, although the principal cause is presently unknown. The triad of elevated blood pressure, proteinuria, and edema is diagnostic; preeclamptic patients with seizures have **eclampsia**. Abnormally formed placentas, kidney changes, vasoconstriction out of proportion to peripheral blood measurements, endothelial dysfunction, and liver abnormalities all play a role in this multisystem disease.[23] Although management of this disorder is best left to experienced obstetricians, several parenteral agents are available for use. Hydralazine, labetalol, and methyldopa are all effective antihypertensives used for this disorder.[24]

Permanent Sequelae

An appreciation for the permanent long-term sequelae of poorly-controlled hypertension, although not imperative for paramedics, provides further insight when evaluating any patient with hypertension. Table 16-5 summarizes the effects of long-standing uncontrolled hypertension.

Table 16-5
The Major Sequelae of Chronic, Poorly-Controlled Hypertension

Hypertension-Related Disorder	Pathophysiology
Atherosclerosis	Supply-demand imbalance
	Acceleration of atherosclerosis
	Vessel damage (?)
Left ventricular hypertrophy	Concentric increase in ventricular mass
Heart Failure	Refer to Chapter 15
Stroke	Most potent risk factor for stroke
	Thickened media of small intracerebral vessels
Intracerebral hemorrhage	Main cause of intracerebral hemorrhage
	Focal damage to small intracerebral arteries
	Lipohyalinosis: leads to vessel occlusion
	Risk factor for subarachnoid hemorrhage

References

1. Joint National Committee. The sixth report of the Joint National Committee on the Prevention, Detection, Evaluation and Treatment of High Blood Pressure (JNC-VI). *Arch Intern Med* 1997; 157: 2413-2446.

2. Burt VL, Whelton P, Roccella EJ, *et al.* Prevalence of hypertension in the U.S. adult population: Results from the third health and nutrition examination survey, 1988-1991. *Hypertension* 1995; 25: 305.

3. Yong LC, *et al.* Longitudinal studies of blood pressure: Changes and determinants from adolescence to middle age: The Dormant high school follow-up study, 1957-1963 to 1989-1990. *Am J Epidemiol* 1993; 138: 973.

4. Calhoun DA. Hypertensive crisis. In: Oparil S, Weber MA (eds.). *Hypertension: A Companion to Brenner and Rector's The Kidney.* Philadelphia: WB Saunders Company, 2000: 715-718.

5. Calhoun DA, Oparil S. Treatment of hypertensive crisis. *N Eng J Med* 1990; 323: 1177.

6. Mathews J. Hypertension. In: Rosen P, Barkin R, *et al.* *Emergency Medicine: Concepts and Clinical Practice.* New York: Mosby, 1997: 1631-1652.

7. Izzo JL. The sympathetic nervous system in human hypertension. *In:* Izzo JL, Black HR. *Hypertension Primer: The Essentials of High Blood Pressure.* 2nd Edition. Dallas: American Heart Association, 1999: 109-112.

8. Houston MC, Meador BP, Schipani LM. *Handbook of Antihypertensive Therapy.* 7th Edition. Philadelphia: Hanly & Belfus Inc., 1997. 58.

9. Weinberger MH. Salt sensitivity of blood pressure in humans. *Hypertension* 1996; 27: 481-490.

10. Pickering TG. Blood pressure measurement and detection of hypertension. *Lancet* 1994; 344: 31-35.

11. Reeves RA. Does this patient have hypertension? How to measure blood pressure. *JAMA* 1995; 273: 1211-1218.

12. Ellestad MH. Reliability of blood pressure recordings. *Am J Cardiol* 1989; 63: 983-985.

13. Kirdendall WM, Feinleib M, Freis ED, Mark AL. Recommendations for human blood pressure determination by sphygmomanometers: Subcommittee of the AHA Postgraduate Education Committee. *Circulation* 1980; 62: 1146A-1155A.

14. Breit SN, O'Rourke MF. Comparison of direct and indirect arterial pressure measurements in hospitalized patients. *Aust N Z J Med* 1974; 4: 485-491.

15. The Sixth Report of the Joint National Committee on Prevention, Detection, Evaluation, and Treatment of High Blood Pressure. *Arch Intern Med* 1997; 157: 2413-2446.

16. Kaplan NM. Management of hypertensive emergencies. *Lancet* 1994; 344(8933): 1335-1338.

17. Grossman E, Messerli HF, Grodzincki T, Kowey P. Should a moratorium be placed on sublingual nifedipine capsules given for hypertensive emergencies and pseudoemergencies? *JAMA* 1996; 276(16): 1328-1331.

18. Nobile-Orazio E, Sterzi R. Cerebral ischaemia after nifedipine treatment. *BMJ* 1981; 283: 948.

19. Wachter RM. Symptomatic hypotension induced by nifedipine in the acute treatment of severe hypertension. *Arch Intern Med* 1987; 147: 556-558.

20. O'Mailia JJ, Sander GE, Giles TD. Nifedipine-associated myocardial ischemia or infarction in the treatment of hypertensive urgencies. *Ann Intern Med* 1987; 107: 185-186.

21. Zangerle KF, Wolford R. Syncope and conduction disturbances following sublingual nifedipine for hypertension. *Ann Emerg Med* 1985; 14: 1005-1006.

22. August P, Lindheimer MD. Pathophysiology of preeclampsia. *In:* Laragh JH, Brenner BM (eds.). *Hypertension: Pathophysiology, Diagnosis, and Management.* 2nd Edition. New York: Raven Press, 1995. 2407-2426.

23. Witlin AG, Sibai BM. Hypertension in pregnancy: current concepts of preeclampsia. *Annu Rev Med* 1997; 48: 115-127.

24. National High Blood Pressure Education Program Working Group Report on High Blood Pressure in Pregnancy. *Am J Obstet Gynecol* 1990; 163: 1691-1712.

Review Questions

1. A female with a history of hypertension complains of severe headache. Blood pressure is found to be 240/130. What is the appropriate diagnosis for this patient?
   A. Hypertensive emergency
   B. Hypertensive urgency
   C. Malignant hypertension
   D. Group C hypertension according to the JNC-VI classification
   E. There is not enough information in the above scenario to determine the exact diagnosis.

Without focal neurologic findings or other obvious evidence of end-organ damage, the appropriate classification of this patient's hypertensive problem cannot be determined. Laboratory and radiologic studies are needed for a complete evaluation. The answer is E.

2. The pathogenesis of a hypertensive emergency is most likely related to which of the following?
   A. Renin-angiotensin-aldosterone inhibition
   B. Excessively high HDL cholesterol levels
   C. Salt insensitivity
   D. Sympathetic hyperactivity
   E. Decreased peripheral insulin resistance

The answer is D.

3. Indirect measurements of blood pressure are complicated by which of the following?
   A. Faint Korotkoff sounds
   B. Inappropriate selection of cuff size
   C. Inappropriate positioning of the patient's arm
   D. Wide intraobserver discrepancies
   E. All of the above are complications of indirect blood pressure measurements

The answer is E.

4. Reasons to avoid administering sublingual nifedipine for hypertensive emergencies include which of the following?
   A. Unpredictable decrease in blood pressure
   B. Steal phenomenon leading to coronary ischemia
   C. Myocardial infarction or ischemia secondary to reflex catecholamine release
   D. Erratic oral absorption
   E. All of the above

The answer is E.

5. Which of the following is the correct triad associated with preeclampsia?
   A. Hypertension, edema, protein in urine
   B. Hypertension, edema, seizures
   C. Hypertension, edema, hypermagnesemia
   D. Hypertension, edema, mental status changes
   E. Hypertension, edema, glucose in urine

The answer is A.

6. Which of the following is believed to be responsible for the pathogenesis of preeclampsia?
   A. Abnormally formed placenta
   B. Excessive vasoconstriction
   C. Liver abnormalities
   D. Kidney abnormalities
   E. All of the above

The answer is E.

Section IV

Shock

Hypovolemic Shock

Shock is a pathologic state characterized by an imbalance between oxygen supply and demand. Shock is generally classified into four broad categories, each having in common the end result of **inadequate blood perfusion to tissues** (Table 17-1).

Throughout this book, each type of shock is fully explained from a pathophysiologic perspective. This chapter is dedicated solely to the pathogenic mechanisms, clinical manifestations, and therapy for **hypovolemic** shock.

Table 17-1
The Four Clinical Shock Syndromes

Type of Shock	Mechanism	Causes
Hypovolemic	Volume loss	Blood, plasma, fluid loss
Cardiogenic	Pump failure	Heart failure (Chapter 15)
Distributive	Increased venous capacitance (i.e., leaky capillaries) or arteriovenous shunting	Septic shock, spinal shock (Chapters 19, 28)
Obstructive (Extracardiac)	Obstruction of blood flow outside of heart	Aortic dissection, pulmonary embolism (Chapter 9), cardiac tamponade

Pathogenic Mechanisms

DEFINITION
Hypovolemic shock results from a reduction in circulating intravascular volume, and can arise from losses of blood (e.g., hemorrhage), plasma, electrolytes, or a combination of all above. Conditions leading to hypovolemic shock include burns, trauma, hemorrhage, and surgery. Hemorrhage and trauma develop when blood is lost externally or internally. Bleeding into affected areas of trauma can lead to surprisingly massive losses of blood; isolated femur fractures can result in the accumulation of over 1 liter of blood. Burns lead to loss of plasma when external protective mechanisms (i.e., skin and blood vessels) are compromised, proceeding to severe losses of plasma, elaborate metabolic changes, and concentration of the circulating blood volume (Table 17-2).

Table 17-2

Causes of Hypovolemia
Hemorrhage
Gastrointestinal losses (third spacing, vomiting, diarrhea)
Trauma
Burns
Surgery

COMPENSATORY MECHANISMS

Blood pressure is determined by the stroke volume multiplied by heart rate.

Cardiac Output = Stroke Volume x Heart Rate

When circulating blood volume is reduced by approximately 10 percent, compensatory mechanisms are activated to sustain cardiac output despite decreased stroke volume.[1] Heart rate increases to sustain blood pressure and tissue perfusion while vasoactive substances such as epinephrine, norepinephrine, and dopamine are released, causing arteriolar vasoconstriction. Vasoconstriction can persist to the point of causing cellular damage when blood is redistributed from the skin, muscles, kidneys, and gastrointestinal tract to the heart, brain, and lungs. As blood volume decreases, the heart must work harder to sustain cardiac output; myocardial ischemia eventually ensues and cardiac output falls. Antidiuretic hormone (ADH) is released and the renin-angiotensin-aldosterone system is activated to increase free water and sodium retention in an effort to sustain intravascular volume.

Anaerobic Compensation

As the oxygen debt increases and compensatory mechanisms fail (*i.e.*, increased heart rate), the body shifts to **anaerobic** metabolism. Glucose is normally converted to pyruvate in the mitochondrial matrix of cells and enters the citric acid cycle as acetyl coenzyme A (Figure 17-1).

Acetyl CoA is oxidized to carbon dioxide and water, yielding approximately two-thirds of the ATP (adenosine triphosphate: the energy currency for human metabolism) produced in the human body. This pathway is disrupted by lack of oxygen because the steps leading to the entry of pyruvate into the citric acid cycle are oxidation reactions (*i.e.*, aerobic reactions). The anaerobic fate of glucose is lactate, a molecule that releases half the energy of glucose when oxidized. Lactate is the final product of all anaerobic glycolysis in human cells. While some organs such as the brain, heart, liver, and skeletal muscle can use lactate as a temporary energy source, the energy yield is less than half of glucose. Lactate accumulation is a cause of metabolic acidosis, a condition that can lead to a decreased pH (**increased** hydrogen ions in the blood). When the pH falls below 7.20, myocardial contraction is severely depressed and peripheral blood vessels become increasingly unresponsive to catecholamines.

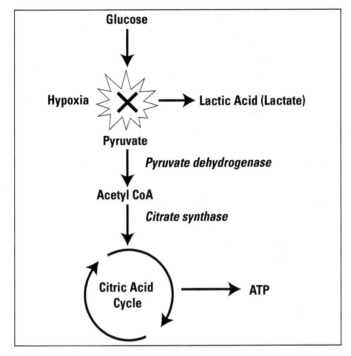

Figure 17-1 The formation of lactate during hypoxia. In the face of hypoxia, pyruvate is converted to lactic acid rather than processed by the citric acid cycle to make ATP.

Cellular Response

In response to hypoxemia, cells swell because of ion pump dysfunction. Cell membranes become hydrolyzed with the release of lysosomal enzymes and cellular death. Inorganic acids, potassium, and other intracellular contents are liberated, exacerbating metabolic acidosis. Sustained global tissue hypoperfusion results in a systemic inflammatory response (SIRS) and can lead to multiple organ dysfunction syndrome (MODS). SIRS and MODS are discussed further in Chapter 19.

Clinical Manifestations

BLOOD PRESSURE, PULSE, MENTAL STATUS CHANGES

The clinical manifestations associated with hypovolemic shock can be explained by the activation of mechanisms aimed at sustaining blood flow in the face of decreased blood volume. The classic finding of a rapid, thready pulse is common and represents maintenance of cardiac output by increased heart rate. It is important to note that tachycardia can be replaced by bradycardia, especially in severe hypovolemia and in patients on beta-blockers. Blood pressure is universally decreased in the later stages of hypovolemic shock, although it may be increased in the early stages because cardiac output is maintained solely by increased heart rate. Decreased blood volume is the most common mechanism, but hypotension also results from increased release of inflammatory mediators such as tumor necrosis factor, interleukins 1,2, and 6, and bradykinins.[1] Metabolites of the arachidonic acid pathway such as thromboxane and prostacyclin may also play a role as well as various endorphins and activation of the complement cascade. Pallor is a common finding and occurs when blood is diverted from the skin to the vital organs during vasoconstriction. Central nervous system changes ranging from disorientation and confusion to coma is the result of decreased cerebral perfusion pressure, a factor dependent on the mean arterial pressure.

**Cerebral Perfusion Pressure = Mean Arterial
Pressure - Intracranial Pressure**

In order for cerebral perfusion pressure to be maintained, the blood pressure must remain stable. The mean arterial blood pressure is equal to the diastolic pressure plus the difference of the systolic and diastolic blood pressures multiplied by one third [**MAP = D + 1/3 (S-D)**].

A summary of the clinical findings in hypovolemic shock is presented in Table 17-3.

HYPERVENTILATION

Lactate production and metabolic acidosis produce abnormal amounts of hydrogen ions, decreasing the pH of the blood, and decreasing the level of bicarbonate. In order to compensate for metabolic acidosis, the respiratory rate is increased. Hyperventilation causes a decrease in the PCO_2 and helps return the pH to a normal level by normalizing the PCO_2 to HCO_3 ratio (Figure 17-2).

ORTHOSTATIC VITAL SIGN CHANGES

When approximately 30% of the intravascular blood volume is depleted, postural vital sign changes can be elicited.[2-4] With the patient supine, record blood pressure and pulse rate. After 5 minutes, seat the patient with the legs dangling over the edge of the stretcher, and note blood pressure and pulse. **Positive postural vital sign changes are indicated by a heart rate increase of over 30 beats per minute or a systolic blood pressure drop over 30 mm Hg in the seated position.**[3] If no postural changes are noted, the clinical state of hypovolemia cannot be excluded for the reason that significant intravascular volume depletion must be present for changes to take place.

Table 17-3
Parameters for the Four Stages of Clinical Shock

Parameter	Class I	Class II	Class III	Class IV
Blood Loss (mL)	<750	750-1500	1500-2000	>2000
Blood loss (%)	<15	15-30	30-40	>40
Pulse	<100	>100	>120	>140
Blood pressure	Normal	Normal	Decreased	Low
Pulse pressure	Normal or increased	Decreased	Decreased	Low
Capillary refill delay	Normal	Positive	Positive	Positive
Respirations	14-20	20-30	30-40	>40
Urine output (ml/hr)	>30	20-30	5-15	Negligible
Mental status	Slightly anxious	Mildly anxious	Anxious, confused	Anxious, lethargic
Fluid replacement*	Crystalloid	Crystalloid	Crystalloid, blood	Crystalloid, blood

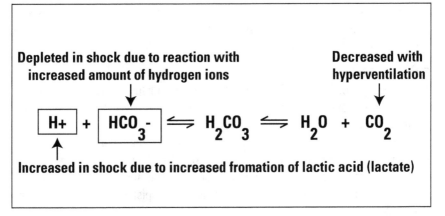

Depleted in shock due to reaction with increased amount of hydrogen ions

Decreased with hyperventilation

$$H^+ + HCO_3^- \rightleftharpoons H_2CO_3 \rightleftharpoons H_2O + CO_2$$

Increased in shock due to increased fromation of lactic acid (lactate)

Figure 17-2 The biochemistry of the bicarbonate buffer system.

Management

ABCS AND V.I.P.

As in all emergencies, the ABCs should be attended to. A useful acronym for the initial management of hypovolemic shock is V.I.P., which stands for **ventilation, infusion, and pump**. Delivery of adequate levels of oxygen should be assured as well as removal of CO_2 with ventilation. Accumulation of CO_2 leads to an unfavorable CO_2 / HCO_3 ratio and intensifies preexisting metabolic acidosis. Infusion of fluids is essential to maintain adequate intravascular volume and is discussed in detail below. The adequacy of the pump function (*e.g.*, the cardiac system) to meet the demands of the body in stress should be addressed. The treatment for all causes of shock is the same regardless, with the understanding that until the underlying cause is corrected, shock continues unabated.

INTRAVENOUS ACCESS

As discussed in Chapter 10, the Hagan-Poiseuille equation explains the physics of blood flow. Blood flow is dependent on blood vessel pressure, radius, length, and blood viscosity. It follows that the rate-limiting factor for fluid and blood infusion is proportional to the radius and length of the catheter used. Thus, the best means of providing rapid, efficient intravenous access for infusion is to **use the shortest catheter with the widest diameter** at two **peripheral** access sites; preferably the veins in the antecubital fossa.

FLUID RESUSCITATION

The survival benefits of aggressive fluid replacement in hypotensive shock remain largely unproved in well-controlled human studies.[5] Indeed, some authors advocate under resuscitation or hypotensive resuscitation to prevent ongoing hemorrhage, a condition that is often worsened by increasing the blood pressure with fluids.[6] Nevertheless, intravenous fluids restore intravascular volume, open closed and contracted capillary blood vessels, and increase tissue perfusion.[5] The choice of which fluid to use continues to be the focus of intense debate among emergency medicine physicians, surgeons, and critical care specialists. The rationale for crystalloids and colloids is discussed below and is reviewed in Chapter 2 of this text.

Crystalloids

The composition of crystalloids is discussed in detail in Chapter 2. Isotonic saline and lactated Ringer's are the two most commonly used preparations in hypovolemic shock. These solutions are administered rapidly and can replace preexisting volume deficits. Because of their tonicity, these fluids redistribute to the interstitial space and eventually lead to expansion of the **interstitial** rather than **intravascular** volume. Patients generally require 20 ml/kg of isotonic crystalloid for each bolus; 3 liters of either isotonic saline or lactated Ringer's should be administered for every estimated liter of blood lost.[5,7]

Colloids

Colloid fluid preparations contain large molecules that cause absorption of fluids into the blood vessels while not readily passing through cell membranes. These fluids theoretically have the potential to expand the intravascular space by increasing the osmotic (sometimes referred to as oncotic) pressure inside the capillaries. To date, no studies have shown a clear benefit of colloids over crystalloids when used for resuscitation in hypovolemic shock.

BLOOD AND BLOOD SUBSTITUTES

Oxygen-carrying capacity is dependent on the number of circulating red blood cells. Hemorrhage can lead to severe, diffuse disruption in the oxygen-supply balance of the human body. Therefore, prompt administration of blood is essential in instances of severe or ongoing blood loss. Once the blood flow is improved by replacing the intravascular volume with intravenous fluids, the oxygen supply-demand imbalance must be addressed. This is accomplished in the emergency department, operating room, or intensive care unit, with the administration of either whole blood or packed red blood cells, both matched according to the patient's ABO and Rh blood type (see Table 17-4).

Table 17-4

The Four Principal Blood Groups, Listed In Descending Order According To Prevalence In The United States Population.
(Note: 85% of all patients in the United States are Rh-positive, therefore making the blood type O Rh-positive the most common blood type in the United States.)

Blood Group	Percent in US Population	Physiology	Clinical Correlation
O	45	Patient has circulating antibodies against A-type and B-type blood	If patient is O-type, can only accept O-type blood; universal donor for all other blood types
A	42	Patient has circulating antibodies against B-type blood	Can accept either A-type or O-type blood only
B	10	Patient has circulating antibodies against A-type blood	Can accept B-type or O-type blood only
AB	3	No circulating antibodies against A-type or B-type blood	Universal recipient

If type-specific blood is not available, O Rh-negative type blood can be administered since this blood type is almost always accepted by patients of any blood type. In many instances, O Rh-positive is the second best choice and is generally more available; approximately 85% of all patients in the United States are Rh-positive.[8]

In recent years, the search for a blood substitute has yielded disappointing results. Stroma-free hemoglobin, pyridoxylated-hemoglobin-polyoxyethylene (PHP), and perfluorocarbons (PFCs) have all been investigated but found to have numerous adverse reactions and short-lived effects. The quest for a viable blood substitute remains an area of active and promising research.

BICARBONATE

Since the treatment of choice for the metabolic acidosis associated with shock is to correct the underlying cause, **the use of bicarbonate is rarely indicated**. Bicarbonate can have a paradoxical effect, exacerbating intracellular acidosis and shifting the oxygen-hemoglobin dissociation curve to the left, impairing oxygen unloading to tissues.[9] When bicarbonate is administered, it combines with hydrogen ions in the blood, elevating the pH and forming carbon dioxide (Figure 17-2).

Carbon dioxide formation then favors a reversal of the equation with the formation of more hydrogen anions, and worsening of the underlying acidosis. Moreover, carbon dioxide is a myocardial depressant and decreases cardiac output.[10] Bicarbonate administered in intravenous lines forms complexes with calcium and deactivates catecholamines. For these reasons, the use of bicarbonate should be reserved for documented severe acidosis, hyperkalemia, tricyclic antidepressant overdose, or prolonged cardiac arrest.[10]

THE PNEUMATIC ANTI-SHOCK GARMENT

The pneumatic anti-shock garret (PASG), known also as medical anti-shock trousers (MAST), or military anti-shock trousers, is still a standard piece of medical equipment on many EMS response vehicles. This device became popular in the 1970s after a series of anecdotal reports of successful use in the Vietnam War. A number of well-designed trials within the last decade have shown that **the PASG does not confer any positive benefit to patients in shock and in some instances may be harmful**.[11-14] The PASG does increase blood pressure by increasing systemic vascular resistance in the lower extremities, but this effect can increase the severity of hemorrhage, especially in patients with chest trauma.[14] Despite its downfalls, the PASG may have a role for use in patients with hemorrhage from pelvic fractures or multiple bilateral lower extremity fractures.[12] In these instances, application of the PASG may help temporarily tamponade actively bleeding vessels until definitive surgical interventions can be conducted.

TRENDELENBURG POSITIONING

The Trendelenburg position, now commonly referred to as the anti-shock position, was introduced in the18th century by the surgeon Friedrich Trendelenburg. The patient is positioned supine with the legs elevated 45 degrees above and the head 15 degrees below the horizontal plane.[15] The proposed beneficial effects include increased cardiac output as a consequence of increased venous return to the heart; however, this assumption has been shown to be untrue.[16,17] Despite a study published in 1967 clearly demonstrating failure of the Trendelenburg position to improve circulatory flow in shock, the technique is still widely taught and practiced in many EMS systems.[16] Trendelenburg positioning actually **decreases cardiac output and does not increase venous return** to the heart.[15-17] Based on the existing evidence, **the use of the Trendelenburg position for patients in hypovolemic shock has not been shown to be beneficial and should be abandoned**.

RESUSCITATION ENDPOINTS

In the past, endpoints such as restoration of blood pressure, normalization of pulse and respirations, and return of urine output were used to guide the administration of fluids in patients with hypovolemic shock. Today, endpoints are widely regarded as purely physiologic changes that can only be recorded in an intensive care setting. Filling pressure of the heart, blood lactate, base deficit, and various oxygen uptake and utilization parameters are a few of the physiologic indicators used by clinicians to signify successful resuscitation of patients in hypovolemic shock.[18]

References

1. Gould SA, *et al.* Hypovolemic shock. *Crit Care Clinics* 1993; 9: 239.

2. Williams TM, Knoop R. The clinical use of orthostatic vital signs. *In:* Roberts JR, Hedges JR (eds.). *Clinical Procedures in Emergency Medicine.* Philadelphia: W.B. Saunders, 1991: 445-449.

3. Moore KI, Newton K. Orthostatic heart rates and blood pressures in healthy young women and men. *Heart & Lung* 1986; 611-617.

4. Committee on Trauma. *Advanced Trauma Life Support.* Chicago: American College of Surgeons, 1989: 57.

5. Dronen SC, Bobek EMK. Fluid and blood resuscitation. *In:* Tintinalli JE, Kelen GD, Stapczynski JS. *Emergency Medicine: A Comprehensive Study Guide.* 5th Edition. New York: McGraw-Hill, 2000. 223-228.

6. Dries DJ. Hypotensive resuscitation. *Shock* 1996; 6: 311.

7. Wagner BKJ, D'Amelio LT. Pharmacologic and clinical consideration in selecting crystalloid, colloid, and oxygen carrying resuscitation fluids. *Clin Pharm* 1993; 12: 335.

8. Vander AJ, Sherman JH, Luciano DS. *Human Physiology: The Mechanisms of Body Function.* 6th Edition. New York: McGraw-Hill, 1994. 729.

9. Cooper DJ, Walley KR, Wiggs BR, Russell JA. Bicarbonate does not improve hemodynamics in critically ill patients who have lactic acidosis. A prospective, controlled clinical study. *Ann Intern Med* 1990; 112: 492.

10. Chameides L, Hazinski MF (eds.) for the Subcommittee on Pediatric Resuscitation, 1994-1997. Pediatric Advanced Life Support. Dallas, TX: American Heart Association, 1997.

11. Maddox KL, Bickell WH, Pepe PE, et al. Prospective randomized evaluation of antishock MAST in posttraumatic hypotension. *J Trauma* 1986; 26: 779.

12. Domeier RM, O'Connor RE, Delbridge TR, Hunt RC. National Association of EMS Physicians Position Paper: Use of pneumatic anti-shock garment (PASG). *Prehosp Emerg Care* 1997; 1: 32.

13. Ali J, Venderby B, Purcell C. The effect of pneumatic anti-shock garment (PASG) on hemodynamics, hemorrhage, and survival in penetrating thoracic aortic injury. *J Trauma* 1991; 31: 846-851.

14. Honigman B, Lwenstein FR, Moore EE, *et al.* The role of the pneumatic shock garment in penetrating cardiac wounds. *JAMA* 1991; 266: 2398.

15. Sing R, O'Hara D. Sawyer MAJ, Marino PL. Trendelenburg position and oxygen transport in hypovolemic adults. *Ann Emerg Med* 1994; 23: 564-568.

16. Taylor J, Weil MH. Failure of Trendelenburg position to improve circulation during clinical shock. *Surg Gynecol Obstet* 1967; 122: 1005-1010.

17. Bivins HG, Knopp R, dos Santos PAL. Blood volume distribution in the Trendelenburg position. *Ann Emerg Med* 1985; 14: 641-643.

18. Porter JM, Ivatury RR. In search of the optimal end points of resuscitation in trauma patients: A review. *J Trauma* 1998; 44: 908.

Review Questions

1. A 44-year-old male with a gunshot wound to the abdomen has the following vital signs: HR 138 RR 24 BP 100/60. Definitive treatment should be aimed at reversing which of the following pathophysiologic mechanisms?
   A. Increased circulating levels of thyroid hormone
   B. Increased circulating levels of glucocorticoids
   C. Inadequate blood perfusion to the tissues
   D. Abnormal circulatory hemodynamics secondary to fluid sequestration and intravascular edema
   E. Increased dromotropic effect on heart by inflammatory mediators

Shock is defined as inadequate perfusion to the tissues and organs. The answer is C.

2. According to the Hagen-Poiseuille equation, which of the following would be the most appropriate catheter(s) for initial intravenous fluid administration in a hypovolemic patient?
   A. Two 16 gauge 1.0 inch catheters
   B. One 14 gauge 1.0 inch catheter
   C. Femoral central line
   D. Subclavian triple-lumen catheter
   E. Two 20 gauge 1.0 inch catheters

The shorter the length (denominator in Hagen-Poiseuille equation) and the larger the radius (numerator), the greater the fluid flow through a vessel or tube. The answer is A.

3. Pathogenic mechanisms for the patient in Question 1 include all of the following EXCEPT:
   A. Increased lactate production
   B. Intravascular blood volume depletion
   C. Increased hydrogen ion concentration (acidosis)
   D. Decreased cerebral perfusion pressure
   E. Decreased oxygen debt

The oxygen debt increases in shock. The answer is E.

4. All of the following statements regarding orthostatic vital sign changes asso-
ciated with hypovolemia are correct EXCEPT:
  A. Five minutes should transpire before the patient sits up for the second
     blood pressure measurement
  B. Positive orthostatic signs include an increase in the heart rate over 30
     beats per minute and a decrease in the systolic pressure by 30 mm Hg
     or more when the patient sits up with the feet dangling off the stretcher
  C. Positive orthostatic signs include an increase in the heart rate over 30
     beats per minute and a decrease in the systolic pressure by 30 mm Hg
     or more when the patient lies supine on the stretcher
  D. When approximately 30% of the intravascular volume is depleted, positive
     orthostatic signs will be elicited
  E. False positive results can occur with patients on vasoactive medications
     such as alpha- and beta-blockers

The answer is C.

5. An 8-year-old female sustains multi-system trauma after a bicycle accident.
Vital signs are: HR 144, RR 32, BP 70/palpation. All of the following are inappro-
priate initial interventions for this patient EXCEPT:
  A. One ampule of bicarbonate intravenously
  B. 20 cc/kg bolus of lactated Ringer's solution, repeated as necessary
  C. Placement of patient in Trendelenburg position during transport
  D. Dopamine infusion titrated to systolic blood pressure over 100 mm Hg
  E. MAST trouser application for hypotension

The answer is B.

The word anaphylaxis means without protection.[1] The current understanding of this disease has revealed that anaphylaxis is an overreaction of the normal immune system as opposed to a delayed or absent response. In the most severe cases, the clinical presentation consists of sudden hypotension with or without bronchospasm or laryngeal obstruction. The differential list is not long and the pharmacologic treatment is straightforward. Patients with anaphylaxis can be assessed and promptly treated before ED arrival. Indeed, the successful recognition and management of anaphylaxis can be extremely rewarding for both patient and provider; in many cases the patient's response to therapy can be quite dramatic.

Gell and Coombs Classification

Anaphylaxis is an immunologically mediated hypersensitivity reaction that occurs when an allergen is introduced to the human body. There are four general types of immunological tissue injury described by the Gell and Coombs classification system.[1] Table 18-1 lists the organs and mechanisms involved in each type of reaction and provides examples for each class.

For the purposes of this chapter, only **type I (anaphylactic) reactions are discussed since this type represents the classical hypersensitivity reaction of anaphylaxis.** When mast cells are activated by non-IgE mechanisms, an **anaphylactoid** reaction ensues.[2] Since the basic pathophysiologic mechanisms and treatment are the same as those in IgE-mediated anaphylaxis, both are considered together in this chapter.

Pathogenesis

Most of the pathophysiologic features of anaphylaxis have much in common with asthma.[3] **Central to the development of anaphylaxis is the release of mediators by mast cells**. For this to take place, IgE antibodies must be produced to sensitize mast cells, providing a bridge for allergens to stimulate additional cells.

Anaphylactic Reactions

IgE-mediated hypersensitivity reactions can result from exposure to a variety of allergens. Stings by insects of the hymenoptera species (hornets, wasps, yellow jackets, honeybees) can illicit a serious anaphylactic reaction in up to five percent of the population.[3] Allergies

Table 18-1

The Gell and Coombs Classification for Hypersensitivity Reactions

Type	Organs Involved	Mechanisms	Examples
I: Anaphylactic	Lung Skin GI Tract	Antibody Mediated; IgE (occasionally IgG)	Asthma Urticaria Gastrointestinal allergies Atopic dermatitis
II: Cytotoxic	Red blood cells White blood cells Platelets	IgG, IgM, Monocytes, Phagocytes, Antibody-mediated Complement Cytolysis	Hemolytic anemia Goodpasture's disease
III: Immune Complex/Serum Sickness	Blood vessels Skin Joints Kidney Lung	IgG Antigen-antibody Complexes	Lupus Serum sickness Glomerulonephritis
IV: Cell Mediated Delayed Hypersensitivity	Skin Thyroid Lung CNS	Sensitized Lymphocytes, Killer T Cells, Macrophages	Tuberculosis Contact dermatitis Thyroiditis
V: Mixed Types (i.e. I&III, III&IV)	Varies	Mixed	Allergic Bronchopulmonary Aspergillosis

to foods such as shellfish, peanuts, nuts, eggs, fruit, and wheat can manifest as gastrointestinal tract disturbances with or without additional systemic signs and symptoms. The beta-lactam class of antibiotics, which includes penicillins and cephalosporins, can cause anaphylaxis; reactions occur in 1 to 5 out of 10,000 administrations of these medications.[3] Allergies to latex-containing materials such as gloves and condoms can precipitate anaphylactic reactions.

Anaphylactoid Reactions

Anaphylactoid reactions are caused by direct mast cell degranulation and are not IgE-mediated. Drugs such as ACE-inhibitors, opiates, aspirin, certain antibiotics, and nonsteroidal anti-inflammatory drugs are the most common cause of anaphylactoid reactions.[2] Radiocontrast media can trigger a reaction.

MAST CELL ACTIVATION

Regardless of how the reaction is initiated (*i.e.*, anaphylactic versus anaphylactoid), the mast cell occupies the central role in the pathogenesis of a hypersensitivity response.[1] When activated by IgE or other stimulants, the mast cell releases histamine, a mediator that can cause bronchoconstriction, urticaria (*i.e.*, hives), and a host of systemic effects. Other activated cells include basophils, B-cells, and T-cells. Mediators released from these cells cause smooth muscle contraction in the airways, increased bronchial mucus secretion, and increased vascular permeability (i.e., leaky blood vessels). Proteases and factors that recruit additional inflammatory cells are also released. B-cells produce the IgE antibodies that are involved in the allergic response. Different types of T-cells release factors (cytokines) that attract additional cells to the site of allergen exposure while also regulating the production of more IgE antibodies. Secondary mediators involved in an anaphylactic reaction include the products of the arachidonic acid pathway (leukotrienes, prostaglandins) as well as interleukins, platelet activating factor, bradykinin, and other factors. These mediators cause further bronchoconstriction, edema, and platelet aggregation.

Clinical Manifestations

Clinical features of anaphylaxis can be explained by the pathophysiologic events that follow exposure to a known allergen. In many patients, a past history of asthma, recent medication use (*e.g.*, antibiotics, ACE-inhibitors, etc.), or previous allergic reactions may help identify predisposing factors. Airway signs include wheezing, chest tightness, or absent breath sounds. Tachycardia is common and may be caused by activation of histamine receptors. In severe cases, hypotension can result from mediator release and increased vascular permeability.

THE LATE PHASE REACTION
A late phase or **biphasic** reaction can occur in some patients, often resembling the initial presentation, 2 to 8 hours or much later after the initial onset of symptoms.[4] This reaction is an immediate type I hypersensitivity reaction caused by a low molecular weight polypeptide produced by mast cells. This polypeptide, known as the **inflammatory factor of anaphylaxis** (IF-A), causes inflammatory cells to migrate to the site of mast cell mediator release. Corticosteroids are capable of blocking the late response by inhibiting the formation of inflammatory mediators.[4]

Management

EPINEPHRINE
Epinephrine is the mainstay of treatment in anaphylaxis; prompt administration can be life-saving.[5] Epinephrine inhibits mediator release from mast cells and basophils, relaxes bronchial smooth muscle through a beta-2 adrenergic effect, and helps increase blood pressure via alpha-1 adrenergic stimulation. It is given subcutaneously, although in severe cases, the intravenous route can be used. For patients in whom epinephrine is contraindicated, (*e.g.*, patients with known cardiac disease, hypertension, pregnancy, or patients on beta-blockers) glucagon can be

substituted.[6] Glucagon, like epinephrine, activates adenylate cyclase, increasing cAMP, inducing smooth muscle contraction (see Chapter 6, Figure 6-5).

ANTIHISTAMINES

Treatment with epinephrine should be followed by administration of histamine receptor blockers (*i.e.*, antihistamines).[7] The two histamine receptors responsible for anaphylactic reactions are the H_1 and H_2 receptors. The H_1 receptor is found in the tissues of coronary arteries, bronchi, blood vessels, and intestinal smooth muscles.[7] Diphenhydramine (Benadryl®) is an effective H_1 receptor blocker and can be given intravenously. H_2 receptors are located in the cardiac and stomach tissue and can be blocked with cimetidine (Tagamet®), ranitidine (Zantac®), or other H_2 receptor antagonists.

STEROIDS

To treat or prevent the late phase reaction, corticosteroids should be administered. Depending on the severity, oral prednisone or intravenous methylprednisolone can be given. Corticosteroids inhibit the synthesis of inflammatory mediators, prevent the migration of inflammatory cells, and prevent mast cells from releasing IF-A.[4]

TREATMENT OF HYPOTENSION

In severe anaphylaxis (*i.e.*, respiratory failure, hypotension not responsive to epinephrine), more aggressive measures should be taken. Several liters of crystalloids may be needed to restore blood pressure in hypotensive patients. Dopamine can be used for patients who remain hypotensive despite treatment with epinephrine and volume repletion.[3,5]

References

1. Sullivan TJ. Systemic anaphylaxis. *In:* Lichtenstein LM, Fauci AS, eds. *Current Therapy in Allergy and Immunology.* St. Louis: Mosby-Year Book, 1988.

2. Claman HN. Allergy and Clinical Immunology. *In:* Schier RW. *The Internal Medicine Casebook: Real Patients, Real Answers.* New York: Little, Brown and Co., 1994.

3. Heilpern KL, Wolfson AB, Fontanarosa PB. The treacherous clinical spectrum of allergic emergencies: Diagnosis, treatment, and prevention. *Emerg Med Reports* 1994; 15: 212-220.

4. Stark BJ, Sullivan TJ. Biphasic and protracted anaphylaxis. *J Allergy Clin Immunol* 1986; 78: 76-83.

5. Bochner BS, Lichtenstein LM. Anaphylaxis. *N Eng J Med* 1991: 324: 1785-1790.

6. Pollack CV. Utility of glucagon in the emergency department. J *Emerg Med* 1993; 11: 195-205.

7. Lieberman P. The use of antihistamines in the prevention and treatment of anaphylaxis and anaphylactoid reactions. *J Allergy Clin Immunol* 1990; 86: 684-686.

Review Questions

1. A 23-year-old female who recently started antibiotics for a urinary tract infection calls 911 and complains of severe trouble breathing. Vitals are: HR 110 RR 28 BP 90/40. Auscultation of the lungs reveals bilateral wheezing. Examination of the skin reveals diffuse urticaria. The patient appears to be in severe distress. According to the Gell and Coombs classification scheme, which type of hypersensitivity reaction is occurring?
   A. Type I
   B. Type II
   C. Type III
   D. Type IV
   E. Type V

The patient is in anaphylactic shock. This is a type I IgE-mediated hypersensitivity reaction. The answer is A.

2. The type of hypersensitivity reaction in Question 1 is caused by:
   A. IgE antibody-mediated mechanisms
   B. IgG, IgM, monocyte, and phagocyte activation with complement activation
   C. Formation of IgG antibody-antigen complexes
   D. Sensitization of lymphocytes and killer-T cell activation
   E. Mixed Type II, IV and IV mechanisms

The answer is A.

3. The principal cell stimulated by the hypersensitivity response in anaphylaxis is the:
   A. Basophil
   B. Eosinophil
   C. Leukocyte
   D. Mast cell
   E. Killer T-cell

The answer is D.

4. All of the following are true about the late-phase reaction of anaphylaxis EXCEPT:
   A. Usually occurs 24 to 48 hours after the initial reaction
   B. Is a type I hypersensitivity reaction
   C. Is caused by a low molecular weight peptide produced by mast cells
   D. IF-A causes migration of inflammatory cells to the site of mast cell mediator release
   E. Can be prevented by corticosteroids

The late-phase reaction can occur 2 to 8 hours after the initial reaction. The answer is A.

5. All of the following medications should be used in anaphylaxis EXCEPT:
   A. H_1-receptor antagonists
   B. H_2-receptor antagonists
   C. Isoproterenol
   D. Epinephrine
   E. Corticosteroids

Isoproterenol is a potent inotrope that is rarely used. This agent has no role for use in anaphylaxis. The answer is C.

Septic shock is a disease process characterized by a persistent, hyperdynamic, hypermetabolic state progressing to a gradual functional deterioration of multiple organs.[1] Shock in general is a syndrome of generalized metabolic failure resulting from inadequate tissue perfusion; in septic shock, inadequate perfusion results from sepsis, bacteremia, or endotoxins. An estimated 400,000 cases occur each year worldwide with 100,000 cases treated in the United States anually.[1] Septic shock is associated with an extremely high mortality: 30% in uncomplicated cases and over 80% in cases associated with multiple organ dysfunction syndrome.[1,2]

Definitions

SEPSIS, SIRS, SEPTIC SHOCK

It is often the case that the prehospital provider does not know whether septic shock, sepsis, or bacteremia is present until after definitive laboratory studies are performed. Since prompt recognition is always necessary to maximize survival, prehospital providers should be well-versed in the nomenclature pertaining to sepsis and related disorders. In an effort to mitigate the confusion regarding sepsis and associated syndromes, the Society of Critical Care Medicine Consensus Conference Committee and the American College of Chest Physicians revised the clinical categorization of sepsis to include SIRS, sepsis, and the varying degrees of septic shock.[2] The revised definitions are explained in Figure 19-1.

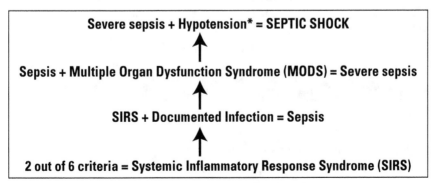

Figure 19-1 The nomenclature for SIRS, sepsis, severe sepsis, and septic shock.
* refers to hypotension refractory to fluid challenge

The term sepsis is misleading and often a point of confusion for prehospital providers and physicians alike. The term is a misconception because it implies infection, but infection is responsible for less than half of cases in the post-traumatic or injury period.[1] An important point for all clinicians to be aware of is that **SIRS and sepsis are not always synonymous with septic shock;** each syndrome is a distinct entity with its own attendant mortality. The diagnosis of SIRS can be suspected in the prehospital care environment with careful examination of the vital signs, but almost always requires laboratory studies including a white blood cell count to be confirmed (Figure 19-2).

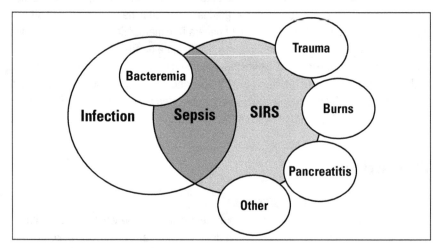

Figure 19-2 The interrelationship of infection, sepsis, and SIRS.

THE SYSTEMIC INFLAMMATORY RESPONSE SYNDROME (SIRS)

The presence of SIRS does not equate to infection; only 25% to 50% of patients with SIRS have an infection.[3,4] SIRS can be caused by infections as well as ischemia, trauma, toxic ingestions, burns, and other causes of shock. For the diagnosis of SIRS to be made, two of six clinical conditions must be met[2] (Table 19-1).

Similarly, septic shock is not always caused by infection; **the diagnosis of septic shock always requires laboratory data before this clinical syndrome can be positively ruled in.**

Table 19-1
The Criteria For SIRS; at Least 2 of the 6 Criteria Must Be Met

Systemic Inflammatory Response Syndrome (SIRS)
1. Temperature > 38°C or < 36°C (>100.4°F or <96.9 F)
2. Heart rate > 100 beats per minute
3. Respiratory rate > 20 breaths/minute
4. White blood cell count > 12,000/mm^3 or <4000/ mm^3
5. Hyperventilation (PaCO$_2$ < 32 mm Hg)
6. Immature neutrophils (bands) > 10%

Pathogenesis

ETIOLOGY

Septic shock can be caused by any condition that can cause a systemic inflammatory response. Burns, trauma, pancreatitis, immune reactions, and ischemia are all possible non-infectious etiologies. Infection by gram negative bacteria is the most common cause of septic shock.[1,5] *Escherichia coli* and *klebsiella-Enterobacter* species of bacteria give rise to more than 60% to 70% of all cases. Other causative gram negative organisms include *pseudomonas aeruginosa, bacteroides* species, *proteus* species, *serratia marcescens,* and *haemophilus* species.[1] Of the gram positive microorganisms, *staphylococcus aureus* and *streptococcal* species are the most commonly implicated.

SOURCES

Table 19-2 lists the most common sources, in order, for bacterial infections leading to sepsis and septic shock. In general, whenever the protective mucosal surfaces of an organ system are disrupted, sepsis may develop. The genitourinary system, when disturbed by catheters, instruments, or even abortions, is the most common source for bacteremia.[1]

Table 19-2
The Infectious Etiologies in Sepsis and Septic Shock

Organ System	Source of Infection	Associated Bacteria
Genitourinary System (#1)	Abortions Instrumentation Indwelling catheters	*E. coli* *bacteroides*
Respiratory System (#2)	Tracheostomies Mechanical ventilation Aspiration	*pseudomonas* *klebsiella-Enterobacter* *serratia* *E. coli*
Gastrointestinal Tract (#3)	Obstructions Perforations Abscesses Hyperalimentation Diverticula	*bacteroides* *E. coli* *klebsiella-Enterobacter* *serratia* *salmonella*
Biliary Tract (#4)	Cholangitis Obstructions	*E. coli* *klebsiella-Enterobacter* *serratia*
Other Causes	Catheters Bacterial endocarditis Mycotic aneurysms Infected grafts Septic thrombophlebitis	All of the above plus gram-positive organisms such as *staphylococcus* and *streptococcus* species

THE TWO-HIT THEORY

A systemic inflammatory response can result from virtually any toxic stimulus and not necessarily from infection in all cases. Clinical observations by critical care researchers have led to the formulation of the two-hit theory of multiple organ dysfunction syndrome (MODS). The systemic inflammatory response can lead to MODS after an initial surgical or traumatic insult occurs. This first hit primes inflammatory cells and white blood cells to turn on metabolic machinery in anticipation of further injury. This stage is not usually clinically apparent. Post-injury infections, toxins, ischemic events, or inflammation cause larger quantities of toxic compounds to be released. Inflammatory substances known as cytokines are the major mediators during this stage, inducing the release of hormones, vasoactive substances, and a host of additional cell-toxic mediators.

MEDIATORS

Endotoxins, the substances released from bacteria, and other bacteria-related toxins play an important role as mediators in the normal stress response to infection and represent one of the best understood mechanisms for the progression to sepsis. The outer surface membrane of gram negative bacteria is comprised of lipopolysaccharides, of which lipid A is commonly implicated as a cause of inflammation.[5] Exposure of macrophages to lipid A causes the release of inflammatory cytokines such as tumor necrosis factor (TNF), interleukins 6 and 8, and granulocyte-monocyte colony stimulating factor (G-M CSF; Figure 19-3).

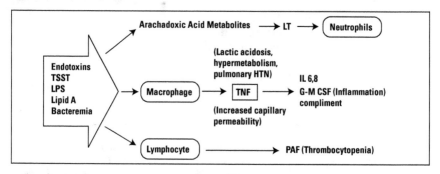

Figure 19-3 A summary of the various mediators implicated in a stress response typical for SIRS, sepsis, and septic shock.

Release of these factors cause increased capillary permeability. Lactic acidosis, pulmonary hypertension, bacteremia, other bacterial toxins, and any hypermetabolic state can also release TNF, inducing the same inflammatory changes. Complement, a substance formed from a variety of precursors, is stimulated and causes infected cells to burst. Lymphocytes release platelet activating factor (PAF), which can lead to an eventual decrease in the number of circulating platelets. Platelets play an important early role in inflammation, migrating to the site of injury and stimulating the release of more cytokines. Arachidonic acid metabolites such as the leukotrienes, also implicated in asthma, lead to the stimulation of neutrophils.

Clinical Assessment

CLINICAL MANIFESTATIONS

The physiologic changes in septic shock are classified as either a **hyperdynamic, hypermetabolic** state, or a **hypodynamic** state. The hyperdynamic, hypermetabolic state is the earliest manifestation of septic shock, and is associated with clinical signs indicating increased metabolic activity. Temperature is increased, as are heart rate and respiratory rate. Mental status changes are typically present, and become evident with decreased alertness, disorientation, or inappropriate behavior. If the hyper dynamic, hypermetabolic state is not corrected, blood pressure decreases.

The hypodynamic state in septic shock is a late response with a mortality of 50% to 80%.[1] Clinical findings include decreased blood pressure, cold, clammy skin, and profound mental status changes (*e.g.*, obtundation). Urine output is absent. The temperature at this stage can be either increased or decreased.

PHYSIOLOGIC CHANGES

The hyperdynamic, hypermetabolic state is marked by increased oxygen uptake (VO_2), increased cardiac output with normal to low cardiac filling pressures. Local microvascular damage ensues as a result of the inflammatory cascade, and results in leaky capillary membranes. Systemic vascular resistance is decreased, leading to decreased blood pressure.

Decreased oxygen uptake, variable cardiac filling pressures, and decreased cardiac output are characteristic of the hypodynamic state of septic shock. Systemic vascular resistance is usually increased in an effort to sustain tissue perfusion in the face of decreased cardiac output, although blood pressure remains low.

LABORATORY FINDINGS

The laboratory findings for hyperdynamic and hypodynamic septic shock are listed in Table 19-3. Lactate, the produce of the abnormal metabolism of glucose, rises steadily in cases of poorly controlled septic shock, reaching levels above 2.0 mm/L in the hypodynamic state. Metabolic acidosis is the end result of disordered cellular metabolism and is present, although to varying degrees, in both states. The white blood cell count is generally high in both states with more immature neutrophils (*i.e.*, left shift) detected as the process progresses.

Table 19-3
Clinical, Physiologic, and Laboratory Findings in the
Hyperdynamic, Hypermetabolic and Hypodynamic
States of Septic Shock.

Hyperdynamic, Hypermetabolic State	Hypodynamic State
Clinical Findings:	
1. Increased temperature	1. Increased or decreased temperature
2. Warm, dry skin	2. Cool skin
3. Decreased blood pressure	3. Decreased blood pressure
4. Tachycardia, Tachypnea	4. Tachycardia, Tachypnea
5. Mental status changes	5. Obtundation
6. Urine output decreased	6. Oliguria (scant urine output)
Physiological Changes:	
1. Increased oxygen uptake	1. Decreased oxygen uptake
2. Filling pressures normal to low	2. Filling pressures variable (usually low)
3. Cardiac output increased	3. Cardiac output decreased
4. A-V O_2 difference normal to low	4. A-V O_2 difference low
5. Systemic vascular resistance decreased	5. Systemic vascular resistance increased
6. Local microvascular damage	
Laboratory Findings:	
1. White blood cells increased	1. White blood cells high or low
2. Metabolic acidosis	2. Metabolic acidosis
3. Lactic acidosis (1.5-2 mM/L)	3. Lactate >2.0 mM/L
	4. Decreased platelet count
	5. Left shift (immature neutrophils/bands)
	6. Hyper- or Hypoglycemia

Management

RESTORATION AND MAINTENANCE OF PERFUSION

The immediate goals for resuscitation of patients in septic shock are aimed at restoring and maintaining tissue perfusion. Increased oxygen consumption during the hyperdynamic state necessitates increased oxygen delivery. An oxygen tension (pO_2) of at least 75 mm Hg should be maintained; this corresponds to a pulse oximetry (SpO_2) reading of greater than 90%. Volume expansion with isotonic crystalloids (*i.e.,* lactated Ringer's or 0.9% isotonic saline) is the initial treatment of choice and helps to increase cardiac output while reopening underperfused areas of microcirculation. Colloids such as albumin can be used to restore the colloid osmotic pressure and may help to restore intravascular blood volume. If volume expansion with isotonic fluids and colloids fails to maintain blood pressure, inotropes and vasoconstrictors such as dopamine, dobutamine, and norepinephrine can be considered.

CONTROL OF HOST RESPONSE TO INJURY

Definitive therapy is aimed at controlling the host response to injury and is accomplished in the intensive care unit. Therapies such as surgical debridement or drainage to remove the devitalized tissue that serves as a nidus for infection and inflammation can be life-saving. Inflammation is controlled by removing infectious agents with broad-spectrum antibiotics as well as controlling the host response with novel therapies such as antioxidants. Antioxidants as Vitamins C, E, and beta-carotene as well as antibodies to cytokines and other agents may play an important role in the future. Steroids are not indicated and are not beneficial for patients with septic shock.[1,6,7]

References

1. Demling RH, Lalonde C, *et al.* Physiological support of the septic patient. *Surg Clin North America* 1994; 74 (3).

2. American College of Chest Physicians/Society of Critical Care Medicine Conference Consensus Committee. Definitions of sepsis and organ failure and guidelines for the use of innovative therapies in sepsis. *Chest* 1992; 101: 1644-1655.

3. Pinsky MR, Matuschak GM. Multiple systems organ failure: failure of host defense mechanisms. *Crit Care Clin* 1989; 5: 199-220.

4. Pittet D, Rangel-Frausto S, Li N, *et al.* Systemic inflammatory response syndrome, sepsis, severe sepsis, and septic shock: incidence, morbidities and outcomes in surgical ICU patients. *Intensive Care Med* 1995; 21: 302-309.

5. Parillo JE. Pathogenetic mechanisms of septic shock. *N Eng J Med* 1993; 328 (20): 1471-1477.

6. Bone RC, Fisher CJ, Clemmer TP. A controlled clinical trial of high-dose methylprednisolone in the treatment of severe sepsis and septic shock. *N Eng J Med* 1987; 317: 653-658.

7. VA Systemic Sepsis Cooperative Study Group. Effect of high-dose glucocorticoid therapy on mortality in patients with clinical signs of systemic sepsis. *N Eng J Med* 1987; 317: 659-665.

Review Questions

1. A 22-year-old patient had a reconstruction of his left anterior cruciate ligament 7 days ago. He complains of fever and a painful, swollen left knee joint. Vitals are: T 104.2°F (40°C) HR 120 RR 24 BP 134/94. What is the most likely diagnosis?
   A. Systemic inflammatory response syndrome (SIRS)
   B. Sepsis
   C. Septic shock
   D. Hypovolemic shock
   E. Toxic shock

In this scenario, the patient has an obvious potential source for infection. A source of infection, combined with the SIRS criteria, equates to sepsis. Since the blood pressure is normal, this patient is not in septic shock. The answer is B.

2. All of the following are potential causes of septic shock EXCEPT:
   A. Burns
   B. Stroke
   C. Pancreatitis
   D. Gram-negative bacteremia
   E. Trauma

Stroke, by itself, is not usually implicated as a cause of septic shock. The answer is B.

3. The initial event for most cases of SIRS or septic shock is:
   A. Disruption of normal mucosal protective surfaces
   B. Fluid overload
   C. Gram-positive bacteremia
   D. White blood cell demargination
   E. Neutrophilia

For example, the most common cause of sepsis in hospitalized patients is urinary tract infection; the most common cause for urinary tract infection is violation of the urinary mucosal surfaces with chronic indwelling catheters. The other answer choices indicate events that take place after this has happened. The answer is A.

4. All of the following play an important role as mediators in sepsis and SIRS EXCEPT:
   A. Complement
   B. Tumor necrosis factor
   C. Platelet activating factor
   D. Platelets
   E. All of the above play important roles

The answer is E.

5. An 84-year-old nursing home resident with a past history of stroke, hypertension, and benign prostatic hypertrophy has the following vital signs: T 102.4°F (39.1°C) HR 100 RR 26 BP 76/palpation. The patient has a urinary catheter with cloudy urine in the bag. Crackles are audible in both posterior inferior lung fields. The nursing staff indicates that the adventitious lung sounds are new. What is the most likely diagnosis?
   A. Systemic inflammatory response syndrome (SIRS)
   B. Sepsis
   C. Septic shock
   D. Hypovolemic shock
   E. Anaphylactic shock

A decreased blood pressure with SIRS criteria and two obvious potential sources for infection (lungs, urinary tract) meets the criteria for septic shock. The urinary tract is the most common source of infection for patients with sepsis; the respiratory tract is the second most common. The answer is C.

6. The decreased blood pressure for the patient in Question 5 is most likely the result of:
   A. Adherence of bacteria to blood vessels
   B. Embolization of bacteria to the heart
   C. *Serratia marcescens* infection
   D. *Salmonella* infection
   E. Leaky capillary membranes secondary to local microvascular damage

The answer is E.

7. Immediate treatment for the patient in Question 5 should include which of the following?
   A. Volume expansion with 0.9% saline or lactated Ringer's solution
   B. Volume expansion with 1000 cc boluses of 0.45% saline
   C. Volume expansion with 5% dextrose in water to supply needed extra calories
   D. Placement of a pulmonary artery catheter
   E. Bronchoscopy to positively diagnose pneumonia

Isotonic fluids are the treatment of choice after the ABCs have been adequately addressed. A chest x-ray can be used to diagnose pneumonia. A pulmonary catheter (*e.g.*, Swan-Ganz catheter) is only placed after initial resuscitative measures are instituted. Hypotonic fluids such as 5% dextrose in water or 0.45% saline can lead to massive fluid shifts out of the vessels into the interstitium and are absolutely contraindicated for patients with sepsis. Added dextrose is abnormally metabolized to lactate, a metabolic toxin. The answer is A.

8. The finding of warm, dry skin in a patient with SIRS criteria and an established source of infection is indicative of:
   A. Hyperdynamic, hypermetabolic state
   B. Lactate level less than 2.0 mm/L
   C. Immature neutrophilia
   D. Decreased partial pressure of carbon dioxide
   E. Decreased oxygen uptake

Choices B-E are characteristics of the hypodynamic state of sepsis. The answer is A.

Section V

Endocrine Disorders

Diabetic Emergencies

Emergency providers are bound to encounter the life-threatening disorders diabetic ketoacidosis (DKA) and hyperglycemic hyperosmolar syndrome (HHS). Aside from the pathogenic mechanisms, the initial management principles are the same for both of these disorders. Since insulin and diabetic drug therapy account for many cases of hypoglycemia in the United States, this condition is also discussed.

Diabetes Mellitus

INCIDENCE

Diabetes mellitus is the most common endocrine disease in the United States, affecting approximately 14 million Americans.[1] 90% of all patients with diabetes have type II diabetes, a condition associated with insulin insufficiency and impaired peripheral glucose utilization. An estimated 8 million patients in the United States (nearly 50% of all patients with type II diabetes) have yet to be formerly diagnosed.[2]

PATHOGENESIS

Diabetes is associated with the production of copious amounts of urine with glucose (glycosuria); hence, the words **diabetes**, which means "running through," and **mellitus**, meaning "sweet," were used by the Greeks over 2000 years ago to describe patients with this disease. The pathophysiology of type I and type II diabetes involves lack of insulin production by the beta cells in the pancreas in addition to other factors preventing the normal metabolism of glucose throughout the tissues of the body. In type I diabetes, antibodies against the beta cells of the islets of Langerhans in the pancreas are formed, destroying the sites for insulin production. Antibodies may also be formed against insulin and essential enzymes for insulin production, rendering a patient with type I diabetes **completely deficient of insulin**. Type II diabetes is associated with a powerful genetic predisposition and is characterized by peripheral insulin resistance as well as insufficient insulin secretion by the beta cells in the pancreas. Since insulin, albeit in lesser quantities, is released in type II diabetes, these patients do not always rely on exogenous injections of insulin for control of blood glucose levels. Both type I and type II diabetes tend to occur more commonly in Hispanic and certain Indian populations; type II diabetes is much more common in obese individuals.[3] High calorie Western diets, infections, and other environmental events continue to be investigated as contributing factors.[4]

Pathogenic Mechanisms in DKA and HHS

DIABETIC KETOACIDOSIS

Epidemiology

Diabetic ketoacidosis (DKA) is the most dangerous complication of diabetes mellitus and represents a true medical emergency. DKA commonly affects patients between 0 and 19 years of age, and accounts for 35% to 40% of children initially diagnosed with type I diabetes; **many patients with type I diabetes do not know they have diabetes until after they present with DKA.**[6,7] DKA is the single most common cause of death in diabetic children.[5] In pregnant patients with DKA, the risk of fetal demise is nearly 50%.[5]

Insulin Deficiency

DKA is characterized by the triad of hyperglycemia, ketosis, and acidosis. DKA can occur in both type I and type II diabetics because the pathophysiology of this disorder is directly related to an **absolute or relative deficiency of insulin**. In normal subjects, insulin plays a vital role as an anabolic hormone; that is, its metabolic effects favor synthesis of glycogen, triacylglycerols, and protein. The disordered physiology encountered with DKA is the result of normal protective mechanisms aimed at sustaining metabolic activity and energy supplies in the face of a profound deficiency of insulin and decreased glucose uptake by muscle, liver, and adipose tissue.

Glucagon Release

The insulin counter regulatory hormones include cortisol, growth hormone, the catecholamines epinephrine and norepinephrine, and glucagon. Glucagon is secreted by the alpha cells of the pancreas, and is the most potent counter regulatory hormone released in DKA (Figure 20-1).

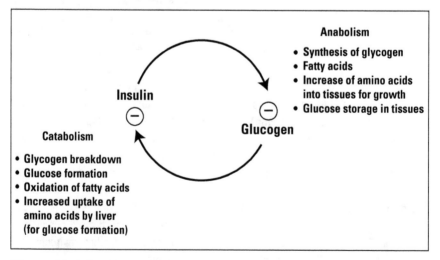

Figure 20-1 The interaction between the hormones glucagon and insulin. High levels of insulin inhibit glucagon release. In the absence of insulin, metabolism is shifted towards catabolism.

Release of this hormone is normally inhibited by circulating insulin; therefore, in the absence of insulin, glucagon levels increase, resulting in increased glucose production by the liver as well as breakdown of fat tissue to release ketoacids.

Ketoacidosis

Due to the glucose-releasing effect of glucagon (catabolism), as opposed to the glucose-storing effect of insulin (anabolism), pyruvate, the end-product of glucose breakdown, is converted to form precursors for free fatty acids. Free fatty acids are not allowed to be processed through the citric acid cycle to produce ATP; rather, they are oxidized to form ketone bodies. The ketoacids acetoacetate, acetone, and 3-hydroxybutyrate are found in the serum and urine of patients with DKA (Figure 20-2).

Ketoacids contribute to the development of metabolic acidosis because the body's alkali reserves are rapidly depleted in their presence. Ketoacids cannot be used as fuels by red blood cells or the liver, whereas the brain can only utilize ketoacids for a limited time.

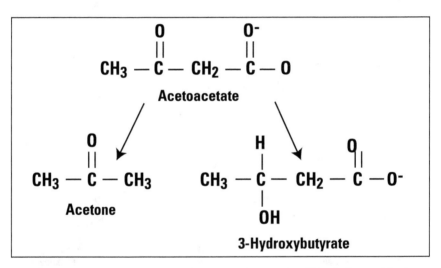

Figure 20-2 The three essential ketoacids formed in diabetic ketoacidosis.

Effect on the Liver

The enzyme lipase is inhibited with normal circulating levels of insulin. This enzyme prevents triacylglycerols from being released from fat cells, but in the absence of insulin, lipid levels increase, releasing more free fatty acids into the circulation. Catecholamines such as epinephrine also raise free fatty acids by promoting triacylglycerol breakdown and release from fat cells. As a result of uninhibited lipase activity and catecholamine release, more ketoacids are produced in the liver. Insulin normally prevents the release of specific prostaglandins from fat cells in the liver, but when absent, prostaglandins PGI_2 and PGE_2 are released, possibly contributing to the nausea, vomiting, and abdominal pain commonly associated with DKA.

Effect on the Peripheral Tissues and Kidney

Insulin resistance, or decreased peripheral glucose uptake by tissues, is due to the action of glucagon and other counter regulatory hormones. Under the influence of glucagon, protein breakdown in muscle takes place, providing amino acids for glucose production. At serum glucose levels over 240 mg/dL, glucose spills into the urine.[7] The kidney serves as a safety valve, excreting glucose as a normal protective mechanism. Excretion of glucose in the urine causes an osmotic diuresis with a variety of electrolyte derangements including hypokalemia, hypomagnesemia, and significant free water loss. Without insulin, potassium cannot move into cells; serum levels may be falsely high when a patient is essentially hypokalemic.

Summary

The disordered physiology of DKA is caused by a lack of circulating insulin. Without insulin, the body attempts to make more glucose rather than store it, and this is accomplished with the breakdown of glycogen and conversion of intermediate metabolites to ketoacids. Ketoacids can only be used temporarily by most tissues (Figure 20-3).

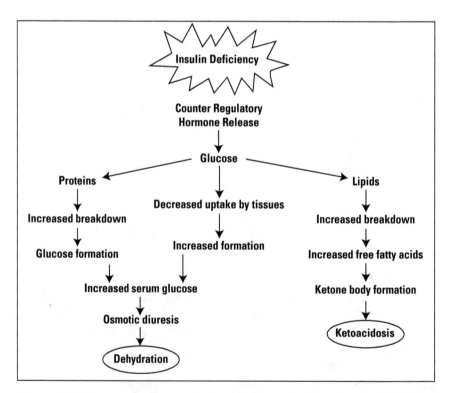

Figure 20-3 Summary of the pathophysiologic mechanisms involved in DKA.

HYPEROSMOLAR HYPERGLYCEMIC SYNDROME

Epidemiology

Uncontrolled hyperglycemia is a common complication in patients with both type I and type II diabetes. The hyperosmolar hyperglycemic syndrome (HHS), known also as hyperglycemic nonketotic coma (HNKC) and a variety of other terms, tends **to occur in elderly patients with poorly controlled type II diabetes** as opposed to DKA, although all patients with diabetes may be affected.[8] HHS occurs in almost a quarter of all patients diagnosed with diabetes mellitus.[8] An associated medical illness, including stroke, myocardial infarction, or pancreatitis is commonly present.[7] In many cases, **considerable overlap with DKA exists** (Table 20-1).

Table 20-1
Diseases Associated with the Development of HHS

Diseases Associated with HHS
Stroke
Subdural hematoma
Myocardial infarction
Pulmonary embolus
Pancreatitis
Intestinal obstruction
Renal failure
Heat stroke
Hypothermia
Severe burns
Thyrotoxicosis

Pathogenic Mechanisms Unique to HHS

The underlying defect in patients who develop HHS is the same as DKA: **insulin deficiency**. As discussed above, the kidney plays an important role in eliminating excess glucose; however, when a patient is dehydrated from another preexisting medical condition, the glomerular filtration rate (GFR) decreases considerably and kidney function is impaired. Severe dehydration and hyperglycemia develop, progressing to hypovolemic shock. The lack of ketoacid production is explained by a blunted rise in the counter regulatory hormones. Moreover, the osmolality of the body fluids increases to a much greater degree than in DKA; the hyperosmolar state itself inhibits the breakdown of fat stores into ketoacid precursors (*i.e.*, free fatty acids).

Clinical Assessment for DKA and HHS

Since many cases of DKA and HHS are precipitated by an underlying illness, diagnosis in children is especially difficult as signs and symptoms overlap with other serious conditions such as sepsis and dehydration. In children, DKA may present as the first manifestation of previously undiagnosed type I diabetes. Considerable overlap exists between DKA and HHS. Table 20-2 summarizes the differential diagnostic considerations for DKA versus HHS.

Establishing a definitive diagnosis can be challenging because other causes of acidosis and **hypo**glycemia can present in a similar fashion. Ultimately, **definitive laboratory studies and physiologic calculations must be evaluated to make the final diagnosis, but prompt treatment is essential if either condition is suspected on clinical grounds alone.**

Table 20-2

Differential Diagnosis of DKA Versus HHS

Characteristics	DKA	HHS
Onset	Takes days to develop in adults, but can develop rapidly in	Typically takes longer to develop than DKA
General appearance and mental status	Acutely ill	25% present in coma, most patients are obtunded
Respirations	Deep and sighing (Kussmaul's Respirations) hyperventilation	Usually normal or tachypneic depending on underlying condition
Glucose level and ketones	> 300 mg/dL Ketones positive in urine and serum	> 600 mg/dL no ketones

Management of DKA and HHS

GOALS

Both DKA and HHS lead to hypovolemic shock. Therefore, the goals for management are the same as in any state of shock and include: restoration of circulating volume and tissue perfusion, resolution of hyperglycemia, normalization of serum osmolarity, and correction of all associated electrolyte and acid-base disorders.

Fluids

The mainstay of initial stabilization is the administration of isotonic fluids to restore intravascular volume and replace total body water. In DKA, patients are typically 5 to 8 liters depleted of total body water; in HHS, patients can be up to 9 liters fluid depleted.[7] Replacement of total body water is best accomplished over the course of 8 hours and is done in either the emergency department, medical ward, or intensive care unit.[6-9] One to two liters of isotonic saline or Ringer's lactate is given over the first hour to augment extracellular fluid volume and to replace the total body water deficit.[7-9] Pediatric patients are managed in a similar fashion, with fluid administration adjusted for weight, and administered with 20 ml/kg boluses repeated as necessary to restore tissue perfusion.[10,11] Fluid administration helps restore intravascular volume, decrease insulin counter regulatory hormones, lower blood glucose, and clear the blood of ketones. Fluid restoration improves insulin sensitivity in peripheral tissues by helping decrease glucagon, allowing glucose to move into cells. Over time, hypotonic solutions may be used, but **initially isotonic saline is the fluid of choice for**

immediate resuscitation. D5W is added in some regimens after resuscitation with fluids and insulin, but has no role in the management of patients with DKA or HHS in the prehospital care arena.[6-9]

Insulin

During or after immediate stabilization, an insulin infusion is initiated at the rate of 0.1 unit/kg/hr in the emergency department.[6-9] This dosage is the same for pediatric patients.[10,11] Intravenous preparations of regular insulin have different pharmacokinetics than subcutaneously administered preparations; intravenous insulin has a much faster onset and shorter duration of action. Some authorities recommend flushing the tubing with approximately 50 cc of regular insulin before starting the infusion as insulin can bind to plastic tubing.[7]

Definitive Care

Definitive management of DKA or HHS can be accomplished on the general medical ward after stabilization in the emergency department. Intensive care is required for patients with hemodynamic instability, inability to protect the airway, severe mental status changes, or inability to closely monitor glucose levels on the medical ward.[7] Bicarbonate, phosphorous, magnesium, and calcium replacement is generally not necessary unless severe deficits exist. Patients must be monitored closely for signs of cerebral edema and the adult respiratory distress syndrome (ARDS). Potassium deficits commonly exist as insulin allows potassium to move back into the intracellular space as excess hydrogen ions from metabolic acidosis are cleared (Figure 20-4).

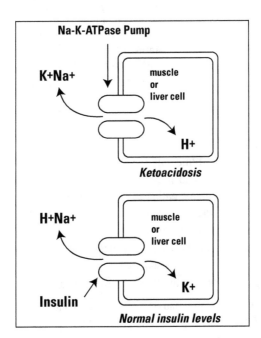

Figure 20-4 The relationship between insulin and potassium homeostasis. In DKA, hydrogen ions are preferentially shifted into cells as potassium is moved into the extracellular space. Insulin stimulates the sodium-potassium-ATPase pump, moving sodium out and potassium into cells in a ration of 3:2.

Hypoglycemia

Hypoglycemia is a common cause of altered mental status for both adult and pediatric patients arriving in the emergency department. This condition is generally defined by **Whipple's triad**: serum glucose level less than 50 mg/dL, symptoms consistent with hypoglycemia, and resolution of symptoms with the administration of glucose.

DIFFERENTIAL DIAGNOSIS

In adults, insulin use and alcohol abuse are the most common causes of hypoglycemia.[12] The differential diagnosis of hypoglycemia is usually not difficult and the list of potential etiologies not long; however, the signs and symptoms of hypoglycemia can be mistaken for a wide variety of other conditions. **In all pediatric and adult patients with altered mental status, hypoglycemia should always be ruled-out** (Table 20-3).

Table 20-3

Common Causes of Hypoglycemia
Insulin excess
Alcohol
Oral sulfonylureas
Toxic drug ingestions
(salicylates, haloperidol, propoxyphene)
Hormonal deficiencies
Fasting
Malnutrition
Heart and renal disease
Liver disease

PATHOGENESIS

The normal glycogen reserve in adults is commonly depleted after 24 to 48 hours of fasting in healthy patients, and possibly earlier in patients malnourished or with underlying disease.[13] In diabetic patients on insulin or glucose-lowering agents such as the sulfonylureas, failure to eat meals at the appropriate time, or increased metabolic needs due to illness or exertion are common etiologic factors. Inhibition of the formation of glucose in the liver by alcohol is a common problem in chronic malnourished alcoholics with low glycogen reserves. Any condition causing metabolic acidosis (*e.g.*, sepsis) can impair the formation of glucose, causing hypoglycemia.

The defense against hypoglycemia is remarkably similar to the defense against hyperglycemia in DKA and HHS. Large amounts of insulin counter regulatory hormones are released to free glucose stores in peripheral tissues, shifting metabolism to an anabolic state, favoring the formation of glucose by the liver. Glucagon and epinephrine are released from the pancreas and adrenal medulla to stimulate hepatic glucose formation, release glucose from glycogen stores, and to limit glucose utilization in peripheral tissues.[13] **In elderly patients, the release of these hormones may be blunted or absent, leaving these patients susceptible to intense hypoglycemia.**

PEDIATRIC CONSIDERATIONS

Like elderly adults, children and infants represent the other end of the spectrum with regards to susceptibility for brain damage or death as the result of hypoglycemia. Although glucose **production** is greater in children than in adults, **utilization** is also greater due to a higher basal metabolic rate.[14] The brain, proportionally much larger in children, uses a higher percentage of glucose and is continuously growing until the end of the second year of life.[14] Children also have far smaller glycogen reserves than adults. Hence, **when glucose levels drop, children and infants may suffer severe permanent brain damage**. Counter regulatory hormone release is often not fast enough to counteract low glucose levels, and ketone body formation takes too long to keep pace with ongoing energy deficits.

DIAGNOSIS AND MANAGEMENT

Rapid screening with bedside glucometers is safe and effective and should be used to evaluate any patient with altered mental status or any patient suspected of having hypoglycemia.[15] Although bedside devices are not as accurate as serum determinations, failure to initiate prompt therapy with dextrose can have catastrophic results. When intravenous access is available, 50% dextrose in water should be administered promptly and repeated to raise the serum glucose level above 100 mg/dL. The response to boluses of 50% dextrose in adults is highly variable and **it is nearly impossible to predict how much the blood glucose will increase for every ampule administered; bedside monitoring or serum samples should be frequently repeated to assess the response to treatment.**[16] If airway protection and profound mental status changes are not an issue, oral glucose loading with orange juice with sugar added, syrup, honey, or glucose paste preparations may be attempted. In infants, 10% dextrose in water should be used since 25% and 50% preparations are hyperosmolar and can cause tissue necrosis and intense pain at the injection site if extravasation occurs. In both adults and pediatric patients who are obtunded without peripheral or central venous access, glucagon administration should be considered, keeping in mind that in patients with depleted glycogen stores, hypoglycemia does not improve with this modality. Likewise, in patients with normal glycogen reserves, the onset of action of glucagon usually takes up to 10 minutes and the effect may be short-lived.

DISPOSITION

The response to glucose in hypoglycemic patients can be dramatic. Profoundly obtunded patients may awaken suddenly and vehemently refuse transport. **It is important for all patients with hypoglycemia to be followed in the emergency department because the effect of immediate treatment in diabetics may be transient.** Furthermore, intravenous glucose can produce hypoglycemia in normal subjects secondary to pancreatic insulin release; this effect may occur hours after the glucose is administered. In children and some adults, the **Somogyi phenomenon** may occur. This phenomenon refers to rebound hyperglycemia after an episode of hypoglycemia and is thought to be caused by counter regulatory hormone release. Hyperglycemia and ketosis can subsequently develop in these patients if serial glucose determinations and insulin dosage adjustments are not made. Therefore, treatment should always be initiated in the ambulance en route to the hospital whenever possible. For all patients with hypoglycemia, the cause of the underlying condition, serial determinations of glucose, and a host of other medical and social factors must be considered before a patient can be safely discharged.

References

1. Centers for Disease Control. Prevention, incidence of diabetes mellitus—United States. *JAMA* 1990; 264: 3126.

2. The Expert Committee on the Diagnosis and Classification of Diabetes Mellitus. Report of the expert committee on the diagnosis and classification of diabetes mellitus. *Diabetes Care* 1997; 20: 1183-1197.

3. Herman WH, Wareham NJ. Diabetes: The diagnosis and classification of diabetes mellitus in nonpregnant adults. *Primary care; Clinics in Office Practice* 1999; 26(4): 755-770.

4. Genuth S, Palmer J, Zimmerman BR, et al. Diabetes: New criteria for diagnosis, screening, and classification. *Patient Care* 1998; 26-39.

5. Keller RL, Rivers CS, Wolfson AB. Update in diabetic ketoacidosis: Strategies for effective management. *Emerg Med Reports* 1991; 12(10): 90-95.

6. White NH. Acute complications of diabetes: Diabetic ketoacidosis in children. *Endo & Metab Clinics* 2000; 29(4): 657-682.

7. Magee MF, Bhatt BA. Endocrine and metabolic dysfunction syndromes in the critically ill: Management of decompensated diabetes. Diabetic ketoacidosis and hyperglycemic hyperosmolar syndrome. *Crit Care Clinics* 2001; 17(1): 75-106.

8. Matz R. Diabetes care update: Management of hyperosmolar hyperglycemic syndrome. *American Family Physician* 1999; 60(5): 1468-1476.

9. Kitabachi AE, Wall BE. Diabetes care update: Management of diabetic ketoacidosis. *American Family Physician* 1999; 60(2): 455-464.

10. Felner EI, White PC. Improving management of diabetic ketoacidosis in children. *Pediatrics* 2001; 108(3): 735-740.

11. White NH. Acute complications of diabetes: Diabetic ketoacidosis in children. *Endocrin Metab Clin* 2000; 29(4): 657-682.

12. Malouf R, Brust JCM. Hypoglycemia: Causes, neurological manifestations, and outcome. *Ann Neurol* 1985; 17: 421.

13. Brady WJ, Harrigan RA. Hypoglycemia. In: Tintinalli JE, Kelen GD, Stapczynski JS (eds.). *Emergency Medicine: A Comprehensive Study Guide.* 5th Edition. New York: McGraw-Hill, 2000. 1327.

14. Pershad J, Monroe K, Atchison J. Childhood hypoglycemia in an urban emergency department: Epidemiology and a diagnostic approach to the problem. *Pediatr Emerg Care* 1998; 14: 268.

15. Brady WJ, Butler K, Fines R, Young J. Hypoglycemia in multiple trauma victims. *Am J Emerg Med* 1999; 17: 4.

16. Balentine JR, Gaeta TJ, Kessler D, et al. Effect of 50 milliliters of 50% dextrose in water administration on the blood sugar of euglycemic volunteers. *Acad Emerg Med* 1998; 5: 691.

Review Questions

1. A 16-year-old presents with abdominal pain. Her mental status deteriorates during evaluation. On exam, the patient appears acutely ill and dehydrated with a fruity odor to her breath. A finger stick reads 298 mg/dL. The underlying pathophysiology of DKA is related to:
   A. Hypoglycemia
   B. Decreased counter regulatory hormone release
   C. Deficiency of glucagon production by the pancreas
   D. Deficiency of glucagon production by the kidneys
   E. Absolute or relative deficiency of insulin production by the pancreas

The answer is E.

2. Type I diabetes is distinguished from type II diabetes by what pathophysiologic process?
   A. Patients with type I diabetes are completely deficient of insulin
   B. Patients with type II diabetes are completely deficient of insulin
   C. Patients with type I diabetes primarily have increased peripheral resistance to insulin
   D. Patients with type I diabetes primarily have increased peripheral resistance to glucagon
   E. Patients with type II diabetes primarily have increased peripheral resistance to glucagons

Patients with type II diabetes are still able to produce insulin. Peripheral resistance to insulin and a relative deficiency of insulin are the principle pathophysiologic factors in type II diabetes. The answer is A.

3. An increase in heart rate, dehydration, and fruity odor to the breath can be explained by all of the processes below EXCEPT:
   A. Increased glucagon release
   B. Increased growth hormone release
   C. Inhibition of epinephrine and norepinephrine release
   D. Overactivity of lipase with increased circulating lipids in the serum
   E. Increased formation of acetoacetate, acetone, and beta-hydroxybutyrate

Epinephrine and norepinephrine are important counter regulatory hormones released in DKA. The answer is C.

5. An elderly patient in a nursing home presents with dry mucus membranes, a heart rate of 110, and a respiratory rate of 20. He does not arouse to sternal rub and brachial pinch. His skin is warm and dry. The nursing staff informs you that he has a history of type II diabetes and was recently treated for an upper respiratory tract infection. Glucose by finger stick is 580 mg/dL. Which of the following would be the most likely condition causing the signs and symptoms in this patient?
   A. Myocardial infarction
   B. Cerebral infarction
   C. Hyperglycemic hyperosmolar syndrome (HHS)
   D. Subdural hematoma
   E. Heat stroke

All of the other answer choices are diseases associated with HHS. The answer is C.

6. The underlying pathophysiologic mechanism for the patient in Question 5 is most likely related to:
   A. Insulin deficiency
   B. Increased CK-MB isozyme levels
   C. Infarction of the brain area supplied by the middle cerebral artery
   D. Exposure to a hot, humid environment
   E. Overstimulation of the thyroid gland

HHS, like DKA, is usually the result of either an absolute or relative insulin deficiency. The answer is A.

7. Initial treatment for both HHS and DKA includes:
   A. Prompt administration of glucagons intramuscularly
   B. Aggressive fluid management with isotonic fluids to restore volume and improve tissue perfusion
   C. Aggressive fluid management with 5% dextrose in water to prevent rebound hypoglycemia
   D. Oral glucose loading regardless of mental status
   E. One ampule of sodium bicarbonate intravenously to reverse metabolic acidosis

After the patient is stabilized, dextrose-containing solutions may be used cautiously to prevent hypoglycemia in patients unable to eat. These solutions are never given to patients with DKA or HHS before insulin is administered. The answer is B.

8. The correct initial treatment in Question 7 is an appropriate management step because this:
   A. Leads to release of extra glucose stores for greater peripheral tissue uptake
   B. Leads to restoration of intravascular volume, decreases insulin counter regulatory hormones, and clears the blood of excess glucose and ketones
   C. Prevents rebound hypoglycemia
   D. Increases epinephrine and norepinephrine, freeing up usable glucose from protein and fat stores
   E. Corrects metabolic acidosis by acting as an intracellular buffer

The answer is B.

9. A 54-year-old patient with a known history of alcohol abuse is transported to the emergency department for the complaint of altered mental status. Glucose by finger stick is 40 mg/dL. What are the two most common causes of hypoglycemia in adults?
   A. Oral sulfonylurea use and malnutrition
   B. Liver disease and hormonal deficiencies
   C. Toxic drug ingestions and alcohol abuse
   D. Alcohol abuse and insulin
   E. Fasting and alcohol use

All of the other answer choices are other potential, but less common causes of hypoglycemia in adults. The answer is D.

10. After one ampule of 50% dextrose in water is given intravenously, the patient proceeds to pull out his intravenous line and asks permission to leave the ambulance. He states, "I feel fine now, thanks." Failure to transport this patient to the emergency department for further evaluation could result in all of the following EXCEPT:
   A. Nothing; hypoglycemia often responds dramatically to intravenous dextrose and patients can often be safely discharged on-scene after treatment
   B. Hyperglycemia and ketosis
   C. Failure to diagnose an underlying medical disorder
   D. Failure to address potentially correctable social factors responsible for the patient's illness
   E. The Somogyi phenomenon

The answer is A.

Adrenal and Thyroid Emergencies

Brief Overview of Adrenal and Thyroid Physiology

ORGANIZATION OF THE ENDOCRINE SYSTEM

The endocrine system is an important communication system in the human body, releasing chemical messengers known as hormones into the blood that have a wide variety of effects on body tissues. For the purposes of this chapter, the focus is solely on the extremes of adrenal and thyroid glands disorders, keeping in mind that there are a large number of other endocrine glands and hormones in nearly every body system. Figure 21-1 provides an overview of the anatomical locations of the major endocrine glands.

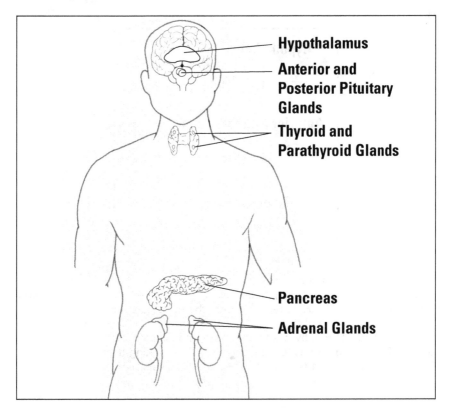

Figure 21-1 Locations of the major endocrine organs.

THYROID PHYSIOLOGY

The thyroid gland is the largest endocrine organ in the body and is composed of two lateral lobes connected by a central isthmus.[1] The thyroid gland is attached to the cricoid cartilage and tracheal rings by Berry's ligament and lies deep to the superficial strap muscles of the neck. The supraoptic and paraventricular nuclei of the hypothalamus in the brain release thyrotropin releasing hormone (TRH), which influences the release of thyroid stimulating hormone (TSH) from the anterior pituitary gland. TSH is secreted from the anterior pituitary and works directly on thyroid tissue to enhance iodine trapping while promoting the release of the active thyroid hormones T_3 and T_4 from thyroglobulin. An active feedback loop exists, regulating the release of TSH from the anterior pituitary; when T_4 and T_3 levels are high, the release of TSH is inhibited by a negative feedback mechanism (Figure 21-2).

The thyroid gland plays an important role in regulating metabolism and growth as well as brain development and function. T_3 and T_4 are the hormones released, binding intracellular receptor complexes to turn on chromosomes and influence the expression of genes. T_4 is inactive and is the precursor for T_3. T_3 has a half-life of approximately 3 days.

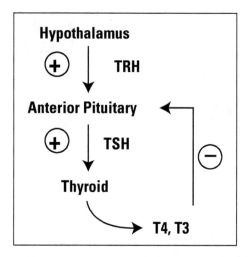

Figure 21-2 Thyroid hormone homeostasis is controlled by feedback loops involving the hypothalamus, pituitary gland, and thyroid gland. Thyrotropin releasing hormone (TRH) is released from the hypothalamus, stimulating the synthesis and release of thyroid stimulating hormone (TSH) from the anterior pituitary gland. TSH activates thyroid hormone synthesis in the thyroid gland. Thyroid hormones, once released and circulating throughout the body, provide negative feedback to TRH and TSH secretion.

ADRENAL ANATOMY AND PHYSIOLOGY

There are two adrenal glands; one is located above each kidney. Each gland releases different hormones from four histologic layers (Figure 21-3). The zona glomerulosa, fasciculata, and reticulosa comprise the adrenal **cortex**; the inner portion of the gland surrounded by the cortex is the adrenal **medulla**.

The adrenal gland is stimulated by adrenocorticotrophic hormone (ACTH) that is released by the anterior pituitary. ACTH stimulates the adrenal cortex to release the steroid hormones cortisol, aldosterone, and androgens (sex hormones). The adrenal medulla is a modified bundle of sympathetic nerves that releases the hormones epinephrine and norepinephrine into the blood rather than conducting electrical impulses. The medulla also secretes small amounts of dopamine and other substances, the significance of which remains unknown.

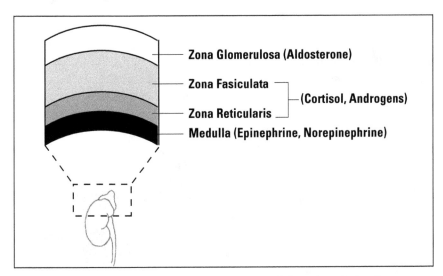

Zona Glomerulosa (Aldosterone)

Zona Fasiculata ┐
                ├ (Cortisol, Androgens)
Zona Reticularis ┘

Medulla (Epinephrine, Norepinephrine)

Figure 21-3 Histology and functional anatomy of the adrenal gland.

Acute Adrenal Insufficiency

PATHOGENESIS

Acute adrenal insufficiency, known in its chronic form as **Addison's disease**, is a life-threatening disorder that is frequently masked by other life-threatening disorders. Cortisol, aldosterone, and the catecholamines released from the adrenal medulla play important roles supporting glucose metabolism and hemodynamic stability. **The most common cause of primary adrenal insufficiency is autoimmune disease of the adrenal glands**, although in critically ill patients there are a host of other precipitating factors, each of which is discussed below.[2]

Anatomical Vulnerability of the Adrenal Glands

The adrenal gland has a rich subcapsular arteriolar plexus that drains into a single vein, making bilateral adrenal hemorrhage an important possible cause of acute adrenal insufficiency in critically ill patients.[2,3] Patients on anticoagulants or with an underlying coagulopathy are especially susceptible to adrenal hemorrhage. In newborn infants, adrenal hemorrhage can be caused by anoxia or sepsis.[4]

Infections

The Waterhouse-Friderichsen Syndrome is a severe form of septic shock commonly associated with *Neisseria meningitidis* and is a known cause of acute adrenal insufficiency.[2] This syndrome is associated with a variety of other bacterial infections including *Streptococcus pneumoniae*, *Pseudomonas aeruginosa*, and *Staphylococcal* infections.[5] In patients with septic shock, over 25% have some degree of adrenal insufficiency.[6] The exact mechanisms of adrenal damage in sepsis are unknown but are likely related to inflammation and vascular instability. Patients infected with the human immunodeficiency virus (HIV) are predisposed to adrenal insufficiency by mechanisms that remain largely unknown. In developing nations such as India, tuberculosis remains a common cause of adrenal insufficiency.[4]

Abrupt Withdrawal of Steroids

Patients with conditions such as systemic lupus erythematosus (SLE), severe asthma, or known Addison's disease, may be receiving chronic courses of exogenous steroids. When steroids are administered, plasma cortisol levels are sensed as being normal and ACTH and cortotropin releasing hormone (CRH) levels decrease by the mechanism of negative feedback, decreasing the amount of natural cortisol production in the adrenal gland. When steroids are withdrawn abruptly, only a small amount of cortisol remains in the circulation, and CRH and ACTH levels rise to stimulate the adrenal gland to secrete cortisol. In essence, exogenous steroids "trick" the body into sensing a normal cortisol level when in fact there is an underlying absence of cortisol production by the adrenals. For this reason, many clinicians argue that **critically ill patients with a recent history of steroid use should be considered adrenally insufficient until proven otherwise**.[2]

Other Causes

Any recent stress, including other acute illnesses or recent surgery, can precipitate acute adrenal insufficiency. **Patients with any history of thyroid or other endocrine disease have a higher frequency of adrenal insufficiency than the general population** because many of these diseases share the common mechanism of autoimmune tissue destruction.[7]

CLINICAL DIAGNOSIS AND MANAGEMENT

The classic signs and symptoms of hyperpigmentation, abdominal pain, muscle weakness, malaise, and poor weight gain, are nonspecific and in some cases, late findings that are not precise enough to support the early diagnosis of acute adrenal insufficiency. The muddy hyperpigmentation of the gums, oral mucosa, palms, and extremities found in patients with Addison's disease is due to the elevation of melanocyte stimulating hormone (MSH) and ACTH, caused by the compensatory activation of the hypothalamus and anterior pituitary in response to low cortisol levels.[4] Of all the signs, acute **adrenal insufficiency is best recognized as severe hypotension that is not responsive to fluids and pressor agents.**[8]

As in any clinical state of shock, fluids should be administered aggressively while other causes of hypotension are considered. If acute adrenal insufficiency is highly suggested, do not delay administration of steroids[2,8] Dexamethasone (Decadron®) can be given in an IV and does not interfere with subsequent tests used to confirm the diagnosis. If dexamethasone is not available, methylprednisolone (Solu-Medrol®) may be administered. The relative dosage strengths of the various steroid preparations available are compared in Table 21-1.

Definitive Care

Confirmation of acute adrenal insufficiency relies on the results of the ACTH stimulation test. This test is usually performed during or after the patient is admitted to the hospital. Since patients with acute adrenal insufficiency are unstable hemodynamically, management in the intensive care unit is preferred. If the condition is recognized promptly and steroids are initiated in a timely manner, the outcome is generally excellent if the underlying condition can be managed successfully.[2]

Table 21-1
Relative Strengths, in Descending Order,
of the Various Steroid Preparations.

Relative Strengths of Various Steroid Preparations
Hydrocortisone 20
Prednisone 5
Methylprednisolone 4
Dexamethasone 0.75

(These preparations are compared to potency of cortisol, thus, hydrocortisone is 20 times more potent than cortisol whereas dexamethasone is only .75 times as potent.)

Thyroid Storm

DEFINITIONS

Thyrotoxicosis and thyroid storm represent exaggerated forms of hyperthyroidism. Although the two terms are frequently used interchangeably, thyrotoxicosis is marked by signs of a hypermetabolic state, while thyroid storm, referred to also as **thyrotoxic crisis**, is best defined as severe thyrotoxicosis with both **fever** in the absence of infection **and** altered mental status.[2]

PATHOGENESIS

The most common cause of hyperthyroidism is Grave's disease, an autoimmune process caused by abnormal IgG antibody binding to TSH receptors. Almost all patients with thyroid storm have a history of decompensated hyperthyroidism. A variety of other precipitating factors exist, including surgery (especially in poorly prepared patients), DKA, and the withdrawal of antithyroid medications.[7] Infections, inflammation (thyroiditis), and various tumors can also lead to thyroid overproduction of T_3 and T_4.

Several hypotheses have emerged regarding the specific mechanisms by which thyroid storm occurs, but to date, the exact pathophysiology remains uncertain. One hypothesis suggests that patients with medical illness and coexisting acidosis have poor hormone binding to carrier proteins in the plasma.[7] Another hypothesis is that target tissues are affected due to metabolic stress with illness, causing a distorted response to sympathetic nervous system stimuli.[7]

CLINICAL DIAGNOSIS AND MANAGEMENT

Since almost all patients with thyroid storm have a strong history of hyperthyroidism, it is important to recognize the signs and symptoms of this disorder. The "10 Ps" is a useful mnemonic for remembering the cardinal features of hyperthyroidism and is summarized in Table 21-2.

Grave's triad of bilateral ophthalmopathy (bulging eyeballs), goiter (swollen, palpable thyroid gland), and thyrotoxicosis (signs and symptoms consistent with disease) may be found in some patients, but all three features may not always be present. Sinus or supraventricular tachycardias, especially atrial fibrillation, are relatively common ECG findings. In cases of thyroid storm, the temperature is usually over 38.5°C (101°F) and confusion, delirium, or frank coma may be observed. Since thyroid function tests in thyroid storm are usually the same for any degree of hyperthyroidism, a careful history, review of medications, and physical examination form the cornerstone for diagnosis.[2,7]

Table 21-2

Clinical Features of Hyperthyroidism
"10 P's"

Pretibial myxedema
Palmar erythema
Palms-sweaty
Peri-orbital swelling
Persistent facial flush
Poor hair growth
Pink papules and plaques
Pigmentation
Proptosis (exophthalmos)
Plummer's nails (spoon-shaped nails)

Therapy for patients with thyroid storm includes supportive care, with strict attention to the ABCs, intravenous fluids, and other medications aimed at lowering circulating thyroid hormones and attenuating the hypermetabolic state.[2] Administration of fluids with dextrose and B-complex vitamins may be considered as patients with hyperthyroidism have the potential to become hypoglycemic. Beta blockade with propranolol can treat many of the signs of thyroid storm and also inhibits the peripheral conversion of T_4 to T_3. Propylthiouracil (PTU) and methimazole (Tapazole®) are commonly used antithyroid hormone preparations. Iodine works more rapidly than anti-thyroid agents, and inhibits release of thyroid hormones from the gland. Consider steroids not only to reduce serum T_4 conversion, but to treat possible concomitant adrenal insufficiency.[2]

DEFINITIVE CARE
Patients with thyroid storm are best managed in the intensive care unit setting. After initial stabilization in the field and emergency department, surgical or radioactive iodine ablation of the thyroid gland is used to treat the underlying hyperthyroidism. Unfortunately, these treatments commonly result in hypothyroidism, requiring the administration of exogenous thyroid hormones.

Myxedema Coma

DEFINITIONS AND INCIDENCE
Hypothyroidism is among the most common disorders in the United States, affecting nearly 8% of all women, and 2% of all men over the age of 50.[7] The most extreme form of hypothyroidism is **myxedema coma**, a rare disorder, but one associated with a significant mortality.

PATHOGENESIS
Myxedema coma is the result of poorly controlled or undiagnosed hypothyroidism. The most common causes of hypothyroidism include previous surgical ablation, autoimmune processes (*e.g.*, Hashimoto's thyroiditis), and previous therapy for hyperthyroidism with radioactive iodine.[2] Drugs such as amiodarone, lithium, narcotics and aminosalicylic acid are also known to cause hypothyroidism. As with Grave's disease and hyperthyroidism, patients with hypothyroidism are also predisposed to adrenal insufficiency.[2,7] Infections, cerebrovascular accidents, or virtually any other cause of increased metabolic stress can exacerbate preexisting hypothyroidism, leading eventually to myxedema coma.

CLINICAL DIAGNOSIS
Although the definitive diagnosis is made on the basis of tests of thyroid function, the clinical features of hypothyroidism are present in patients with myxedema coma and can be remembered by the mnemonic listed in Table 21-3. As always, **a good history and focused physical examination remain the best tools with which to diagnosis hypothyroidism**.[2] By definition, myxedema coma represents the extreme

form of hypothyroidism and patients are typically found to be hypothermic and in a stuporous state. In awake patients, verbal responses are slowed and inappropriate. Hypoxia is common due to decreased ventilatory drive and carbon dioxide narcosis. Bradycardia, the result of poor cardiac contractility, is the most common ECG finding. The term **myxedema** refers to the accumulation of hydrophilic mucopolysaccharides in the ground substance of the dermis of the skin and other tissues leading to thickening, and should not be confused with the pretibial myxedema found in hyperthyroidism nor the generalized edema found in heart failure or other conditions.

Table 21-3

Clinical Features of Hypothyroidism
"COLD MAN"
Coarse hair
Orange-yellow palms
Large tongue
Dry skin
Myxedema, menorrhagia
Alopecia (especially the lateral third of the eyebrows)
Nails-brittle

DEFINITIVE MANAGEMENT

The treatment for myxedema coma is directed at replacing thyroid hormone, treating the underlying predisposing condition, and supportive care.[7] Hypothermia should be addressed immediately and is treated best with ordinary blankets while keeping the room temperature warm. Warming blankets are contraindicated because they induce vasodilation, which may lead to hemodynamic collapse. Intubation and mechanical ventilation may be required in patients with decreased ventilatory drive. Oxygen should be administered to maintain the SpO_2 above 95%. Hypoglycemia, usually the result of coexisting adrenal insufficiency, should be addressed immediately with either 50% dextrose injections or dextrose-containing fluids, although any intravenous fluid should be administered judiciously because heart failure is a common consequence of severe hypothyroidism. On the other hand, isotonic fluids and pressors should not be withheld if the patient is profoundly hypotensive. Steroids should be given to cover for possible life-threatening adrenal insufficiency. Definitive care with thyroid hormone replacement and identification and treatment of the underlying disorder is accomplished in the intensive care unit (Table 21-4).

Table 21-4

Clinical Comparison of Thyrotoxicosis, Thyroid Storm, and Myxedema Coma

Parameter	Thyrotoxicosis	Thyroid Storm	Myxedema Coma
Temperature	Normal	High	Hypothermia
Mental Status	Normal, agitation, hyperactivity	Obtundation, confusion, coma	Delirium, lethargy, coma
Vital Signs	Tachycardia	Tachycardia	Bradycardia
	Hypertension	Hyper- or hypotension	Hypotension
	Hyperventilation	Hyper- or hypoventilation	Hypoventilation
ECG	Sinus tachycardia	SVT, atrial fibrillation	Sinus bradycardia, bradydysrhythmias
Diagnostic Clues	See text	Table 21-2	Table 21-3

References

1. Brunt LM, Halverson JD. The endocrine system. *In:* O'Leary JP (ed.). *The Physiologic Basis of Surgery.* Philadelphia: Williams and Wilkins, 1993. 376-381.

2. Martinez FJ, Lash RW. Intensive care unit complications: Endocrinologic and metabolic complications in the intensive care unit. *Clinics in Chest Medicine* 20(2); 1999: 401-421, xi.

3. Rao R, Vagnucci A, Amico J. Bilateral massive adrenal hemorrhage: Early recognition and treatment. *Ann Intern Med* 1989; 110: 227-235.

4. Ten S, New M, Maclaren N. Addison's disease 2001. *J Clin Endo Metabol* 2001; 86(7): 2909-2922.

5. Siegel L, Grinspoon S, Garvey G, *et al.* Sepsis and adrenal function. *Trends in Endocrinology Metabolism* 1994; 5: 324-328.

6. Soni A, Pepper GM, Wyrwinski PM, *et al.* Adrenal insufficiency occurring during septic shock: Incidence, outcome, and relationship to peripheral cytokine levels. *Am J Med* 1995; 98: 266-271.

7. Ringel MD. Endocrine and metabolic dysfunction syndromes in the critically ill: Management of hypothyroidism and hyperthyroidism in the intensive care unit. *Crit Care Clin* 2001; 17(1): 59-74.

8. Chin R. Adrenal crisis. *Crit Care Clin* 1991; 7: 23-42.

Review Questions

1. A 33-year-old male with a past medical history of hypothyroidism recently underwent surgery for repair of an inguinal hernia. You are called to his residence for the chief complaint of weakness and lethargy. Vital signs are as follows: HR 110 RR 24 BP 80/palpation. The patient is in moderate distress. During prolonged transport, the blood pressure remains 80/palpation despite several fluid boluses of isotonic saline and a dopamine infusion. The most likely problem with this patient is:
   A. Cushing's disease
   B. Thyrotoxicosis
   C. Myxedema coma
   D. Acute adrenal insufficiency
   E. Atrial fibrillation with normal rate

The hallmark of acute adrenal insufficiency is hypotension unresponsive to fluids and pressor agents. The answer is D.

2. Potential lifesaving treatments for this patient would include all of the following EXCEPT:
   A. Intravenous dexamethasone
   B. Oxygen as needed to maintain pulse oximetry above 95%
   C. Fluids to increase the blood pressure
   D. Pressor agents such as dopamine and norepinephrine to maintain blood pressure
   E. Thyroid hormone preparations intravenously

The answer E.

3. In critically ill patients, which of the following increases the susceptibility for acute adrenal insufficiency?
   A. Increased susceptibility of bilateral adrenal hemorrhage in critical illness
   B. Infection with *Neisseria meningitidis*
   C. Abrupt cessation of steroids
   D. Infection with human immunodeficiency virus
   E. All of the above

The answer is E.

4. All of the following are true statements about acute adrenal insufficiency EXCEPT:
   A. Critically ill patients with a history of steroid use should be considered adrenally insufficient until proven otherwise.
   B. Patients with thyroid disease have an increased risk of acute adrenal insufficiency.
   C. Of all the signs, acute adrenal insufficiency is best recognized as hypotension responsive to pressors.
   D. The most common cause of primary adrenal insufficiency is autoimmune disease.
   E. Recent surgery or other metabolic stressors can precipitate acute adrenal insufficiency.

The answer is C.

5. You are called to the scene of a physical rehabilitation center for a 70-year-old with a history of thyroid problems. The patient is obtunded with the following vital signs: T 104.0°F (40°C) HR 110 RR 24 BP 100/72. The ECG monitor shows atrial fibrillation with a rapid ventricular response. Upon physical examination, you would expect to find all of the following EXCEPT:
   A. Dry skin and coarse hair
   B. Red palms (palmar erythema)
   C. Spoon-shaped fingernails (Plummer's nails)
   D. Bulging eyes (exophthalmos)
   E. Sweaty palms

All of the other answers are clinical characteristics of hyperthyroidism. The patient in this scenario is likely to be suffering from thyroid storm. The answer is A.

6. Treatment for the patient in Question 5 should include:
   A. Intravenous propylthiouracil (PTU) in the field
   B. Thyroid hormone intravenously in the field
   C. Oxygen, intravenous beta-blockers, intravenous insulin
   D. Supportive care, intravenous fluids, intravenous dextrose as needed
   E. Supportive care, intravenous fluids, intravenous insulin as needed

Patients with thyroid storm are usually hypoglycemic, so glucose can be given as needed as well as intravenous fluids and B-vitamins. PTU and other anti-thyroid medications are reserved for use when the patient arrives at the hospital. The answer is D.

7. You are called to the scene of a 59-year-old for the complaint of decreased mental status. The patient's daughter informs you that the patient was once diagnosed with "some kind of Japanese-sounding disease of the thyroid." The patient is usually noncompliant with her medications. Vital signs: HR 52 RR 10 BP 90/60. The skin appears thickened and swollen in some areas. Upon further physical examination of the patient you would expect to find all of the following EXCEPT:
   A. Large tongue
   B. Loss of hair, especially over the lateral aspect of the eyebrows
   C. Periorbital swelling and bulging eyes
   D. Coarse hair and thickened dry skin
   E. Brittle nails and orange-yellow palms

All other answer choices are signs of hypothyroidism. The patient is likely to be in myxedema coma. The patient's hypothyroidism is probably the result of Hashimoto's thyroiditis. The answer is C.

8. Treatment for the patient in Question 7 should include:
   A. Oxygen, intubation for decreased ventilatory rate
   B. Warming blankets
   C. Rapid infusion of intravenous fluids to maintain blood pressure at 120/80 mm Hg
   D. Insulin infusion to correct hyperglycemia
   E. Beta-blockers to prevent atrial fibrillation

Fluids must be administered judiciously since heart failure commonly coexists in patients with myxedema coma. Intubation is often required to protect the airway and prevent hypoxia. The answer is A.

Section VI

Gastrointestinal Emergencies

According to the U.S. National Center for Health Statistics, in 1996, abdominal pain was listed as the single most frequently mentioned complaint for patients seen in the emergency department.[1] Providers compare the painful abdomen to the dark side of the moon: a nebulous and enigmatic terrain.[2] While definitive care can only be accomplished in the hospital by surgeons and other specialists, the prehospital care provider plays a critical role in assessing and transporting patients to the appropriate facility.

This chapter is limited to a discussion of the pathophysiology of acute abdominal pain as it relates to various clinical manifestations, and is not meant to be comprehensive. Indeed, entire volumes have been written on the topic. Abdominal pain in children, trauma patients, and women in the third trimester of pregnancy is purposely excluded. Adult and pediatric trauma life support courses cover these topics in much greater detail.

Definitions

ACUTE ABDOMINAL PAIN
According to the American College of Emergency Physicians' clinical policy statement for nontraumatic abdominal pain, **acute** abdominal pain is defined as pain of less than 1 week's duration.[3] This definition neglects prepubescent patients, women in the third trimester of pregnancy, and trauma patients.

THE ACUTE ABDOMEN
The acute abdomen is the extreme manifestation of acute abdominal pain, and is defined by most surgeons as abdominal pain requiring immediate surgical intervention. Many surgeons prefer the term **acute surgical abdomen**. This term should be used sparingly in the prehospital environment as this condition is best diagnosed by the emergency department physician or surgical specialist. Once stabilized in the field, all patients with a suspected acute abdomen should be transported rapidly, regardless of the suspected cause.

The Physiology of Abdominal Pain

VISCERAL PAIN
Dull, aching, or colicky pain, usually without guarding or tenderness on physical exam, is referred to as visceral pain. Visceral pain is more of a symptom than a sign. This type of pain is mediated by sympathetic nerve fibers in the walls of hollow organs or the capsules of solid organs, and is caused by the stretching of these fibers, usually accompanied by ischemia and the release of inflammatory mediators. Pain follows a distribution according to the segments of the thoracolumbar (sympathetic) nervous system. Since intraperitoneal organs are embryologically derived from the sympathetic fibers on both sides of the spinal cord, pain is usually felt in the midline. Likewise, visceral pain can occur in different topographic segments of the abdomen, depending on which organs are involved. For instance, stomach, biliary tract, or duodenal pathology typically manifests as epigastric pain whereas pathology of the small bowel, appendix, or cecum manifests as periumbilical pain.

PARIETAL PAIN
Parietal pain, known also as somatic pain, is caused by irritation of nerve fibers in the peritoneum: the thin fibrous abdominal layer that overlies the intra-abdominal organs. Parietal pain is usually more well-localized than visceral pain because pain signals are sent directly from specific parts of irritated peritoneum. As opposed to visceral pain, parietal pain is more often a sign rather than a symptom, and manifests as tenderness, guarding, and rigidity, of the abdomen on physical exam.

REFERRED PAIN
Referred pain, like visceral pain, produces symptoms more often than signs, and is a pattern of pain based on the embryological origins of organs and tissues.[4] Referred pain exists when pain is felt in a location away from the actual affected area of the abdomen. For example, since the testes and urinary tract are anatomically contiguous organs with the same embryological origin, kidney stones (nephro- or urolithiasis) may present with referred pain to the testicle and groin. Other examples include infrascapular pain associated with biliary tract disease, as well as jaw and arm pain associated with myocardial infarction.

Clinical Correlation: Appendicitis
To further understand the interrelationship of visceral, parietal, and referred pain, consider the example of acute appendicitis. Appendicitis is inflammation of the appendix, a vestigial organ located in the right lower quadrant of the abdomen (although the tail of the appendix can extend into other abdominal quadrants; Figure 22-1).

When the lumen of the appendix is occluded by food matter, adhesions, or lymphoid hyperplasia, the intraluminal pressure increases while mucosal secretions continue. Visceral pain occurs at this stage as the lumen of the appendix and cecum become stretched and irritated. Increased intraluminal pressure obstructs venous and lymphatic drainage, resulting in congestion, mucosal breakdown, and bacterial invasion by normal bowel flora. As the intraluminal pressure and inflammation increase, the contents of the appendix eventually spill into the peritoneum, causing parietal pain, commonly in the right lower quadrant of the abdomen.

Intra-abdominal Pain

ABDOMINAL TOPOGRAPHY

The sources of intra-abdominal pain can be remembered as the 3 Gs: **gastrointestinal**, **genitourinary**, and **gynecological**. A fourth category includes the potentially devastating group of vascular emergencies: abdominal aortic aneurysm (AAA) and mesenteric ischemia or infarction. An appreciation of physiologic pain patterns, combined with a basic understanding of anatomy, can assist with localizing the source of abdominal pain.

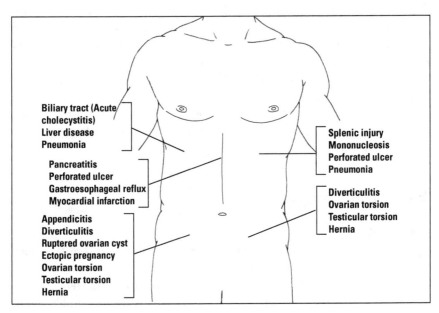

Biliary tract (Acute cholecystitis)
Liver disease
Pneumonia

Pancreatitis
Perforated ulcer
Gastroesophageal reflux
Myocardial infarction

Appendicitis
Diverticulitis
Ruptered ovarian cyst
Ectopic pregnancy
Ovarian torsion
Testicular torsion
Hernia

Splenic injury
Mononucleosis
Perforated ulcer
Pneumonia

Diverticulitis
Ovarian torsion
Testicular torsion
Hernia

Figure 22-1 Abdominal topography and localization for common causes of acute abdominal pain.

PERITONEAL INFLAMMATION

Peritoneal inflammation, or peritonitis, can be either primary or secondary, the latter being the more common of the two. Primary peritonitis, known also as **spontaneous** peritonitis, is most likely to be caused by infection with bacteria such as *E. coli, Streptococcus, Pneumococcus,* or *Mycobacterium tuberculi.* Secondary peritonitis is most often caused by pelvic or abdominal trauma, and by disease in organs such as the gallbladder, appendix, and pancreas. The bacteria found in these infections closely resembles the bacteria found in the bowel as normal flora. The patient typically complains of sharp, constant, and sometimes cramping pain, which may be limited to a specific abdominal quadrant, with localization dependent on the source of the infection or parietal irritation. With peritonitis, the pain usually stays where it starts.

OBSTRUCTION OF HOLLOW VISCUS

Some of the most common sources of abdominal pain include obstruction of the ureter, biliary tract, or intestine.[5] The source of the obstruction can include calculi, adhesions, tumor, volvulus, or intussusception.[6] In any patient presenting with abdominal pain and a history of previous abdominal surgery, the clinical suspicion of intestinal obstruction secondary to adhesions should be ruled out.

VASCULAR DISORDERS

Patients with vascular disorders usually have either a ruptured or rapidly dissecting abdominal aortic aneurysm (AAA) or an ischemic or infarcted bowel. Mesenteric ischemia should be suspected in any patient with a history of atherosclerotic heart disease (ASHD), previous deep vein thrombosis (DVT), pulmonary embolism (PE), or underlying bleeding disorder associated with cancer, oral contraceptive use, or pregnancy. In patients with abdominal pain progressing to signs and symptoms consistent with septic shock, bowel infarction or ischemia is possible. Dissecting AAA pain is often described as tearing in nature, and may be accompanied by back pain. A pulsatile mass may occasionally be palpated on physical exam.

Extra-abdominal Pain

THORAX

In the thorax, PE, pneumonia, pneumothorax, esophageal disease, and myocardial infarction or ischemia can present with upper quadrant or epigastric abdominal pain. Epigastric or left upper quadrant pain associated with gastroesophageal reflux disease (GERD) can mask an underlying cardiac etiology; in these cases a normal 12-lead ECG, which may still be normal in a patient with atypical chest pain, is at least reassuring.[2] Pneumonia, as well as PE, can refer pain to the abdomen and shoulders when the diaphragm is irritated.

ABDOMINAL WALL

Abdominal wall pain is most commonly related to either soft tissue infection or trauma. Light palpation is the most valuable technique to help with differentiating abdominal wall lesions from deeper abdominal structure involvement; Carnett's sign is another useful test that can be rapidly performed (Table 22-2).[7] Abscesses noted near the umbilicus should always be of concern since the abdominal wall in this region is thin, predisposing patients to the greater potential for intra-abdominal infection. Trauma can include muscle strains, contusions, hematomas, and penetrating wounds.

While abdominal wall injury may present with a mild appearance, it can be associated with underlying organ tears, rupture, or contusions. A penetrating wound may be small in nature and not easily seen, particularly if bleeding at the surface is absent; however, detection of penetrating wounds to the abdomen is essential for proper referral to level I trauma centers for mandatory surgical exploration. In abdominal trauma, the spleen is the most commonly injured organ, especially in blunt trauma, but the onset of symptoms can be immediate or delayed.

Any patient with possible blunt trauma to the abdomen should have orthostatic blood pressure measurements taken if possible, as well as careful palpation and examination of the abdomen. Nontraumatic splenic rupture is often associated with Epstein Barr virus infection (*i.e.*, infectious mononucleosis); therefore, if this disease is being considered, the history should include questions about recent sore throat and fatigue, and an examination of the cervical lymph nodes for lymphadenopathy should be performed.

PELVIS

In the female pelvis, important sources of abdominal pain include ectopic pregnancy, ovarian torsion, spontaneous or threatened abortion, and ovarian cyst rupture. A woman with a history of pelvic inflammatory disease (PID) is at risk for ectopic pregnancy as a result of previous tubal scarring from infection. Ectopic pregnancy can cause unilateral or generalized abdominal pain with or without vaginal bleeding, with abdominal pain usually noticeable early in the course. Ectopic pregnancy can also present with syncope alone. A history of a previous ectopic pregnancy increases the odds of subsequent ectopic pregnancies.

Signs and Eponyms

Prehospital providers and emergency department personnel may be aware of the use of eponyms by physicians and surgical specialists to describe certain pathognomonic features of disorders causing acute abdominal pain. It is helpful, but not essential, to be familiar with these terms. Table 22-1 lists some commonly used signs and eponyms for patients with acute abdominal pain.

Table 22-1

Commonly Used (and Not-So-Commonly Used) Eponyms
Used to Describe the Features of Selected Known
Causes of Acute Abdominal Pain

Eponym or Sign	Condition
McBurney's Point	Located 1/3 of the distance from the anterior superior iliac spine to the umbilicus; location of parietal pain associated with acute appendicitis
Murphy's Sign	Inspiratory arrest by the patient when palpating the right upper quadrant; associated with acute cholecystitis
Rosvig's Sign	Referred pain in the right lower quadrant when the left lower quadrant is palpated; usually found in acute appendicitis
Obturator Sign	Pain with flexion and internal rotation of the right lower extremity; caused by irritation of the obturator internus muscle by an inflamed appendix
Cough Test	Examiner asks patient to cough, looking for post-tussive abdominal pain; highly sensitive clinical test for peritonitis
Kehr's Sign	Referred left subscapular pain ("shoulder strap") associated with an injured spleen; caused by irritation of the diaphragm by splenic leakage of blood
Right Subscapular Referred Pain	Associated with biliary tract disease
Carnett's Sign	Increased tenderness to palpation when the abdominal muscles are contracted (e.g. when patient lifts head and/or legs off bed); highly sensitive test for abdominal wall pain

Dangerous Mimics

Since the physical exam, history, and even laboratory and radiologic studies may not be reliable in every case of acute abdominal pain, providers should always formulate a differential diagnosis, keeping in mind the dangerous mimics (see Table 22-2).

Table 22-2

True Diagnosis	Misdiagnosis
Appendicitis	Gastroenteritis, Pelvic inflammatory disease (PID), Urinary tract infection (UTI)
Ruptured AAA	Urologic stone disease, Diverticulitis
Bowel Obstruction	Constipation, Gastroenteritis
Diverticulitis	Constipation, Gastroenteritis, Kidney Infection
Ectopic Pregnancy	PID, UTI, Ovarian cyst
Incarcerated or Strangulated Hernia	Bowel obstruction
Mesenteric Ischemia	Gastroenteritis, Constipation, Bowel obstruction
Perforated Viscus	Peptic ulcer disease, Pancreatitis
Shock or Sepsis from Perforation or Abdominal Infection	Pneumonia, Sepsis from other causes

Definitive Care

Definitive care is administered after specific tests and serial examinations of the patient are performed. As mentioned previously, the acute surgical abdomen always requires early assessment by a surgical specialist. The recommended tests for the definitive diagnosis of selected causes of abdominal pain are listed in Table 22-3.

Table 22-3
Diagnostic Tests for Various Causes of Acute Abdominal Pain

Intra-abdominal Causes

Condition	Diagnostic Tests
Appendicitis	Usually a clinical diagnosis!
Biliary Tract Disease	Ultrasound (US)
Diverticulitis	US or Computed Tomography (CT) scan
Bowel Obstruction	Plain abdominal radiographs, US, CT
Intestinal Ischemia/Infarction	CT, Magnetic Resonance Imaging (MRI), Angiography (*very difficult diagnosis—must have strong clinical suspicion)
Pancreatitis	CT, serum amylase and lipase
Urinary Stone Disease	Helical (spiral) CT, US + Kidney, Ureters, Bladder (KUB) radiographs, Intravenous Pyelogram (IVP)
AAA	MRI, US, CT, Angiography

Extra-abdominal Causes

Condition	Diagnostic Tests
Ectopic Pregnancy	US, serum or urine beta-hCg level
Testicular Torsion	US with color flow Doppler
Pelvic Inflammatory Disease	US, White Blood Cell Count (WBC), Erythrocyte Sedimentation Rate (ESR), C-Reactive Protein (CRP)
Ovarian Torsion	US with color flow Doppler

* Indicates accepted gold standard test.

References

1. McCaig LF, Strussman BJ. *National Hospital Ambulatory Medical Care Survey: 1996 Emergency Department Summary. Advance data from vital and health statistics*, no 293, p 8. Hyattesville, MD: National Center for Health Statistics, 1997.

2. Colucciello SA, Lukens TW, Morgan DL. Assessing abdominal pain in adults: A rational, cost-effective, and evidence-based strategy. *Emergency Medicine Practice* 1999; 1(1): 1-20.

3. American College of Emergency Physicians' Clinical Policies Committee: Clinical policy for the initial approach to patients presenting with a chief complaint of nontraumatic acute abdominal pain. *Ann Emerg Med* 1994; 23:906.

4. Gallagher EJ. Acute abdominal pain. In: Tintinalli JE, Kelen GD, Stapczynski JS. *Emergency Medicine: A Comprehensive Study Guide.* New York: McGraw-Hill, 2000. 497-498.

5. Spiro HM. An internist's approach to acute abdominal pain. *Medical Clinics of North America, Gastroint Emerg* 1993; 77(5): 964-970.

6. Murtagh J. Acute abdominal pain: a diagnostic approach. *Aus Fam Phys* 1994; 23(3): 359-361.

7. Thompson WHF, Dawes RFH, Carter S. Abdominal wall tenderness: A useful sign in chronic abdominal pain. *Br J Surg* 1991; 78: 223-225.

Review Questions

1. A 23-year-old male with no previous past medical history presents with peri-umbilical abdominal pain for 2 hours. The patient reports loss of appetite and a low grade fever. Palpation of the abdomen reveals tenderness in the umbilical area. Which of the following is the most likely pathophysiologic explanation for this patient's abdominal pain?

A. Inflammation of nerve fibers in the parietal peritoneum
B. A referred pain pattern based on the embryological origin of the kidney
C. Leakage of bowel contents into the pelvic cavity
D. Irritation of sympathetic nerve fibers in the hollow organs
E. Obstruction of the ureters by a stone

Visceral pain is most often associated with the early symptoms of acute appendicitis. Pain is diffuse, and more of a symptom than a sign. Pain is caused by irritation of sympathetic fibers by increased intraluminal pressure in the inflamed appendix. The answer is D.

2. Refer to Question 1; while in the emergency department, the patient's pain pattern changes from periumbilical pain to pain in the right lower quadrant. Physical examination reveals tenderness to light palpation in the right lower quadrant, one-third of the distance from the iliac spine to the umbilicus. Which of the following best explains the likely pathophysiology for this patient's pain?

A. Inflammation of nerve fibers in the parietal peritoneum
B. A referred pain pattern based on the embryological origins of the kidney
C. Leakage of bowel contents into the pelvic cavity
D. Irritation of sympathetic nerve fibers in the hollow organs
E. Obstruction of the ureters by a stone

Parietal pain in acute appendicitis results from irritation of the peritoneum as the disease progresses. The answer is A.

3. A 19-year-old female had laparoscopic surgery 3 days ago for possible endometritis. You are called to the scene to evaluate her complaint of redness and swelling at the incision site near the umbilicus. The patient has a fever and complains of general malaise for the past several days. To differentiate an abdominal wall lesion from deeper abdominal pathology, the most valuable bedside technique would be:
   A. Deep palpation in all quadrants to identify the location of the pain
   B. Light palpation over the area affected
   C. Tapping the patient's back to check for costovertebral angle tenderness
   D. Bimanual exam to check for cervical motion tenderness
   E. Auscultation to check for hyperreactive bowel sounds

The answer is B.

4. A 22-year-old female with a history of pelvic inflammatory disease and a prior ectopic pregnancy is 7 weeks pregnant and complaining of mild vaginal bleeding with right lower quadrant abdominal pain for 8 hours. One of the most important diagnoses that should be considered for this patient given her history is:
   A. Gallbladder rupture
   B. Splenic abscess
   C. Perforated peptic ulcer
   D. Rectal carcinoma
   E. Ectopic pregnancy

The answer is E.

5. A 55-year-old is involved in a motor vehicle accident. The patient complains of diffuse abdominal pain. Bowel sounds are decreased. The abdomen is rigid and diffusely tender upon palpation. Vital signs: HR 112 RR 24 BP 122/92. In blunt trauma, which of the following is the most commonly injured organ in adults?
   A. Spleen
   B. Heart
   C. Gallbladder
   D. Bladder
   E. Small bowel

The answer is A.

Gastrointestinal Bleeding

Gastrointestinal bleeding requires a careful assessment and appropriate resuscitation. Upper gastrointestinal (GI) bleeding is more common than lower, and males are affected more than females.[1,2] While it is impossible to determine the exact etiology in the prehospital care environment, a focused history and physical examination can provide important clues for determining the severity and location of the bleeding. This chapter focuses on the identification of common causes of gastrointestinal hemorrhage with a brief discussion concerning definitive diagnosis and management.

Definitions

The source of GI hemorrhage can originate in either the upper or lower GI tract. The anatomical division of the upper and lower GI tract is made at the ligament of Treitz, the suspensory muscle of the duodenum. This musculotendinous structure is derived from the crus of the left diaphragm, and is located at the junction between the fourth anatomical segment of the duodenum and the beginning of the small bowel (Figure 23-1).

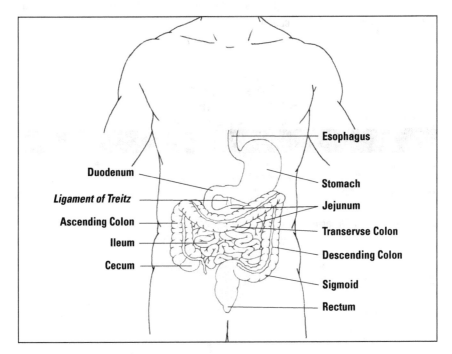

Figure 23-1 Anatomical location of the ligament of Treitz.

Gastrointestinal bleeding can originate from either the upper or lower GI tract and may be overt or occult. **Hematemesis** is the term used to describe the vomiting of blood and is almost always a sign of bleeding from a source above the ligament of Treitz. **"Coffee grounds"** emesis is the result of slowed upper GI bleeding, and is caused by the conversion of red hemoglobin to brown hematin by gastric acid in the stomach. **Hematochezia** refers to the passage of gross blood through the rectum, and is also described as **bright red blood per rectum**, often abbreviated BRBPR. **Melena** is the passage of black tarry stools, and typically occurs with upper GI bleeding, although small bowel or right colon bleeding can also be the cause.

Pathogenesis of Upper GI Bleeding

Bleeding above the ligament of Treitz can usually be attributed to one of six major causes. Table 23-1 lists a useful mnemonic created by medical students at the University of Virginia Medical School.[3]

The most common causes of upper GI bleeding are ulcers and gastric erosions (*i.e.*, hemorrhagic gastropathy).[4] Duodenal or peptic ulcers are usually caused by infection with the microorganism *Helicobacter pylori*, a urease-producing gram negative bacteria.[5] Excessive alcohol intake or chronic use of nonsteroidal anti-inflammatory drugs (NSAIDs) such as ibuprofen is often the grounds for inflammation of the esophagus, duodenum, and stomach. NSAIDs inhibit the production of protective prostaglandins for the gastric mucosa. Mallory-Weiss tears are longitudinal mucosal tears at the cardioesophageal region caused by protracted vomiting or retching, and in some cases, forceful bouts of coughing or generalized seizures.

Table 23-1
Mnemonic to Remember the Major Causes of
Upper GI Bleeding

"UVA-MED"

U- Ulcers

V- Varices

A- Angiodysplasia/ arteriovenous malformations

M- Mallory-Weiss tears

E- Esophagitis, gastritis

D- Duodenitis

Esophageal varices are dilated blood vessel segments in the esophagus, and when ruptured, can lead to abrupt and massive upper GI hemorrhage. These lesions are usually the result of portal hypertension secondary to cirrhosis of the liver. Cirrhosis is characterized by replacement of the hepatic cells by fibrous tissue. Fibrous tissue prevents blood from draining into the liver through the right and left hepatic veins, with blood backing up into the left gastric vein and other venous tributaries, leading to bulging and eventual rupture of these vessels.

Pathogenesis of Lower Gastrointestinal Bleeding

A helpful mnemonic to remember the five major sources of bleeding below the ligament of Treitz is presented in Table 23-2.

Table 23-2
Mnemonic to Remember the Major Causes of
Lower GI Bleeding

"NADIR"
N- Neoplasms
A- Angiodysplasia/ arteriovenous malformations
D- Diverticulosis, drugs (NSAIDs)
I- Inflammatory bowel disease, infection
R- 'Rhoids (hemorrhoids)

The most common cause of what may appear to be lower GI bleeding is usually upper GI bleeding; brisk bleeding from a source in the upper GI tract may masquerade as a major lower GI bleed.[6] Arteriovenous malformations (*i.e.,* angiodysplasia) and diverticulosis are the two most common causes of **true** lower GI bleeding. Diverticulosis, as opposed to diverticulitis, is caused by erosion of an arterial vessel into a diverticulum (mucosal outpouching) of the GI tract and presents as painless lower GI bleeding. Hemorrhoids are a major cause of lower GI bleeding in the United States population, although massive hemorrhage is the exception rather than the rule. Inflammatory bowel disease refers to either Crohn's disease or ulcerative colitis, and these disorders rarely cause severe GI bleeding. Some infectious causes of diarrhea can cause GI hemorrhage; a mnemonic to remember the common causes of bloody diarrhea is summarized in Table 23-3. Bloody diarrhea is thought to result from the invasive properties of these microorganisms.

Table 23-3
Mnemonic for the Common Causes of Bloody Diarrhea

"CHESS"
C- *Campylobacter*
H- *Hemorrhagic E. coli* (0157:H7)
E- *Entamoeba histolytica*
S- *Salmonella*
S- *Shigella*

Diagnosis

HISTORY

The history and physical exam usually provide valuable clues to the etiology of the bleeding, even before a definitive diagnostic evaluation. In patients with a history of epigastric pain relieved by the ingestion of food or antacids, peptic ulcer disease should be highly suspected; however, many patients with bleeding ulcers do not have pain. GI bleeding after protracted vomiting or retching suggests a possible Mallory-Weiss tear. A history of anorexia, weight loss, and other systemic symptoms is often consistent with malignancy. In patients with fever, abdominal pain, and bloody diarrhea, inflammatory bowel disease or infection is likely. Patients with diverticulosis or arteriovenous malformations may present with massive painless GI bleeding.

PHYSICAL EXAMINATION

Based on the vital signs, GI bleeding can be assessed as major or minor. If orthostatic vital sign changes are present, such as a heart rate increase of over 30 beats per minute or a systolic blood pressure drop over 30 mm Hg when the patient is moved from the supine to a seated position, major blood loss has clearly occurred.[7,8] The classic signs and symptoms of hypovolemic shock are often present in major GI hemorrhage; these signs and symptoms are reviewed in Chapter 17. Evidence of trauma to the head, chest, or abdomen should be sought. Enlargement of the spleen and liver, ascites, jaundice, and spider angiomas on the skin, is consistent with cirrhosis. If stool is present, the color and consistency should be observed.

DEFINITIVE DIAGNOSIS

While often not feasible in the field, when the patient with GI bleeding is evaluated in the emergency department, nasogastric aspiration should be performed. Recovery of blood in the nasogastric tube is highly suggestive of a source above the ligament of Treitz, but not all upper GI bleeds have a positive aspirate. Coffee grounds emesis recovered during aspiration suggests slowed or stopped upper GI bleeding.

The examination of choice to determine the exact cause of either upper or lower GI bleeding is **endoscopy**. This procedure enables the operator, either a surgeon or gastroenterologist, to carefully examine the esophagus, stomach, duodenum, rectum, or colon with a flexible endoscope. When performed in the lower GI tract up to the sigmoid colon, the procedure is known as a **flexible sigmoidoscopy**. GI x-rays, CT scans, and bleeding scans are other options to determine the exact source of the bleed.

Management

As with all conditions causing hypovolemic shock, attention to the ABCs with appropriate fluid resuscitation takes precedence over all other measures during the immediate stage of treatment. Blood should be taken for immediate type and crossmatch. The patient should be transported expeditiously to a facility with full surgical capabilities.

Effective drug therapies include somatostatin, octreotide, and proton pump inhibitors. Somatostatin, and its longer-acting derivative octreotide, are hypothalamic hormones that reduce bleeding from varices and ulcers, but are reserved for use in either the emergency department or intensive care unit.[9,10] These agents reduce portal pressure, inhibit intestinal secretion and motility, inhibit enzyme secretion, and reduce splanchnic blood flow.[9,10]

In patients with bleeding peptic ulcers and signs of recent bleeding, treatment with the proton pump inhibitor omeprazole (Prevacid®) decreases the rate of further bleeding and the need for surgery.[11] Since the function of platelets is severely impaired at a low pH, and since pepsin digests blood clots overlying ulcer craters, neutralization of the gastric pH with a proton pump inhibitor helps stabilize clots and stop bleeding. Intravenous preparations of proton pump inhibitors are effective as well.[12]

Specific therapy depends on the bleeding site, and although infrequently required, surgery may be necessary to control severe, acute bleeding. In many cases, endoscopic coagulation of the bleeding site with electrocoagulation, injection of epinephrine, or laser coagulation, stops the bleeding. Many cases of lower GI bleeding stop without intervention, but in cases of ongoing hemorrhage, surgery is definitely indicated. Minor bleeding caused by hemorrhoids can be surgically managed on a elective basis, but lower GI bleeding always deserves a careful approach since less common, but potentially devastating causes such as neoplasms, infections, or angiodysplasia, can have catastrophic consequences if not fully investigated.

References

1. Longstreth GF. Epidemiology of hospitalization for acute upper gastrointestinal hemorrhage: A population-based study. *Am J Gastroenterol* 1995; 90:206.

2. Longstreth GF. Epidemiology and outcome of patients hospitalized with acute lower gastrointestinal hemorrhage: A population-based study. *Am J Gastroenterol* 1997; 92:419.

3. Bergin JA, Nadmarni CP (eds.). *Medicine Recall.* Philadelphia: Williams & Wilkins, 1997.

4. Epstein A, Isselbacher KJ. Gastrointestinal bleeding. In: Fauci AS, Braunwald E, Isselbacher KJ, *et al. Harrision's Principles of Internal Medicine.* 14th ed. New York: McGraw-Hill, 1998. 246-249.

5. NIH Consensus Development Panel. *Helicobacter pylori* and peptic ulcer disease. *JAMA* 1994; 272: 65.

6. Overton DT. Gastrointestinal bleeding. *In:* Tintinalli JE, Kelen GD, Stapczynski JS (eds). *Emergency Medicine: A Comprehensive Study Guide.* New York: McGraw-Hill, 2000. 520-523.

7. Williams TM, Knoop R. The clinical use of orthostatic vital signs. *In:* Roberts JR, Hedges JR (eds.). *Clinical Procedures in Emergency Medicine.* Philadelphia: W.B. Saunders, 1991: 445-449.

8. Moore KI, Newton K. Orthostatic heart rates and blood pressures in healthy young women and men. *Heart & Lung* 1986; 611-617.

9. Avgerinos A, Nevens F, Raptis S, *et al.* Early administration of somatostatin and efficacy of sclerotherapy in acute oesophageal variceal bleeds: The European Acute Bleeding Oesophageal Variceal Episodes (ABOVE) randomized trial. *Lancet* 1997; 250: 1495.

10. Imperiale TF, Birgisson S. Somatostatin or octreotide compared with H2 antagonists and placebo in the management of acute nonvariceal upper gastrointestinal hemorrhage: A meta-analysis. *Ann Intern Med* 1997; 127: 1062.

11. Khuroo MS, Yattoo GN, Javid G, *et al.* A comparison of omeprazole and placebo for bleeding peptic ulcer. *N Eng J Med* 1997; 336: 1054-1058.

12. Lau JYW, Sung JJY, Lee KKC, *et al.* Effect of intravenous omeprazole on recurrent bleeding after endoscopic treatment of bleeding peptic ulcers. *N Eng J Med* 2000; 343: 310-316.

Review Questions

1. You are called to a nursing home to evaluate a 52-year-old male with a past medical history of Huntington's chorea. The nursing staff reports that the patient has been vomiting coffee grounds-colored emesis for the past 2 days. Vitals: HR 110 RR 24 BP 100/70. The patient cannot communicate because of his neurologic condition. Which of the following is the most common cause of gastrointestinal bleeding?
   A. Ulcer or gastropathy
   B. Duodenitis
   C. Neoplasms
   D. Angiodysplasias/arteriovenous malformations
   E. Esophageal varices

The answer is A.

2. The proper initial treatment for the patient in Question 1 would be:
   A. Ensure patency of the airway
   B. Intravenous proton pump inhibitor
   C. Octreotide infusion
   D. Blood transfusion
   E. Nasogastric tube lavage

The ABCs always take precedence above all other measures. The answer is A.

3. A 62-year-old with a history of alcohol abuse is vomiting bright red blood. Physical examination of the skin reveals jaundice and spider angiomas. What is the most likely pathophysiology of this disorder?
   A. Inhibition of prostaglandins that protect the gastric mucosa
   B. Infection of the duodenum with the microorganism *H. pylori*
   C. Longitudinal tears in the esophagus from protracted vomiting
   D. Fibrosis of the liver leading to rupture of dilated blood vessels in the esophagus
   E. Infection with enterohemorrhagic *E. coli*

The answer is D.

4. Which of the following would indicate major GI bleeding?
   A. Decrease in systolic blood pressure by 10 mm Hg and increase in heart rate by 10 beats per minute when the patient stands from a seated position
   B. Recovery of coffee grounds-colored emesis from a nasogastric tube aspiration
   C. Decrease in systolic blood pressure by 30 mm Hg and increase in heart rate by 30 beats per minute when the patient sits up from a supine position with the feet dangling over the stretcher or exam table
   D. Spider angiomas and jaundice
   E. Resting heart rate greater than 100 beats per minute

Positive postural vital sign changes (orthostatic vital signs) may indicate a 30% or greater loss of intravascular volume. The answer is C.

5. The procedure of choice to precisely determine the etiology of lower or upper gastrointestinal bleeding is:
   A. Hemoglobin and hematocrit level
   B. Endoscopy
   C. Nasogastric tube lavage
   D. Computed tomography (CT scan)
   E. Abdominal radiographs

The answer is B.

Section VII

Infectious Diseases

Pneumonia

Sir William Osler once referred to pneumonia as the "captain of the men of death," and "the old man's friend."[1,8] Despite advances in diagnostic techniques and advances in pharmacotherapy, pneumonia remains a common and potentially serious illness. In the United States, pneumonia is the sixth leading cause of death and the number one cause of death from infectious disease.[2] In the elderly, pneumonia is the fourth overall leading cause of death and is the leading infectious cause of death in persons over 65 years of age.[3] Mortality ranges from 1% to 5% for patients treated on an outpatient basis, but increases to 12% for patients requiring hospitalization; patients with hospital-acquired pneumonia have a mortality of 50% to 90%.[2,4]

Risk Factors

Patients with coexisting illnesses are most prone to develop pneumonia. Patients with chronic renal insufficiency, diabetes mellitus, COPD, coronary artery disease, malignancy, chronic neurological disease, and chronic liver disease have a higher incidence of developing pneumonia (Table 24-1).[2]

Factors indicating a poor prognosis for patients with diagnosed pneumonia are summarized in Table 24-2.

Table 24-1

Factors Increasing Susceptibility to Pneumonia
Age > 65
Antibiotic therapy within past 3 months
Alcoholism
Immune-suppressive illness (including therapy with steroids)
Exposure to children in day care setting
Residence in a nursing home
Underlying cardiopulmonary disease
Malnutrition

Table 24-2

Poor Prognostic Factors for Patients with Pneumonia

Age > 65

Coexisting disease:
Diabetes, heart failure, COPD, alcoholism,
malignancy, hospitalization within 1 year, immunosuppression

Clinical Findings:
Respiratory rate > 30 breaths/min
Fever > 38.3 C (101∞F)
Systolic BP < 90 or diastolic < 60 mm Hg
Altered mental status

Pathogens:
Streptococcus pneumoniae
Legionella

Pathogenesis

DEFINITIONS

Pneumonia is defined as inflammation of the lung tissue (parenchyma) caused by infection from a microbial agent.[1] Various terms are used to describe the development of pneumonia according to age and environment. Some of these classifications include community-acquired, nosocomial (hospital-acquired), nursing home, ventilator-associated, and aspiration pneumonia. The term **aspiration pneumonia** is somewhat of a misnomer as all pneumonias share the common mechanism of micro-aspiration of microbial agents into the lung parenchyma; this term is reserved for describing instances of pneumonia that result from the **gross** aspiration of gastric contents into the pulmonary system. The term atypical pneumonia is also potentially misleading since the term refers to particular pathogens, and not a different clinical syndrome.[2] This chapter is limited to a discussion of community-acquired and nursing home pneumonia, as these are the types most frequently encountered by prehospital providers.

MICROBIOLOGY

Although the responsible microbial agent is identified in less than 50% of all cases, across all age groups, the most commonly isolated pathogen is the gram positive bacteria *Streptococcus pneumoniae*, also referred to as pneumococcus.[1,3] Reportedly, 9% to 20% of all cases of adult pneumonia are caused by this agent.[1,2] Other important causes in adults include *Mycoplasma pneumoniae*, *Chlamydia pneumoniae*, *Haemophilus influenzae*, and other bacteria. Viruses cause approximately 3% to 4% of all pneumonias in adults according to several studies, but are responsible for almost all cases of pneumonia in toddlers and preschoolers, with the respiratory syncytial virus (RSV) being the most common.[1,6] Table 24-3 summarizes the common microbial agents that cause pneumonia in different age groups.

Haemophilus influenzae is the name given to both the virus and its subtypes as well as the gram-negative bacteria; vaccinations are available for both. The diagnosis of atypical pneumonia is made when there is evidence of infection by *Mycoplasma pneumoniae, Chlamydia pneumoniae,* and *Legionella* species of bacteria.[2] When sputum samples are cultured and analyzed in the hospital, only about 50% show evidence of infection with a specific microorganism.[1]

Table 24-3
Causative Microbial Agents for Pneumonia, Grouped by Age.

Adults*	Newborns	Infants (1-3 mo. old)	Toddlers & Preschoolers	Children & Adolescents
S. Pneumoniae (65%)	Group B. Strep.	Chlamydia (25%)	Viral	Atypical Agents
H. Influenza (12%)	Listeria	Ureaplasma (21%)	Atypical agents	Same pathogens as adults
Atypical agents (12%)		Cytomegalovirus (20%)		
Viral (4%)		Pneumocystis (18%)		

* Community-acquired pneumonia

PULMONARY DEFENSE MECHANISMS

Pneumonia is the consequence of a deficiency in the normal mechanisms of pulmonary defense, such as abnormal swallowing, bypass of the upper airway, immune deficiencies, and clearance of mucus.[6] The upper airway acts as a filter for infectious agents, and when bypassed by intubation or tracheostomy, serves as a direct passage into the pulmonary parenchyma. The use of antitussive agents or neurologic conditions that impair cough can inhibit the lung's ability to clear infectious particles from the airways. Cigarette smoke and exposure to pulmonary irritants such as noxious fumes inhibits the ability of cilia to transport mucus up and out of the airways. Any immunodeficiency (*e.g.*, acquired immunodeficiency syndrome) disorder predisposes patients to pneumonia.[6]

INFECTIOUS DROPLETS

Droplets laden with microbial agents reach the pulmonary parenchyma by either the bloodstream or the airways.[6] When pneumonia spreads to the pleural space, empyema, pleural effusion, or pleuritis is the likely end result. Viruses and *Mycoplasma pneumoniae* are known to be highly contagious; *Mycoplasma* alone can infect up to 75% of all household contacts.[6] These infections tend to occur more often in children and young adults.

INFLAMMATION AND EDEMA

As with any injury to tissue, inflammation and edema play an important role not only in terms of patient recovery and microbial eradication, but also in terms of expected complications. Microbes and the products of the inflammatory response are engulfed by macrophages and coughed up or swallowed with deactivation in the highly acidic environment of the stomach.[6] In complicated pneumonias, organization of the inflammatory reaction typically occurs within 1 to 2 weeks with enzymatic degradation of remaining white blood cells.[6]

VENTILATION-PERFUSION MISMATCH

Unventilated, infected and edematous portions of the lung often remain perfused in the face of normal perfusion, causing a ventilation-perfusion (V/Q) mismatch. Hypoxemia is the result of poorly oxygenated blood entering the circulation after passing through poorly ventilated sections of the lung (Figure 24-1).

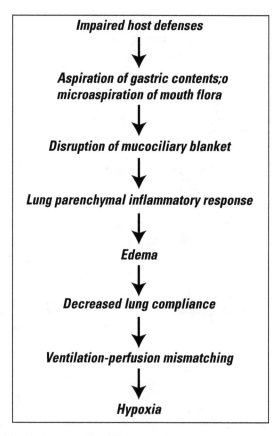

Figure 24-1 The Pathogenesis of Pneumonia.

Clinical Manifestations

Patients with pneumonia generally have cough, fever, sputum production, and in some instances, chest pain related to coughing or deep inspiration (pleurisy). Nonspecific signs of systemic illness such as loss of appetite, night sweats, vomiting, fatigue, and aching of the joints are common.[1]

COUGH

Cough is nearly a universal finding in patients with pneumonia, but it may not always be productive. Green-tinged sputum is a likely sign of a bacterial infection, but clinical assessment of sputum alone is unreliable in terms of determining the etiology. In children, cough is often productive, although expectoration is rare.[6] Lower respiratory infections such as pneumonia typically cause cough that lasts day and night, whereas upper respiratory infections are generally more productive at night. Asthma may be an important cause of cough, especially after exertion, or in upper respiratory infections, may be more pronounced at night.

VITAL SIGN ABNORMALITIES

Early in the infection, the acute inflammatory stage causes the lungs to become stiff and less distensible (compliant). The response to decreased compliance is an increase in the respiratory rate. **An increased respiratory rate is one of the earliest and most consistent signs of respiratory disease.** Observation and counting for less than 1 minute is far less accurate than auscultation and counting for a full 60 seconds.[6]

The normal respiratory rates for all age groups are listed in Table 24-4.

Table 24-4
Normal Respiratory Rates for Infants, Children, and Adults

Age	Respiratory Rate (breaths/minute)
< 2 months	<60
2-12 months	<50
1-5 years	<40
6-8 years	<30
8-adult	<20 (average: 12-16)

AUSCULTATORY FINDINGS

Adventitious (*e.g.*, added) breath sounds are common in pneumonia and can be found in up to 80% of all affected patients.[1] The term **crackles** has replaced **rales** and is describes miniature explosions when closed airways are opened suddenly, allowing pressure upstream and downstream to equalize.[6] The loudness, pitch, timing, and location, as well as persistence from breath to breath, should be recorded.[7]

Wheezing is an adventitious lung sound generated by the movement of air through narrowed airways.[6] Wheezing can be described as either homophonous (*e.g.*, monophonic) or heterophonous (*e.g.*, polyphonic), depending the characteristic sounds auscultated. **Homophonous** wheezing sounds like a single musical note and can be heard equally across the entire chest. This type of wheezing is common when large airways, such as the trachea, are narrowed and can sometimes be heard during inspiration and expiration without a stethoscope. **Heterophonous** wheezing sounds like many different musical notes and varies in intensity and pitch across different lung fields. Heterophonous wheezes occur in bronchiolitis, asthma, pulmonary edema, and pneumonia because this type of wheeze is generated when the smaller airways are obstructed. In small infants, detecting wheezing can be difficult; wheezing can be detected by squeezing the chest in the anterior-posterior direction upon exhalation.[6] This technique is common referred to as "squeezing the wheeze."

HYPOXEMIA

While cyanosis is generally a late sign of hypoxemia, and is often noticed most readily only in children, pulse oximetry should be used to detect decreases in oxygenation.[6] Once in the emergency department, an arterial blood gas analysis can be used to accurately assess the degree of hypoxemia as well as any coexisting acid-base disorders.

PEDIATRIC CONSIDERATIONS

In addition to the caveats described above for adult patients, there are a number of critical signs of respiratory distress that should be checked in infants and young children suspected of having pneumonia.

Retractions

When compliance of the lung is decreased due to edema and inflammation, a greater negative intrathoracic pressure must be generated to achieve proper ventilation. Drawing in of the chest, more commonly known as retractions, is the physical manifestation of an infant or child's attempt to increase lung volume and generate more negative intrathoracic pressure. Since the diaphragm moves in an anterior and posterior direction during these circumstances, abdominal contents are pushed forward, resulting in the characteristic see-saw breathing pattern.[6] In some instances, head-bobbing may occur due to the contraction of the sternocleidomastoid muscles. **The combination of tachypnea and retractions is the most sensitive sign for pneumonia in infants and children.**[6]

Grunting

Grunting is the result of vocal cord approximation or narrowing and is a frequent finding in infants who have either bronchiolitis or pneumonia. When the vocal cords approximate, expiratory pressure increases and provides positive pressure to be transmitted into the airways. Grunting is a means for infants to prevent airway collapse and V/Q mismatches, but it is an ominous finding and should prompt both expeditious transport and further evaluation by a pediatric specialist.

GERIATRIC CONSIDERATIONS

Sir William Osler once stated, "In old age, pneumonia may be latent, coming on without chill; the cough and expectoration are slight, the physical signs ill defined."[8] This statement holds true because elderly patients often have suppressed cough reflexes, decreased mucociliary clearance, and a decreased ability to mount a proper inflammatory response and fever. Patients may present with confusion, decreased life activities, falls, or other nonspecific signs and symptoms. In one study, only 56% of all elderly patients with pneumonia had at least one of the signs of fever, cough, or shortness of breath.[9] This study, as well as many others, underscores the fact that many of the findings typical for adults are absent in geriatric patients.

Definitive Diagnosis and Treatment

DIAGNOSIS

Although some clinicians argue that crackles or signs of lung consolidation on physical exam are sufficient to make the diagnosis of pneumonia, virtually all studies and expert panel recommendations caution against diagnosing pneumonia on clinical grounds alone.[1,2,10] A chest x-ray should be performed on any patient suspected of having pneumonia, with the exception of toddlers and preschoolers since these patients usually have a self-limiting viral pneumonia.[1,2,6,10] The Centers for Disease Control (CDC) published criteria for establishing the diagnosis of hospital-acquired pneumonia (Table 24-5).[10]

Table 24-5

CDC Criteria for Hospital-Acquired Pneumonia
Change in character of sputum
Isolation of pathogen from blood cultures
Isolation of pathogen from protected bronchial specimen
Presence of diagnostic antibody titer(s)
Histologic evidence of pneumonia (lung biopsy)
Presence of new infiltrate on chest radiograph

In addition to chest x-rays, recommended studies include arterial blood gas analysis, blood cultures, complete blood count, chemistry profile, sputum Gram's stain and culture, and pleural fluid analysis if a pleural effusion is present.[1]

TREATMENT

With the exception of toddlers and preschoolers, all patients with pneumonia are treated with antibiotics having a broad antimicrobial spectrum. Some patients meeting specific criteria may be treated as outpatients with oral beta-lactam, macrolide, or fluoroquinolone antibiotics, but for patients requiring hospitalization, combination or monotherapy with parenteral antibiotics is recommended.[1,2]

References

1. Bartlett JG. *Management of Respiratory Tract Infections.* New York: Lippincott Williams & Wilkins, 1998. 1-116.

2. Niederman MS, Mandell LA, Anzueto A, *et al.* for the American Thoracic Society ad-hoc subcommittee of the Assembly on Microbiology, Tuberculosis, and Pulmonary Infectious. Guidelines for the management of adults with community-acquired pneumonia: Diagnosis, assessment of severity, antimicrobial therapy, and prevention. *Am J Respir Crit Care Med* 2001; 163: 1730-1754.

3. Chan ED, Welsh CH. Geriatric respiratory medicine. *Chest* 1998; 114(6): 1713-1718.

4. Fagon JY, Chatre J, Hance AJ, *et al.* Detection of nosocomial lung infection in ventilated patients: Use of a protected specimen brush and quantitative culture techniques in 147 patients. *Am Rev Respir Dis* 1988; 138: 110.

5. Fine MJ, Smith DN, Singer DE. Hospitalization decision in patients with community-acquired pneumonia. *Am Med J* 1990; 89: 713.

6. Schidlow DV, Callahan CW. Pneumonia. *Pediatr Rev* 1996; 17(9): 300-309.

7. Bates B, Bickley LS, Hoekelman RA. *A Guide to Physical Examination and History Taking.* 6th edition. Philadelphia: J.B. Lippincott Co., 1995. 242-257.

8. Osler W. *Principles and practice of medicine.* New York: Appleton and Co., 1984.

9. Harper C, Newton P. Clinical aspects of pneumonia in the elderly veteran. *J Am Geriatr Soc* 1989; 37: 867-872.

10. Garner JS, Jarvis WR, Emori TG, et al. CDC definitions for nosocomial infections, 1988. *Am J Infect Control* 1988; 16: 128-140.

Review Questions

1. A 1-year-old is transported to the emergency department with fever, cough, tachypnea, and moderate intercostal retractions. You later learn that the patient was hospitalized for pneumonia and underwent an uneventful recovery after a week in the pediatric ward. Pneumonia is an infectious disease process best defined as:
   A. Inflammation of the airways due to acquired immune deficiency
   B. Layering of fluid in the pleural space as the result of infection
   C. Necrosis of lung tissue secondary to infection
   D. Inflammation of the large airways as the result of infection
   E. Inflammation of lung tissue as the result of infection

D describes bronchitis. B describes pleural effusion. The answer is E.

2. All of the following are true statements about the pathophysiology of pneumonia EXCEPT:
   A. All pneumonias share the common mechanism of micro-aspiration of microbes into lung tissue
   B. Aspiration pneumonia should always be considered a distinct pathophysiologic entity
   C. Atypical pneumonias indicate atypical pathogens, not necessarily atypical symptoms
   D. *S. Pneumoniae* is the most common bacterial pathogen in adults
   E. Droplets laden with microorganisms can reach the lung by either the bloodstream or airways

All pneumonias share the common mechanism of micro-aspiration of infectious microbial agents into the lung parenchyma, although pneumonia can also be caused by pathogens in the blood; hence, the term aspiration pneumonia is somewhat of a misnomer with regards to the pathophysiology of pneumonia. The answer is B.

3. Which of the following is (are) condition(s) predisposing a patient to pneumonia?
   A. Bypass of the upper airway with a tracheostomy
   B. Immunodeficiency states
   C. Antitussive medications
   D. Cigarette smoking
   E. All of the above

The answer is E.

4. Hypoxemia associated with pneumonia is caused by:
   A.Ventilation of edematous, infected segments of lung tissue with normal perfusion
   B. Blockage of airways by microorganism sediment
   C. Decreased blood perfusion to the lung due to sepsis-induced vasodilation
   D. Rerouting of blood away from the lungs into the heart and brain as the result of infection
   E. Persistent cough with decreased inhalation

The answer is A.

Match the type of wheezing with the correct auscultatory findings:
   A. Heterophonous
   B. Homophonous
   C. Heterozygous
   D. Homozygous
   E. Monosyllabic

5. Sounds like a single musical note throughout the entire chest; commonly found when the large airways are narrowed due to inflammation and edema

6. Sounds like many different musical notes, varying in intensity and pitch across several lung fields; found in bronchiolitis, asthma, pulmonary edema, and pneumonia

5. The answer is B.

6. The answer is A.

Infectious Disease Emergencies

Infectious diseases can present initially as situations requiring rapid assessment, expeditious transport, and immediate care. This chapter provides information on the salient features of several important infectious disease emergencies with which every emergency care provider should be familiar. The most extreme manifestation of any infectious disease is septic shock. This topic is covered extensively in Chapter 19.

Toxic shock syndrome, a variant of septic shock, is discussed separately at the end of this chapter.

Nervous System Infections

MENINGITIS
Bacterial meningitis is defined as inflammation from infection of the tissue layers surrounding the brain and spinal cord (meninges) and is the most common serious infection of the central nervous system.[1] The mortality rate of meningitis is approximately 100% without proper treatment, and even with optimal therapy, the disease is still fatal in over 5% of all cases with over 30% of all survivors suffering permanent neurologic damage.[1] While there are several causes of meningitis including viruses, fungi, and mycobacteria (*e.g.*, tuberculosis), bacterial meningitis has the greatest potential for a fulminant course; hence, the pathophysiology of bacterial meningitis is the focus of this section.

Pathogenesis
Bacterial meningitis begins with bacterial invasion of the host with subsequent spread to the central nervous system. Most bacterial pathogens are transmitted by the respiratory route, leading to colonization of the nasopharyngeal mucus layers with bacteria.[1] Colonization is more common after viral illnesses or in dry climates when the nasal and oral mucosal epithelium becomes denuded, increasing the risk for bacterial invasion. The most common bacteria responsible for meningitis in adults are *Neisseria meningitidis*, *Haemophilus influenzae*, and *Streptococcus pneumoniae*. Pathogens differ according to age; a useful method for remembering the important pathogens is summarized in Table 25-1.

Bacteria that cause meningitis possess the ability to break down naturally-occurring antibodies such as IgA, allowing invasion of the small epithelial blood vessels and passage beyond the blood-brain barrier into meninges[1] (Figure 25-1).

Table 25-1

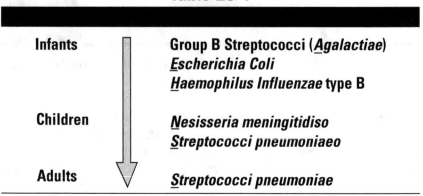

Infants	Group B Streptococci (_A_galactiae) _E_scherichia Coli _H_aemophilus Influenzae type B
Children	_N_esisseria meningitidiso _S_treptococci pneumoniaeo
Adults	_S_treptococci pneumoniae

Encapsulation of _N. meningitidis, H. influenzae_, and _S. pneumoniae_ is a survival factor for these bacteria in the blood stream. Protective capsules prevent these bacteria from becoming destroyed by the immune system. The normal host defense against encapsulated organisms is destruction of bacterial cells by the alternative complement system. **This system is impaired in individuals with sickle-cell disease and patients without a functioning spleen; therefore, patients with these disorders are at greater risk for developing meningitis**. In cases of middle ear infection (otitis media), inflammation of the mastoid bone (mastoiditis), sinusitis, trauma, or neurosurgery, the blood-brain barrier can be bypassed, allowing nonhematogenous spread of microorganisms into the brain.

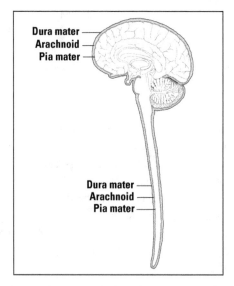

Figure 25-1 The blood-brain barrier. The brain and spinal cord are surrounded by three layers: the pia mater, arachnoid, and dura mater. Tight junctions between the capillaries within these layers permit very little passive transport. While water and CO_2 can pass through this barrier freely, other substances cannot.

The brain is especially vulnerable to infection when bacteria pass beyond the blood-brain barrier because brain cells have fewer antibodies, neutrophils, complement components, and other mechanisms to mount the immunological response found elsewhere in the body.[1] Tumor-necrosis factor, interleukins, and other proinflammatory cytokines and chemokines are released in response to the presence and breakdown of bacteria. These molecules trigger a potent inflammatory response that leads to inflammation of the meninges, the layer of cells that cover the brain. Reactive oxygen species such as superoxide anion radicals are formed in greater quantities as the inflammatory cascade continues, and these molecules cause oxidative damage, potentiating cerebral ischemia.[1] Other damaging molecules released during the inflammatory cascade include nitric oxide and matrix-metalloproteinases, both of which further compromise the blood-brain barrier.

If meningitis is not treated promptly with antibiotics, the consequence is permanent damage to brain tissue, which leads to either death or inevitable neurologic damage. Cerebral palsy, mental retardation, deafness, blindness, and seizure disorders are all possible complications of meningitis.[1]

Clinical Manifestations
Most patients with meningitis present with the triad of headache, neck stiffness (meningismus), and high fever, although variations often exist. In acutely ill children with a recent rash, infection with *N. meningitidis* should strongly be considered; any delay seeking treatment will result in death. **Kernig's sign** is elicited by flexing the patient's leg at both the hip and knee, and then straightening the knee. Pain and increased resistance to this maneuver constitutes a positive sign and suggests meningeal irritation.[2] When the neck is flexed and the patient flexes the hips in response, this is a positive **Brudzinski's sign**, and is suggestive of meningeal irritation.[2]

Definitive Diagnosis and Treatment
The diagnosis of meningitis rests on the results of a cerebrospinal fluid (CSF) examination. The CSF is typically analyzed for the presence of bacteria, white blood cells, protein, neutrophils, and protein. Delay of antibiotic administration can have catastrophic results, and antimicrobial agents must be started promptly. The choice of antibiotic depends on the clinical situation, local bacteriology, and CSF findings. According to one study, hypotension, altered mental status, and seizures were found to be predictive for poor outcome.[3]

ENCEPHALITIS
Encephalitis is the acute infection of the brain tissue (parenchyma) and is a rare complication of viral infections.[4]

Pathogenesis
Many viruses are capable of causing encephalitis, but in the United States most cases are the result of infection with herpes simplex virus (HSV types 1 and 2) or rabies virus.[4] Arthropod-borne viruses, including Eastern equine encephalitis, St. Louis encephalitis, Japanese B encephalitis, and other rare viruses such as enteroviruses

cause sporadic cases of encephalitis. The tick-borne rickettsial infection that causes Rocky Mountain spotted fever can occasionally cause encephalitis. Immunocompromised patients, such as patients with the acquired immune deficiency syndrome, organ transplant recipients, and patients with chronic disease can develop encephalitis as a result of cytomegalovirus, Epstein-Barr virus, varicella-zoster virus, or other viruses.[5]

Encephalitis secondary to HSV (type 1) infection usually begins in the oropharyngeal mucosa and is asymptomatic.[5] As lesions spread to the oral mucosa, the virus is spread along the trigeminal (fifth cranial nerve) nerve and replicates in the trigeminal ganglion. In the newborn, HSV (type 2) can be contracted from parents or relatives with herpes, but is usually acquired by intrapartum contact of the fetus with maternal genital secretions infected with HSV.[5] HSV can replicate in the nasal mucosa and can spread to the brain via the olfactory bulb and tract. After primary infection, reactivation of the virus leads to further spread of infection. HSV has a predilection for the temporal lobes of the brain.[5]

Arthropod-borne encephalitis follows an insect bite with local replication of the virus at the skin site.[4] The reticuloendothelial system, including the liver, lymph nodes, spleen, and muscle become seeded with virus, leading to eventual spread to the central nervous system. Virus tends to spread from cell to cell, with a predisposition for cortical gray matter, the brain stem, and thalamus.[5] The response to infection is composed of macrophages, leukocytes, plasma cells, and lymphocytes; all lead to progressive inflammation and pathologic changes.

Rabies is caused by bites from animals infected with the virus. If infection occurs, it is invariably fatal. Bites from animals such as raccoons, foxes, bats, and skunks can lead to infection as these animals are the primary carriers of the virus in the United States.[4] Following an incubation period of days to months, the central nervous system can become infected, with the pathognomonic formation of Negri bodies in the brain parenchyma.[4]

Clinical Manifestations
Encephalitis is characterized by the acute onset of fever with headache, altered consciousness, disorientation, and behavioral and speech abnormalities.[4] Hemiparesis and seizures are more commonly seen in encephalitis than in meningitis although meningismus and findings consistent with meningitis may be present in many cases. Because HSV has a predisposition for infecting the temporal lobe, **the clinical findings of aphasia (inability to speak), anosmia (inability to smell), and seizures should prompt a strong suspicion for infection with this virus.**[4]

Definitive Diagnosis and Treatment
The work-up for encephalitis is similar to the work-up for meningitis. Examination of the CSF is essential, as well as neurodiagnostic tests such as electroencephalography (EEG), computed tomography (CT), and magnetic resonance imaging (MRI).[4] New diagnostic assays based on advanced molecular biological techniques can detect specific antibodies against viruses andare both sensitive and specific. Brain biopsy is rarely indicated, but has a sensitivity and specificity of over 96% for diagnosing HSV encephalitis.[5]

Treatment depends on the responsible viral or microbial agent. For HSV encephalitis, acyclovir (Zovirax®, Avirax®) is the treatment of choice and improves survival from 72% to 92%.[4] Treatment for arthropod-borne encephalitis is mainly supportive with antiepileptics for seizures and other agents for increased intracranial pressure. Clinical trials for effective antiviral treatments for arthropod-borne encephalitis are ongoing. Administration of rabies vaccine can be lifesaving if given promptly and before the end of the incubation period.

Upper Airway Infections

EPIGLOTTITIS
Epiglottitis is a true medical emergency that has long been recognized as a feared catastrophic disease of children between the ages of 2 and 8.[6,7] Due to the availability and administration of the *Haemophilus influenzae* type B vaccine, epiglottitis in children has decreased dramatically and is now more common in adults.[6] In fact, one of the earliest reported cases was described in the late 1700s when President George Washington awoke with a sore throat that rapidly progressed to stridor and hoarseness made more severe when lying supine.[6,8] He died the same day after losing more than 2 liters of blood during a bloodletting procedure.[8] Today, despite improved diagnostic techniques, airway management interventions, and antimicrobial therapy, epiglottitis continues to have a mortality of 6% to 20% in adults.[6]

Pathogenesis
Epiglottitis is inflammation, usually due to infection, of the epiglottis. For this reason, some authors refer to this condition as **supraglottitis**. *H. influenzae* is the most common agent responsible for epiglottitis in children and adults.[6,7] Other less common causes include the bacteria *streptococci* and *Staphylococcus aureus*, and the fungus *Candida albicans*. In the majority of cases, no definite bacterial pathogen can be identified.[6] *H. influenzae* commonly colonizes the airways of children and can seed into the bloodstream, leading to bacteremia. The epiglottis is normally thin and curved when viewed laterally with radiographs, but when inflamed, becomes thick and obstructs the upper airway.

Clinical Manifestations
Patients with epiglottitis invariably have high fever, difficulty swallowing, stridor, drooling, and respiratory distress. Signs and symptoms develop rapidly, often less than 24 hours, with rapid progression to severe illness. The 4 Ds describe the common symptoms of epiglottitis and include dysphagia, dysphonia, dyspnea, and drooling.[7] **Although never recommended outside of a controlled setting (*i.e.*, operating room with anesthesiology and surgical experts readily available)**, the inflamed epiglottis has an edematous and cherry red appearance. **Lying the patient down exacerbates respiratory distress**; most patients position themselves in the sitting position, leaning forward with the mouth open and head extended, with rapid and shallow respirations.[7]

Definitive Diagnosis and Treatment

Epiglottitis is a true medical emergency. Airway maintenance before complete respiratory obstruction is of paramount importance.[7] Once the diagnosis is entertained, both surgical and anesthesia personnel should be summoned immediately for a double set-up. Patients are taken to the operating room for controlled intubation or immediate formal tracheostomy or cricothyrotomy. It is of the utmost importance to never agitate the patient by forcing a supine position or airway exam with a tongue depressor or laryngoscope; doing so can lead to irreversible airway closure and death if a surgical airway cannot be placed immediately. Once the airway is secured, antibiotic treatment is initiated and the patient is monitored in a critical care setting. Most children are extubated within 48 to 72 hours if treated promptly.

VIRAL CROUP

The word croup means to "cry aloud." Croup is a common illness in children and has the potential for causing severe respiratory distress. Croup accounts for more than 15% of all respiratory tract disease in children and is most common between the ages of 1 and 6.[9] Various terms are used to describe croup. The terms **laryngotracheitis** and **laryngotracheobronchitis** are commonly used to characterize the extent of airway involvement. **Spasmodic** croup is a variant with different pathophysiology and is used to describe an allergic reaction to viral infection.[9]

Pathogenesis

Parainfluenza viruses types 1, 2, and 3 are responsible for most cases of croup.[9] Other viruses implicated include adenovirus, influenzae A and B, respiratory syncytial virus, and measles.[9] Infection usually begins in the nasopharynx and spreads along the respiratory mucosa to the larynx, trachea, and bronchi. The vocal cords become inflamed and mobility becomes impaired, leading to the characteristic hoarseness associated with croup. In children, the airway is narrowest below the trachea, and swelling in this area can lead to significant airflow restriction and audible inspiratory stridor[9] (Figure 25-2).

As infection and inflammation continues, exudates form at the level of the vocal cords and below the trachea, leading to further airway compromise. Edema and infiltration of immune cells such as polymorphonuclear leukocytes, plasma cells, and lymphocytes may extend into the bronchi and precipitate a secondary bacterial infection.

The pathophysiology of spasmodic croup differs from viral croup because there is no direct viral involvement of the respiratory mucosa in the trachea.[9] Edema and inflammation develop, but are thought to be mediated by an allergic reaction to viral antigens rather than infection.

Clinical Manifestations

Croup is typically preceded by several days of a nonspecific upper respiratory tract infection with runny nose, mild sore throat, cough, and low-grade fever. A barking cough, stridor most notable during inspiration, and hoarseness may develop rapidly, although the presentation is almost never as severe as epiglottitis. The respiratory rate may be slightly increased and a low-grade fever may persist, but unlike epiglottis,

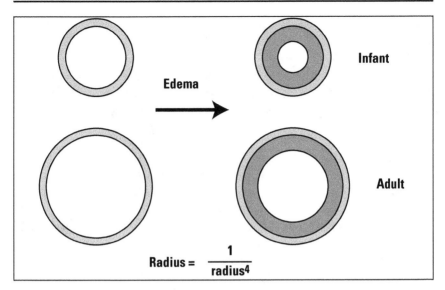

Figure 25-2 Airway diameter differences between adults and children. Small amounts of edema can lead to severe narrowing of the airway in infants since resistance to flow is inversely proportional to the fourth power of the airway radius. In other words, for adults and infants with the same amount of edema in the upper airway, infants have far greater airway closure and increased work of breathing because the diameter is so much smaller.

patients with croup are usually able to lay supine without difficulty. Spasmodic croup tends to occur at night in children between 3 months and 3 years of age with improvement of symptoms after exposure to either warm or cool mist.[9]

Definitive Diagnosis and Treatment

The diagnosis of croup may be assisted by radiographs of the neck that demonstrate the classic steeple sign of subglottic narrowing, but clinical signs and symptoms alone are sufficient to make an accurate diagnosis.[9] As with epiglottitis, the mainstay of treatment is airway management, although children only need intubation or hospitalization for croup if symptoms cannot first be controlled with a trial of medications. Once in the emergency department, racemic or l-isomer epinephrine nebulizer treatments may be used to assist with fluid reabsorption in the respiratory interstitial space and decrease laryngeal edema.[9] A potential rebound effect can occur with reappearance of symptoms after use; therefore, all patients receiving racemic epinephrine treatments should be observed for a minimum of 3 to 4 hours after treatment.[9] Corticosteroids decrease laryngeal edema and improve signs and symptoms of croup in children.[9] Dexamethasone is the most common agent utilized. In some emergency departments, helium-oxygen mixtures (Heliox®) are used to improve air flow and decrease the mechanical work of breathing. Helium is an inert gas that is able to move through obstructed airways due to its low viscosity and density. When combined with oxygen, blood oxygenation is improved and intubation may be averted.[9] Since most cases result from viral infection, antibiotics are generally not indicated.

Infections of the Heart

PERICARDITIS

Pericarditis is inflammation of the pericardium, the tough inelastic sac that surrounds the heart. This disorder has many causes, ranging from connective tissue diseases and cardiac injury, to trauma or infection with bacteria, viruses, or fungi. This disorder can be life-threatening if not recognized and treated promptly.

Pathogenesis

The pericardium normally contains 15 to 50 ml of fluid that serves to lubricate the heart surface.[10] When the pericardium becomes inflamed from infection, trauma, or other causes, the fluid in the sac increases and causes an effusion. Pericardial effusions can raise the defibrillatory energy requirement, cause pericardial tamponade, and lead to heart failure.[9] Tamponade results in hypotension and circulatory collapse when a pericardial effusion compresses the chambers of the heart, increasing filling pressures, and decreasing venous return (Figure 25-3).

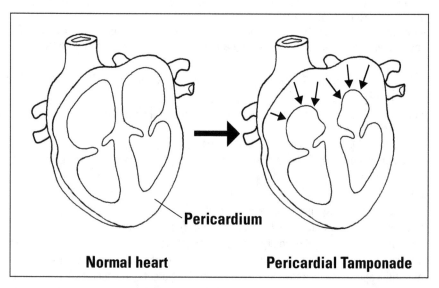

Normal heart   **Pericardial Tamponade**

Figure 25-3 The pathophysiology of pericardial tamponade. The normally elastic pericardium, when filled with fluid, compresses the chambers of the heart. The right and left atrium are affected the most since these chambers are thinner than the ventricles. Because blood can not enter the right atrium normally, systemic venous pressure becomes elevated, leading to increased hepatic congestion, ascites, and paradoxical jugular venous distention with inspiration (Kussmaul's sign).

Clinical Manifestations

A viral illness with muscle aches and low-grade fever is common before pericarditis develops. Pleuritic chest pain, or chest pain that increases with respiratory excursions, and an audible friction rub are common. The friction rub of pericarditis is heard best at the left lower sternal border with the diaphragm of the stethoscope and is described as scratchy or "Velcro-like."[10] Radiation of pain to the trapezius muscle is specific for pericarditis.[10] In patients with a pericardial effusion and tamponade, Beck's triad of jugular venous distension (increased systemic venous pressure), hypotension, and muffled heart sounds may be accompanied by orthopnea, dyspnea, peripheral edema, enlargement of the liver, or ECG changes.

Definitive Diagnosis and Treatment

The ECG has characteristic findings in pericarditis that may suggest the diagnosis. These changes include diffuse ST-segment elevations in all leads except aVR and V1 and diffuse PR-segment depression, most prominent in lead II.[10] Definitive diagnosis is made when the chest radiograph and echocardiogram findings are reviewed.

If pericarditis is strongly suspected and hemodynamic compromise is imminent, give an infusion of isotonic fluids. This action helps to maintain cardiac output by increasing preload. If pericardial tamponade is present, pericardiocentesis should be performed. Definitive care of patients with pericarditis is accomplished in the critical care unit with a multidisciplinary team comprised of intensivists, cardiologists, and cardiothoracic surgeons.

ACUTE INFECTIVE ENDOCARDITIS

Acute infective endocarditis is infection of the heart valves and endothelium by microorganisms.[11] The overall mortality of infectious endocarditis can be over 20%, and over 60% in patients with infected prosthetic valves.[10] Risk factors include intravenous drug use, diabetes, alcoholism, immunocompromised states, and infections elsewhere in the body.[11]

Pathogenesis

The formation of vegetation on the endothelial lining of the heart or valves is the initiating event in endocarditis. Patients with abnormally thickened valves, mechanical damage, rheumatic heart disease, or mitral valve prolapse are at greatest risk. When the endothelium is injured, a platelet-fibrin complex forms, as in the pathogenesis of acute coronary syndromes.[10] The complex is colonized by bacteria or other microorganisms, leading to valvular insufficiency and progressive systemic infection. The most common infectious agents are the *Staphylococci* and *Pseudomonas* species.[10,11]

Clinical Manifestations

Fever is the most common sign in infective endocarditis, and the disorder should be strongly suspected in any patient with risk factors for valvular disease, a new murmur, and lack of any obvious source for the fever. Up to 90% of all patients with acute infectious endocarditis will have a new or changed murmur at some point during the disease, but many patients present initially without a detectable murmur.[11] The commonly described findings of splinter hemorrhages, petechiae, and other lesions are quite rare.[10,11] Osler's nodes are tender, reddened nodules seen on the pulp of digits and represent vascular inflammation that results from immune complex deposition.[10] Janeway lesions are nontender flat, reddened lesions found on the palms, soles, and ears, and are thought to result from septic emboli or inflammation of end arteries.[10] Both lesions are found in less than 5% of all patients, but if seen, are fairly specific for endocarditis.[11]

A different but similar syndrome that shares a similar pathophysiology is subacute infectious endocarditis. This disease differs from acute endocarditis insofar as patients are not acutely ill and usually do not have a fever.[11] The agents that cause subacute endocarditis are generally less virulent than those causing acute endocarditis, but the classic peripheral findings described above are more common.[11]

Definitive Diagnosis and Treatment
Echocardiography and blood cultures provide the most information for diagnosing acute infectious endocarditis. Transesophageal echocardiography is the most sensitive technique for demonstrating valvular abnormalities and vegetations.[11] Cardiopulmonary stabilization is the first step in management, and after this is accomplished, antibiotic therapy is implemented to eradicate the responsible microorganism. In some cases, cardiothoracic surgery to repair or replace damaged prosthetic valves may be needed.

Skin and Soft Tissue Infections
Skin and soft tissue infections are rarely life-threatening upon initial presentation, yet awareness of the pathophysiology of serious infections is important not only for the patient, but also to protect the provider from inadvertent contamination and infection. Early recognition of serious infections can facilitate timely definitive care and improved outcomes in many cases.

CELLULITIS
Cellulitis is an infection of the dermis caused by streptococcal and staphylococcal species.[12,13] Patients typically present with a history of a minor skin injury that progresses to an area of redness, warmth, and swelling with symptoms of fever and malaise. This infection is more common in immunocompromised patients (*e.g.*, those with diabetes mellitus, AIDS, chronic steroid therapy). Cellulitis can be confused with other disorders such as heart failure that present with swelling of the extremities. Cellulitis is usually not a true medical emergency and is managed in many cases with outpatient oral antibiotics. Periorbital cellulitis requires immediate evaluation and hospitalization with parenteral antibiotics because septic cavernous thrombosis, meningitis, and blindness can result if treatment is delayed.

NECROTIZING SKIN AND SOFT TISSUE INFECTIONS

Necrotizing soft tissue infections, including necrotizing fasciitis, are a group of potentially life-threatening infections of the skin, often resulting in massive tissue damage, progressive gangrene, shock, and in some cases, death.[13] The popular media reported several instances as cases of flesh-eating bacteria in 1994, raising public awareness for the potential seriousness of these infections.[14] Many organisms are responsible including *Clostridium*, streptococci, *Bacteroides*, and other Gram-negative species of bacteria.[13] Predisposing conditions include trauma, surgery, diabetes mellitus, renal failure, malignancy, alcoholism, and other immunosuppressive conditions.[12] Diabetes mellitus is the most common risk factor for necrotizing fasciitis.[13]

Necrotizing fasciitis is pathologically characterized by widespread necrosis of the fascia and deep subcutaneous tissues; the skin is often initially spared.[12] A painful area of cellulitis may develop over the underlying infection, evolving gradually to frank gangrene.[12] The extremities are most often affected, but any soft tissue area is susceptible. The injury pattern is believed to be due to the release of bacterial toxins and the presence of superantigens. Surface M proteins of streptococci allow bacteria to adhere to, invade, and multiply in soft tissue. Treatment includes wide surgical excision and debridement, antibiotic therapy, and supportive care.[12]

MUCORMYCOSIS

The term **mucormycosis** refers to a variety of infections caused by fungi of the order Mucorales.[13] Fungi such as Absidia, Mucor, and Rhizopus are airborne and invasive. These fungi have the potential for causing severe infections. As with other soft tissue infections, diabetes mellitus, high-dose steroid therapy, and other states of immunosuppression are important risk factors. Cutaneous mucormycosis is a fungal infection of both the epidermis and dermis and may present initially as cellulitis.[13] Over time, the lesion develops into a black necrotic area with a margin of redness and swelling. In many cases, extensive surgical debridement is the only effective treatment; amputation of an involved extremity is occasionally necessary to prevent the infection from spreading to additional fascial compartments. Antibiotics and hyperbaric oxygen are additional modalities used in conjunction with surgery for definitive care.

Toxic Shock Syndromes

DEFINITIONS

In the late 1970s and early 1980s, several fulminant infections associated with shock and multiple organ failure were described and termed collectively as the **streptococcal toxic shock syndrome**.[15] Investigators later learned that staphylococci species as well as streptococci were the bacteria responsible for the disease. Toxic shock syndrome was once recognized to occur primarily in menstruating females and was strongly associated with tampon use, but it is now understood that this disorder can occur in patients with influenza, sinusitis, tracheitis, intravenous drug use, HIV infection, cellulitis, and other diseases.[12]

PATHOGENESIS: SUPERANTIGENS

The toxic shock syndromes are described as a classic example of **superantigen** infection. Antigens are immunological substrates produced by bacteria or other foreign substances and recognized by cells of the immune system (Figure 25-4).

Antigens are normally processed after being engulfed by an antigen-presenting cell (*e.g.*, macrophage) and form an immune complex with appropriate activation of cells directed to destroy the antigen. Superantigens are capable of bypassing several steps necessary for normal antigen processing and destruction.[15] This can lead to massive cytokine release and large-scale activation and premature death of immune cells.[13] A single bacterial toxin, acting as a superantigen, can induce a severe inflammatory response with fever, hypotension, tissue injury, and shock.[13]

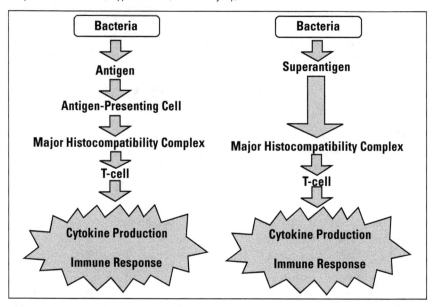

Figure 25-4 The pathophysiology of the superantigen in toxic shock syndrome. Superantigens bypass certain steps of the immunologic sequence, leading to an abrupt, massive cytokine release and immune response.

CLINICAL MANIFESTATIONS

Physical signs suggestive of toxic shock syndrome include rash, a strawberry tongue, redness and swelling of the hands, and desquamation of the palms.[13] By the time the patient is admitted, fever and hypotension are nearly universal findings.[13] In some cases of streptococci-mediated disease, evidence of soft tissue infection such as cellulitis, open sores, or blistering lesions provide a clues to the likely portal of entry.

DEFINITIVE DIAGNOSIS AND TREATMENT

Therapy for toxic shock syndrome is primarily supportive, with hydration, intensive care monitoring, vasopressors, broad-spectrum antibiotics, and surgical debridement of infected areas. Renal, pulmonary, and other systemic involvement is common, and managed accordingly with dialysis, ventilatory support, and other intensive care modalities. The mortality rate is approximately 5% overall, but has been reported to be as high as 30% to 40% in some cases.[13]

Fever in Immunocompromised Patients

An underlying theme in this chapter is the importance of obtaining a focused history with specific questions about the immune status of any patient with a possible life-threatening infection. In some instances, the patient's condition may deteriorate prior to emergency department admission, and the prehospital provider's history may serve as an invaluable piece of information. Table 25-2 lists several important conditions of immunosuppression mentioned periodically throughout this chapter. Knowledge of the patient's immune status plays a significant role in determining the potential severity and likely organisms involved.

In normal adults, body temperature varies from 37.2°C (98.9°F) in the morning to 37.7°C (99.9°F) in the afternoon.[16] In immunocompromised patients, a significant fever is defined by a temperature elevation above 38°C (100.4°F).[16]

A thorough history is essential when evaluating fever in an immunocompromised patient. Specific questions about immune status including questions about use of chemotherapeutic agents, malignancy, prior use of antibiotics, and other conditions listed in Table 25-2 should be asked. The degree and duration of known neutropenia (low neutrophil count) should be elicited because a low neutrophil count is an important determinant of bacterial infection.[16]

Immunocompromised patients with fever should be transported with full infection control measures not only to protect the provider, but to protect the patient from further infection. Immunocompromised patients with fever undergo an extensive work-up when admitted, and are started on broad-spectrum antibiotics with a multidisciplinary approach and supportive care. If the infection is treated without delay, the outcome is usually excellent.

Table 25-2
Immunocompromised States

Diabetes mellitus

Human immunodeficiency virus infection (HIV/AIDS)

Chronic corticosteroid use

Malignancy

Chemotherapy

Bone marrow or organ transplantation

Primary hereditary immunodeficiency

References

1. Leib SL, Tauber MG. Pathogenesis of bacterial meningitis. *Infectious Disease Clinics of North America* 1999; 13(3): 527-544.

2. Bates B, Bickley LS, Hoekelman RA. *A Guide to Physical Examination and History Taking.* 6th edition. Philadelphia: J.B. Lippincott Co., 1995. 533-534.

3. Aronin SI, Peduzzi P, Quagliarello VJ. Community-acquired bacterial meningitis: Risk stratification for adverse clinical outcome and effect of antibiotic timing. *Ann Intern Med* 1998; 129: 862.

4. Whitley RJ, Kimberlin DW. Viral encephalitis. *Pediatrics in Review* 1999; 20(6): 192-198.

5. Roos KL. Central nervous system infections: Encephalitis. *Neurologic Clinics* 1999; 17(4): 813-833.

6. Carey MJ. Epiglottitis in adults. *Am J Emerg Med* 1996; 14(4): 421-424.

7. Millan SB, Cumming WA. Community-acquired respiratory infections in children: Supraglottic airway infections. *Primary Care; Clinics in Office Practice* 1996; 23(4): 741-758.

8. Lewis FO. Washington's last illness. *Ann Med History* 1932; 4: 245-248.

9. Malhotra A, Krilov LR. Viral croup. *Pediatrics in Review* 2001; 22(1): 5-12.

10. Pawsat DE, Lee JY. Inflammatory disorders of the heart: Pericarditis, myocarditis, and endocarditis. *Emergency Medicine Clinics of North America* 1998; 16(3): 665-681, ix.

11. Cunha BA, Gill MV, Lazar JM. Acute infective endocarditis: Diagnostic and therapeutic approach. *Infectious Disease Clinics of North America* 1996; 10(4): 811-834.

12. Manders, SM. Toxin-mediated streptococcal and staphylococcal disease. Journal of the American Academy of Dermatology. 1998; 39(3): 383-398.

13. Hill MK, Sanders CV. Infections in critical care II: Skin and soft tissue infections in critical care. *Critical Care Clinics* 1998; 14(2): 251-262.

14. Stone DR, Gorback SL. Necrotizing fasciitis: The changing spectrum. *Dermatol Clin* 1997; 15: 213-220.

15. Stevens DL. Infectious disease emergencies: The toxic shock syndromes. *Infectious Disease Clinics of North America* 1996; 10(4): 727-746.

16. Donowitz GR. Fever in the compromised host. *Infectious Disease Clinics of North America* 1996; 10(1): 129-148.

Review Questions

1. A 29-year-old with no significant past medical history presents with the complaint of headache, fever, and neck stiffness for one day. As you check the patient's pupils with a penlight, the patient complains that the headache gets worse. A fine, red rash is noted during the physical examination. The patient complains of pain and stiffness in the cervical spine area when the neck is flexed. What is the most likely diagnosis for this patient?
   A. Migraine headache
   B. Pericarditis
   C. Bacterial meningitis
   D. Cellulitis
   E. Acute endocarditis

The answer is C.

2. The pathophysiology of the disorder in Question 1 is most likely related to:
   A. Imbalance of neurotransmitters in the brain
   B. Leakage of cerebrospinal fluid from the spinal canal
   C. Inflammation of the meninges by bacteria
   D. Infection of the dermis in the neck area by bacteria
   E. Viral infection of the respiratory mucosa

The answer is C.

3. The most important historical questions to ask the patient in Question 1 include all of the following EXCEPT:
   A. History of human immunodeficiency virus (HIV) infection?
   B. History of recent steroid use?
   C. History of sickle cell disease?
   D. History of recent antitussive medication use?
   E. History of splenectomy?

The answer is D.

4. If a patient presents with the same symptoms as the patient in Question 1 but develops seizures, an inability to smell, or loss of speaking ability, which of the following would be the most likely diagnosis?
   A. Group A streptococcal pharyngitis
   B. Acute viral bronchitis
   C. Acute pericarditis
   D. Subacute bacterial endocarditis
   E. Encephalitis

The answer is E.

5. A 20-year-old complains of high fever, sore throat, loss of voice, difficulty breathing, and drooling for 6 hours. As the patient lies down on the stretcher, he becomes more dyspneic. Which of the following is the most likely diagnosis?
   A. Epiglottitis
   B. Viral croup
   C. Group A streptococcal pharyngitis
   D. Acute bronchitis
   E. Pneumonia

The answer is A.

6. The pathophysiology of the condition in Question 5 is related to:
   A. Inflammation of the epiglottis by bacterial infection
   B. Viral infection of the vocal cords by parainfluenza virus
   C. Colonization of the tonsils by staphylococcal bacteria
   D. Inflammation of the bronchi and bronchioles by infection with adenovirus
   E. Inflammation of the lung parenchyma by streptococcal bacteria

The answer is A.

7. You are called to the scene of a 3-year-old complaining of a barking cough for 2 days. The cough is worse during the night. The child has inspiratory stridor, low-grade fever, and is in moderate respiratory distress. Lung sounds are clear to auscultation bilaterally. Skin is warm and dry. The parents report that the child has had a cough with a low-grade fever and runny nose for the past week. Which of the following is the most likely diagnosis?
   A. Acute epiglottitis
   B. Viral croup
   C. Pneumonia
   D. Streptococcal pharyngitis
   E. Asthma

The answer is B.

8. The pathogenesis of the condition in Question 7 is most likely related to:
   A. Infection of the epiglottis with *H. Influenzae*
   B. Inflammation of the lung parenchyma with streptococci species
   C. Airway narrowing of the trachea secondary to viral infection and inflammation
   D. Infection of the posterior oropharynx with streptococci bacteria
   E. Airway inflammation secondary to mold allergy

The answer is C.

9. A 60-year-old male with a history of recurrent mild upper respiratory infections complains of chest pain. A friction rub is heard upon cardiac auscultation, although heart sounds are muffled. Jugular venous distention is noted. Vitals: BP 90/62 HR 100 RR 24. Which of the following ECG changes would you expect for this patient?
   A. Biphasic T-waves in I, V_1, V_6
   B. ST-segment depression in II, aVR
   C. Increased R waves in V_{1-3}
   D. Diffuse ST-segment elevation in nearly all leads with PR-segment depression in lead II
   E. Q waves in leads I, V_6

Diffuse ST-segment elevation is common in pericarditis, although leads aVF and V1 may be unrevealing. Diffuse PR-segment depression is also quite common, and is usually seen best in lead II. Beck's triad of JVD, muffled heart sounds, and narrowed pulse pressure is evident in this case. The answer is D.

10. Which of the following would be likely to differentiate the condition in Question 9 from acute infective endocarditis?
   A. Lack of fever and few other peripheral signs
   B. Positive Valsalva test and widened pulse pressure
   C. Tracheal deviation and subcutaneous emphysema
   D. Hyperresonance upon percussion of the thorax
   E. Peripheral edema and a loud S3 heart sound

Infective endocarditis usually presents as a new heart murmur with fever. Peripheral signs, while often unreliable, can be highly specific for this disorder. The answer is A.

Section VIII

Neurological Disorders

Acute Cerebral Infraction

Ischemic stroke is a leading cause of morbidity and mortality in the United States, affecting more than 400,000 people at a cost of $23 billion annually.[1] According to several surveys on stroke, the incidence increases with age, affecting 3% to 5% of all men and women over the age of 55 with an aggregate lifetime cost of approximately $40.6 billion.[2,3]

Stroke is a syndrome characterized by a sudden central neurologic deficit caused by intracranial hemorrhage or ischemia.[4] Until recently, no approved therapy existed to reverse or terminate the pathophysiologic changes resulting from the cessation of cerebral blood flow that leads to neurological impairment. With recent advances in neuroradiologic imaging and improved pharmacotherapy, this debilitating disease is now treatable when recognized promptly.

This chapter concentrates on the pathophysiology of thrombotic and embolic strokes with a brief discussion of hemorrhagic strokes. The use of the term cerebrovascular accident (CVA) is avoided in this chapter because it does not accurately describe the current understanding of the pathophysiology of cerebral ischemia and infarction. Some authors jokingly accept the term CVA to mean "cursory vascular analysis." The use of appropriate terminology in this chapter underscores the importance of understanding and describing the underlying pathophysiology rather than using poorly descriptive terms.

Pathogenesis of Acute Ischemic Stroke

ARTERIAL OCCLUSION

Arterial occlusion accounts for more than 80% to 85% of acute strokes.[4,7] Clot formation, in addition to progressive vessel narrowing or alterations in the lining of blood vessels, limits cerebral blood flow, leading to ischemia and infarction of brain tissue. Since the brain does not store energy, a continuous nutrient supply from the blood is mandatory to meet metabolic demands. Any limitation of blood flow results in ischemia and brain injury by restricting the flow of oxygen and glucose to regions of the brain. The amount of residual blood flow depends on the vessel involved and the availability of collateral blood flow[6] (Figure 26-1).

The greatest risk factor for stroke is atherosclerotic disease.[8,9] The process of atherosclerosis in the larger arteries of the brain is the process that occurs in the coronary arteries (see Chapter 12). Fibrolipid plaques lead to progressive luminal narrowing and platelet adhesion, leading to thrombosis, or complete occlusion of blood vessels in the brain. Other conditions such as sickle cell disease, vasculitis, and hypercoagulable states can initiate the process of atherosclerosis.

Hypertension is one of the most potent risk factors for stroke.[8,9] Hypertension accelerates atherogenesis and causes hypertrophy and thickening of the media of small intracerebral arteries.[8,9] Hypertension is also a major cause of intracerebral hemorrhage and is a risk factor for the rupture of berry aneurysms and subarachnoid hemorrhage.[8] Some investigators suggest that approximately 50% of all strokes can be eliminated by effective control of hypertension.[9]

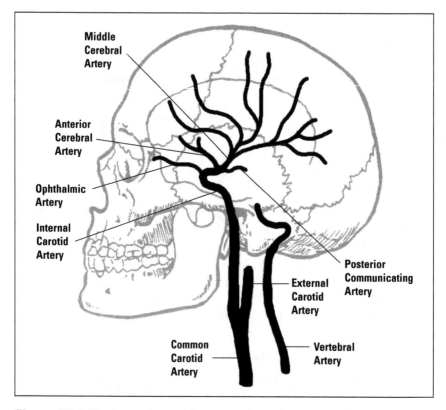

Figure 26-1 The internal carotid system: the major source of blood supply to the brain.

Emboli

Emboli arise either from the blood vessels or heart and lead to transient or permanent cerebral arterial occlusion.[9] Heart defects such as a patent foramen ovale or ventricular septal defect can cause a paradoxical embolism. Paradoxical emboli pass from the right atrium into the left atrium, bypassing the lungs, causing distal embolization in the cerebral circulation. Cardiac sources include thrombi, tumors, or vegetations on the valves. Patients with atrial fibrillation are especially prone to intracardiac thrombi that can embolize when a normal sinus rhythm is rapidly restored; it is for this reason that it is never recommended to cardiovert a patient with atrial fibrillation, whether electrically or pharmacologically, if the condition has existed for over 48 hours.[4]

THE ISCHEMIC PENUMBRA

In the area of ischemia, the central core is surrounded by an area of marginal blood flow. This area is referred to as the ischemic penumbra, border-zone, or watershed area.[6,9] The cerebral blood flow in the penumbra is usually 25% to 50% of normal, and is sufficient to temporarily support metabolic processes and tissue viability for a period of 6 to 8 hours.[6] Over a short period of time, this area becomes dependent on perfusion as autoregulation is lost, and any precipitous drop in blood pressure can extend the area of ischemia with eventual infarction.[6] Without a normal blood supply in the affected area, irreversible brain cell injury (infarction) occurs, expanding the distribution of the original ischemic core (Figure 26-2).

Cerebral infarction is not an all-or-nothing process as once thought. Rather, the evolution of cerebral infarction undergoes a dynamic course when slight reductions in blood supply can cause temporary loss of function without injury, and may be reversible if blood flow is promptly restored. Successful treatment with thrombolytics and neuroprotective agents appears to be dependent on the presence of an ischemic penumbra in patients with potential cerebral infarction.[9]

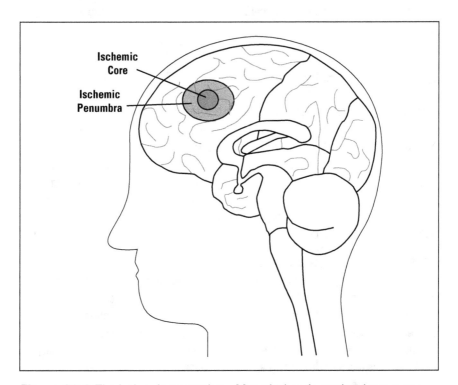

Ischemic
Core

Ischemic
Penumbra

Figure 26-2 The ischemic penumbra. Many ischemic strokes have a central core of severe reduction of blood flow with permanent infarction surrounded by a rim of brain tissue with moderate reduction of blood flow in which the dysfunction is potentially reversible. The surrounding area is referred to as the ischemic penumbra or watershed area.

CYTOTOXIC EDEMA

Brain edema plays a major role in the pathophysiology of cerebral ischemia and infarction.[10] Cortical water content increases significantly when the cerebral blood flow is reduced below the critical level of 10 to 15 ml/100 g/min.[10] This uptake of water is accompanied by additional complications relating to sodium and potassium redistribution. Brain edema causes progressive microcirculatory compression and further aggravates the ischemic insult. After approximately one hour of ischemia caused by the osmotic and ionic gradients resulting in the accumulation of water, reperfusion of the affected area does not lead to resolution and may exacerbate the spread of the edema.[11]

HEMORRHAGIC STROKE

Whereas 80% to 85% of ischemic strokes are caused by arterial occlusion, the remaining 15% to 20% of strokes are caused by hemorrhage.[4,5,7] Intracerebral hemorrhages involve rupture of blood vessels and bleeding directly into brain tissue. Risk factors include chronically high blood pressure, Asian or African-American race, tobacco and alcohol use, thrombolytic or anticoagulant use, vascular malformations, cocaine use, and amyloidosis.[12] Subarachnoid hemorrhage is discussed separately at the end of this chapter.

Clinical Manifestations

NEUROANATOMIC CONSIDERATIONS

The vessels most commonly affected during acute cerebral ischemia are derived from branches of the internal carotid artery. The ophthalmic artery is the first branch off the internal carotid artery, and when occluded, can cause sudden painless blindness (amaurosis fugax). This syndrome is described by patients as a shade coming down over the eye, and may be an early sign of impending infarction. Table 26-1 lists the anatomical distribution and clinical consequences of occlusion for the three main branches of the internal carotid artery.

PREHOSPITAL STROKE SCALES

An in-depth neurological examination is difficult, if not impossible, to perform in the prehospital environment. Moreover, patients with acute ischemic stroke should be transported immediately if consideration for effective treatment is an option. Assessment devices have been designed to assist EMTs and paramedics to correctly identify stroke and transient ischemic attack in the majority of patients.[4] The Cincinnati Prehospital Stroke Scale is a simple device for early identification of stroke (Table 26-2).

If any one of three signs is abnormal, the probability of a stroke, whether ischemic or hemorrhagic, is 72%.[13] The Los Angeles Prehospital Stroke Screen (LAPSS) is a more in-depth and potentially more sensitive and specific screening device (Table 26-3).[14,15]

Table 26-1

The Three Main Branches of the Internal Carotid Artery: Anatomical Distribution and Clinical Correlations

Artery	Distribution	Supplies	Clinical
Middle cerebral	Internal capsule	Primary motor	Contralateral paralysis (face and arm)
	Frontal lobes	Premotor cortex	Contralateral hemianopsia (bilateral visual fields)
	Parietal lobes	Language (Left)	Global aphasia
	Temporal lobes	Inferior frontal gyrus (Broca's area)	
		Geniculocalcarine tract	
Anterior cerebral	Head of caudate	Head of caudate	Contralateral paralysis with sensory loss (leg and perineum)
	Putamen	Putamen	Urinary incontinence
	Internal capsule	Medial frontal and parietal lobes	Contralateral face, tongue, upper limb weakness
	Medial frontal and parietal lobes	Corpus callosum	Ipsilateral anosmia
		Olfactory tracts and bulbs	Confusion, dysphagia
Posterior cerebral	Temporal and occipital lobes	Splenium	Contralateral blindness
	Splenium	Primary visual cortex	Memory impairment
	Hippocampus	Hippocampus	Alexia and homonymous hemianopsia
		Choroid plexus	
		Thalamus	
		Fornix, Tectum (midbrain)	

If all five criteria are checked yes or unknown, and if any of the three exam categories under the sixth criteria are checked, 93% of patients will have a stroke (93% sensitivity; 97% specificity).[14,15] Prehospital screening devices for stroke can only be used for the evaluation of acute, nontraumatic, noncomatose patients.[4,13-15] It is important to remember that those patients not meeting specific criteria with these screening devices may still have a stroke.[4]

Table 26-2

The Cincinnati Prehospital Stroke Scale

I. Facial Droop (have patient smile)
Normal   Both sides of face move equally
Abnormal   One side of face does not move as well as the other side

II. Arm Drift (patient closes eyes and hold both arms out straight for 10 seconds)
Normal   Both arms move the same or both arms do not move at all
Abnormal   One arm does not move or one arm drifts down

III. Abnormal Speech (have patient say "you can't teach an old dog new tricks")
Normal   Patient uses correct words with no slurring
Abnormal   Patient slurs words, uses the wrong words, or is unable to speak

Table 26-3

The Los Angeles Prehospital Stroke Screen (LAPSS) [14,15]			
	Yes	No	Unknown
1. Age >45 years	O	O	O
2. No history of seizures or epilepsy	O	O	O
3. Symptoms duration <24 hours	O	O	O
4. Patient not wheelchair bound or bedridden at baseline	O	O	O

5. Obvious asymmetry in any of three exam categories below:

	Equal	Right weak	Left weak
Facial smile/grimace	O	O	O
Grip	O	O	O
Arm strength	O	O	O

NATIONAL INSTITUTES OF HEALTH (NIH) STROKE SCALE

The NIH stroke scale (NIHSS) is a 15-item neurologic evaluation used by physicians to provide an estimate of infarct volume and evaluation of a given patient over time.[16] This focused neurologic exam is divided into six major categories: level of consciousness, visual assessment, motor function, sensation and neglect, cerebellar function, and cranial nerves. If the total NIHSS is over 22, a severe stroke is likely, and patients are excluded from thrombolytic therapy.[16,17]

NONSPECIFIC SYMPTOMS

Cerebral ischemic events are generally marked by the sudden onset of specific neurologic findings such as weakness, loss of sensation, or inability to speak. Headache in stroke is not a universal finding; only 30% of all patients with acute ischemic stroke present with this complaint.[6] Seizures are reported to occur in up to 5% of all patients with acute ischemic stroke.[6]

TRANSIENT ISCHEMIC ATTACK

A transient ischemic attack (TIA) is a brief episode of cerebral ischemia followed by rapid spontaneous resolution and prompt clinical improvement. This entity can mimic acute cerebral ischemia and infarction because the pathophysiology of TIAs is thought to be the same. Carotid atherosclerotic plaques are an important risk factor for TIAs and should be suspected if a bruit is auscultated over the common carotid artery in the neck. TIAs are regarded as incomplete ischemic events, analogous to angina in the spectrum of acute coronary syndromes, and are a diagnosis of exclusion from the prehospital perspective. Up to 80% of patients with a TIA usually have complete resolution of symptoms within one hour; 50% of patients improve within 30 minutes, and 25% improve within 5 minutes.[6,17] TIAs are associated with a 30% increased risk for stroke over 5 years.[6]

Definitive Diagnosis and Management

INITIAL MANAGEMENT

Prehospital care for stroke patients involves securing the airway, providing oxygen supplementation only if needed (*i.e.*, using pulse oximetry), and maintaining an intravenous line. Isotonic fluids should be given at a rate to keep the vein open (20-30 cc/hr) and dextrose-containing solutions such as D5W should be avoided. Dextrose solutions promote increased production of lactic acid and may induce the formation of toxic oxygen metabolites.[18] Since hyperglycemia has been shown in animal models of cerebrovascular occlusion to increase the infarct size, not only should dextrose-containing solutions be avoided, but insulin should be administered if the serum glucose is over 300 mg/dL.[4,19] If the patient is malnourished or a chronic alcoholic, thiamine may be administered. Thiamine plays an important role in decarboxylation of pyruvate and other substrates for normal energy metabolism in cells and a deficiency can result in decreased ATP production and Wernicke-Korsakoff syndrome. Febrile patients should be treated with acetaminophen (Tylenol™), not aspirin, until further studies are performed because aspirin cannot be administered with thrombolytics.[4] If the patient is at risk for aspiration, nothing should be given by mouth.

Heparin has been associated with worse outcomes in acute ischemic stroke and is no longer recommended.[6] Aspirin should be withheld until the decision to use thrombolytics is made; aspirin is contraindicated when t-PA is administered for acute ischemic stroke.[4,6,17]

BRAIN IMAGING

Early thrombolysis for acute ischemic stroke is an effective therapy only when clinical information and neuroradiologic findings are considered together in a timely fashion. Imaging in patients presenting with the symptoms of acute ischemic stroke has two objectives: assessment of the immediate pathophysiologic state of the cerebral circulation and tissue and assessment of the underlying disease.[20] Although magnetic resonance (MR) imaging appears to offer greater sensitivity and specificity, all major clinical trials continue to use computed tomography (CT) as the means to guide treatment.[6,17,21-26] Advantages of CT include lower financial cost, shorter examination time, and superior access of clinicians to the patient during the examination. The success of thrombolysis within a given window of opportunity for treatment is closely linked with the initial CT findings.

THROMBOLYSIS FOR ACUTE ISCHEMIC STROKE

Several recent studies have shown improved outcome in stroke patients given thrombolytic therapy.[6,17,21-24,26] Despite these findings, the American College of Emergency Physicians agreed to the 1996 American Academy of Neurology recommendations with reservations, and many emergency physicians continue to question the safety of thrombolytic use in stroke patients.[27] Despite the skepticism, the American Heart Association, the American Academy of Neurology, and the American College of Chest Physicians all strongly endorse the use of tissue plasminogen activator (t-PA) for the treatment of acute ischemic stroke in properly selected patients.[6,25]

The Evidence For and Against t-PA Use

The safety profile of t-PA has been assessed in numerous studies. Both the National Institute of Neurological Diseases and Stroke (NINDS) recombinant tissue plasminogen activator (rt-PA) trial and a follow-up study at the University of Texas showed 35% to 39% of all stroke patients treated with rt-PA to have a near-complete or complete recovery as measured by the modified Rankin scale and other neurologic measures.[22,26] Symptomatic intracerebral hemorrhage, the most feared complication of t-PA therapy, was determined to occur in 6.4% of all patients in part 2 of the NINDS trial with a fatality rate of 3% for patients without CT evidence of an initial intracranial hemorrhage.[22,26] The Standard Treatment with Alteplase to Reverse Stroke (STARS) study was the largest prospective cohort performed to date in 2000.[25] For 296 patients treated with t-PA within 3 hours of stroke onset, very favorable outcomes were observed in 35% of all patients followed for a 30-day period.[25] Although the methods for assessment of ICH differed from the NINDS study, the rate of symptomatic intracerebral hemorrhage was found to be lower at 3.3%.[25] The investigators involved in the above studies concluded that t-PA can be an effective therapy when administered according to strict protocols by properly trained physicians.

Despite the clear benefits that have been shown in several major clinical studies, some investigators argue that little is known regarding the outcomes for patients treated with t-PA outside of a trial setting. In a 29-center study in Cleveland, Ohio, 70 acute stroke patients admitted and treated with t-PA were followed.[24] The total rate of intracerebral hemorrhage was 22% for patients receiving t-PA; of those patients, 15.7% were symptomatic, and 6 expired from fatal intracerebral hemorrhage.[24] Another study found an 11% rate of symptomatic intracerebral hemorrhage within 10 days of treatment for patients treated within 0 to 6 hours of presentation.[28]

Notable downfalls in the aforementioned studies include numerous protocol violations, including the most common violation, treatment outside of the 3-hour window established by the NINDS investigators. Authors in nearly every study involving t-PA for acute ischemic stroke acknowledge that protocol deviations are very common worldwide. Nevertheless, when used in carefully selected patients within the 3-hour window, the risk of symptomatic intracerebral hemorrhage appears to be outweighed by the potential advantage of a full or near-full recovery.

The risk of thrombolytic therapy is similar to that of other treatments for stroke. The complication rate for carotid endarterectomy is approximately 5% to 6%; the risk of hemorrhagic complications from Coumadin therapy is 1.5% per year.[6] Table 26-4 summarizes the results of several pivotal clinical studies involving t-PA for the treatment of acute ischemic stroke.

Conclusions

The NIH consensus guidelines and the American Heart Association recommend a door-to-needle time of 60 minutes or less for use of thrombolytics with acute stroke patients.[4,16] Today, the majority of acute ischemic stroke patients remain ineligible for thrombolytic therapy because of delays in obtaining treatment. When strategies devised to reduce the time to treatment are widely implemented, more patients will become eligible for therapy that can potentially lead to complete reversal of symptoms. Comprehensive strategies addressing issues of access, transport, education, and diagnosis, combined with a strong institutional commitment, will conceivably lead to the potential benefit of patients afflicted by this debilitating, and now treatable, disease.

Table 26-4
The Results of Several Landmark Studies on the
use of T-PA for Acute Ischemic Stroke

Study	Number of Patients	Percentage of Patients with Symptomatic Intracerebral Hemorrhage	Comments
NINDS	312	6	First major study to define proper use of t-PA for ischemic stroke
STARS	296	3	Largest prospective cohort performed to date (as of this writing)
Cleveland	70	15.7	Numerous protocol violations
Multicenter survey	189	6	Retrospective survey

Subarachnoid Hemorrhage

Subarachnoid hemorrhage is not a clinical stroke syndrome per se, but deserves special mention due to the high mortality when treatment is delayed. In the United States, the annual incidence of subarachnoid hemorrhage is 6 to 25 per 100,000.[30] The incidence increases with age and is more common in African-Americans, alcohol abusers, females, and smokers.[31] An estimated 10% to 15% of all patients die before reaching the hospital and mortality rates reach as high as 40% within the first week.[30] More than one third of survivors have major neurological deficits.[30] Patients with a family history of subarachnoid hemorrhage in a first or second degree relative are roughly four times more likely to have suffer from the disorder.[30,31]

PATHOGENESIS

The most common cause of nontraumatic subarachnoid hemorrhage is hemorrhage from an intracranial aneurysm.[32] Saccular aneurysms and arteriovenous malformations in the blood vessels of the brain are the two most common pathologic entities causing subarachnoid hemorrhage.[32] Other causes include trauma, blood and coagulation disorders, vascular malformations, tumors, and infection. A ruptured aneurysm below the arachnoid layer of the brain causes leakage of blood into the brain parenchyma with resultant compression of critical areas of the brain. Blood supply becomes disrupted when an artery ruptures and brain tissue becomes ischemic, leading to eventual infarction.

19. de Courten-Meyers G, Meyer RE, Schoolfield L. Hyperglycemia enlarges infarct size in cerebrovascular occlusion in cats. *Stroke* 1988; 19: 623-630,

20. von Kummer R, Weber J. Brain and vascular imaging in acute ischemic stroke: The potential of computed tomography. *Neurology* 1997; 49 (Suppl 4): S52-S55.

21. Hacke W, Kaste M, Fieschi C, *et al.* Intravenous thrombolysis with recombinant tissue plasminogen activator for acute hemispheric stroke: The European cooperative acute stroke study (ECASS). *JAMA* 1995; 274: 1022-1024.

22. The National Institute of Neurological Disorders and Stroke rt-PA Stroke Study Group. Tissue plasminogen activator for acute ischemic stroke. *N Eng J Med* 1995; 333: 1581-1587.

23. Kwiatkoski TG, Libman RB, Frankel M, *et al.* Effects of tissue plasminogen activator for acute ischemic stroke at one year. *N Eng J Med* 1999; 340: 1781.

24. Katzan IL, Furlan AJ, Lloyd LE, *et al.* Use of tissue-type plasminogen activator for acute ischemic stroke: The Cleveland area experience. *JAMA* 2000; 283(9): 1151-1158.

25. Albers GW, Bates VE, Clark WM. Intravenous tissue-type plasminogen activator for treatment of acute stroke: The standard treatment with alteplase to reverse stroke (STARS) study. *JAMA* 2000; 283(9): 1145-1150.

26. Chiu D, Krieger D, Viallar-Cordova C, *et al.* Intravenous tissue plasminogen activator for acute ischemic stroke: Feasibility, safety, and efficacy in the first year of clinical practice. *Stroke* 1998; 29: 18-22.

27. ACEP Newsletter Editorial Staff. ACEP agrees with reservations to new stroke guidelines. *ACEP News* 1996; 3: 3.

28. Wayne C, Albers GW, Madden KP, *et al.* for the Thrombolytic Therapy in Acute Ischemic Stroke Study Investigators. The rt-PA (Alteplase) 0- to 6-hour acute stroke trial, part A (A0276g): Results of a double-blinded placebo-controlled, multicenter study. *Stroke* 2000; 31(4): 811-816.

29. Tanne D, Bates VE, Verro P, *et al.* Initial clinical experience with IV tissue plasminogen activator for acute ischemic stroke: A multicenter survey. *Neurology* 1999; 53: 424-427.

30. Inagawa T. What are the actual incidence and mortality rates of subarachnoid hemorrhage? *Surg Neurol* 1997; 47(1): 46-52.

31. Sawin PD, Loftus CM. Diagnosis of spontaneous subarachnoid hemorrhage. *Am Fam Physician* 1997; 55(1): 145-156.

32. Ojemann RG, Ogilvy CS, Heros RC, *et al.* (eds.). *Surgical Management of Cerebrovascular Disease.* Third edition. Baltimore: Williams & Wilkins, 2002.

33. Weaver JP, Fisher M. Subarachnoid hemorrhage: An update of pathogenesis, diagnosis, and management. *J Neurol Sci* 1994; 125(2): 119-131.

Review Questions

1. A 65-year-old female with an unknown past medical history presents with right sided facial droop, aphasia, and decreased finger grip strength. The diagnosis of stroke is considered. All of the following are risk factors for stroke EXCEPT:

   A. Atherosclerotic disease
   B. Hypercoagulable states
   C. Sickle cell disease
   D. Aspirin use
   E. Hypertension

The answer is D.

2. Reduction of cerebral blood flow due to thrombosis of major blood vessels in the brain leads to all of the following EXCEPT:

   A. Increased cortical edema
   B. Brain injury or infarction
   C. Sodium and potassium redistribution
   D. Progressive ischemia of brain tissue
   E. Atrial fibrillation

Atrial fibrillation is a potential cause, not a result of, cessation of blood flow to brain tissue. The answer is E.

3. The potential use of thrombolytics for the patient in Question 1 is predicated on what pathophysiologic principle?

   A. Presence of an ischemic penumbra in patients with potential infarction
   B. Need to increase sodium and potassium levels in order to keep up with ongoing brain losses of these electrolytes
   C. Need to rapidly correct atrial fibrillation first to prevent embolization of clots
   D. Use of diuretics first to decrease cortical water content
   E. Presence of irreversible brain death

The answer is A.

4. 80% to 85% of all strokes are caused by:
   A. Arterial occlusion
   B. Intracerebral hemorrhage
   C. Rupture of Berry aneurysms
   D. Rupture of vessels branching off the external carotid artery
   E. Hypertensive emergencies

The answer is A.

5. For thrombolytics to work for the patient in Question 1, provided all criteria for safe use are met (*i.e.*, no contraindications), the recommended door-to-needle time is:
   A. Less than 6 hours
   B. Less than 10 minutes
   C. Less than 24 hours
   D. Less than 48 hours
   E. Less than 60 minutes

Studies have shown the best results for carefully selected patients treated with thrombolytics within 60 minutes of onset of symptoms. Brain imaging must be completed before thrombolytics can be given. The answer is E.

6. A 51-year-old female with a history of smoking and hypertension presents with "the worst headache of my life." The headache is described as diffuse with an acute onset. En route, the patient becomes less responsive. The patient's speech is clear and there is no muscular asymmetry. Which of the following is the most likely diagnosis?
   A. Acute ischemic stroke
   B. Subarachnoid hemorrhage
   C. Hypertensive urgency
   D. Epilepsy
   E. Pseudoseizures

Stroke does not usually present with severe headache. A patient with stroke would be expected to have focal neurologic findings (*e.g.*, facial droop, slurred speech, decreased motor ability). The answer is B.

7. The most common event leading to the condition in Question 6 is:
   A. Arterial occlusion by emboli
   B. Infection of the meninges by bacteria
   C. Rupture of saccular aneurysms or arteriovenous malformations
   D. Abnormalities in dopamine or serotonin levels in brain
   E. Prolonged hypotension

The answer is C.

8. Initial care for the patient in question 6 should include which of the following?
   A. ABCs and prompt transport to a hospital with neurosurgical capabilities
   B. Intravenous thrombolytics
   C. Beta-blockers and calcium channel blockers for hypertension
   D. Sedation with haloperidol to prevent reemergence phenomena
   E. Prophylactic administration of fosphenytoin to prevent seizures

The answer is A.

27

Status Epilepticus

Status epilepticus (SE) is classically defined as a epileptic seizure that is repeated and prolonged so as to create a fixed and lasting condition.[1] The World Health Organization defines status epilepticus as "a condition characterized by an epileptic seizure that is sufficiently prolonged or repeated at sufficiently brief intervals so as to produce an unvarying and enduring epileptic condition."[2] This disorder has been recognized since the 7th century BC, and still occurs in nearly 195,000 cases per year in the United States.[3,4] An understanding of the pathophysiology of this disorder accentuates the importance of proper early management.

Epilepsy and seizures are the most common neurologic disorders affecting all ages.[1] **Epilepsy** is defined as a condition in which an individual is predisposed to recurrent seizures because of a central nervous system disorder.[1] This chapter is limited to a discussion of the pathophysiology, clinical manifestations, and early management of status epilepticus.

Pathogenesis

THE RULE OF THIRDS
The imperfect rule of thirds describes the three categories of causative factors for SE.[5] The rule is imperfect because significant overlap exists between groups. One-third of all episodes of SE occur in patients with a known underlying seizure disorder and roughly another third occur as the initial manifestation of an underlying seizure disorder.[5] **For patients with known seizure disorders, SE is most often the result of poor compliance with previously prescribed anticonvulsant medications.** The remaining third of patients with SE have underlying medical, toxicologic, or structural abnormalities causing seizures. Hypoxia, stroke, tumors, infections, drugs, and metabolic abnormalities cause SE in these patients.

PRECIPITANTS
The causes of SE can be classified as either a predisposition or precipitant. A predisposition is an unchanging condition that increases the likelihood of SE in patients exposed to a precipitant. Precipitants are events such as infection, tumor, or intoxication, that can produce SE in most normal individuals, but more commonly affect those with a history of seizures.[6]

Factors precipitating SE vary according to age. In children, most episodes of SE are caused by underlying epilepsy.[6] The second most common cause in children is an atypical febrile convulsion. Meningitis, encephalitis, and other causes include intoxication, metabolic abnormalities (*e.g.*, electrolyte disturbances), tumor, anoxia, or complications relating to drugs or intoxications.[6]

In adults, most patients with SE have a known or previously undiagnosed seizure disorder. Other common causes of SE in adults in descending order are: stroke, withdrawal from antiepileptic drug therapy, alcohol withdrawal, anoxia, and metabolic disorders.[6]

Some authors identify adults with SE as part of two broad groups (Table 27-1).[1,17] Group I patients with SE have no new structural central nervous system lesion. These patients usually have a preexisting seizure disorder or have SE caused by drug intoxications. The prognosis for Group I patients is excellent if treatment is initiated promptly.[17] Group II patients have structural lesions such as tumor, infection, or hemorrhage. Prognosis in these patients is generally poor.

Drug intoxications and exposure to toxic substances can cause seizures leading to SE. The most commonly reported drugs responsible for causing SE are listed in Table 27-2.

Table 27-1
Static And Acute Pathological Precipitants Of Status Epilepticus

Group I (static)

- Exacerbation of seizures in patient with epilepsy
- Withdrawal from drugs
- Alcohol or drug abuse
- Undetermined causes

Group II (acute)

- Anoxic encephalopathy
- Stroke
- Brain tumor
- Head trauma
- Metabolic encephalopathy
- Meningitis, encephalitis

Table 27-2
Drugs and Toxins Commonly Associated with Seizures

Cocaine
Alcohol
Lidocaine
Tricyclic antidepressants
bupropion
Theophylline
Isoniazid
Imipenem
Phencyclidine

PHYSIOLOGIC EFFECTS OF SE

In general, SE is a condition of neuronal hyperexcitation caused by nearly simultaneous activation of the entire cerebral cortex. As such, markers of physiologic parameters tend to be increased. Although body temperature can vary during SE, hyperpyrexia is most common. Hypertension, tachycardia, cardiac dysrhythmias, and hyperglycemia are the initial systemic effects caused by the increased amount of circulating catecholamines that coincides with SE.[5] Prolonged SE can lead to hypotension, hypoglycemia, permanent brain damage, and cardiac arrest.

Ion Channels

Ion channel disturbances play a central role in the pathogenesis of SE. Excitatory amino acids circulate during a seizure and open NMDA, AMPA, and metabotropic ion channels, raising intracellular calcium to toxic levels within the neurons of the brain.[6] These effects increase the osmolarity of neurons, leading to cellular edema. If seizures are allowed to continue, neuronal swelling leads to neuronal death and permanent biochemical alterations in the brain. Excitotoxic mechanisms involving glutamate and aspartate have also been postulated; the end result of both is increased calcium entry into the neuron.[5]

Cellular Damage

During SE, the neurons in the brain are overwhelmed by intense cellular activity. Oxygen and glucose are rapidly depleted and blood flow initially increases. After approximately 20 minutes, energy reserves are depleted and local catabolism in the brain is called on to provide energy for the ion pumps.[6] The intrinsic systems in the brain that terminate seizures include the GABAergic interneurons and inhibitory thalamic neurons; these systems are overwhelmed in SE. The hippocampus is a crucial area in the brain for memory, and contains the neurons most susceptible during SE.[6]

Systemic Effects

Seizures cause increased blood pressure and elevations of epinephrine and cortisol levels. Excessive muscular activation leads to further depletion of energy stores and increased lactate production. A combined respiratory and metabolic acidosis results and is often associated with hyperkalemia. Hyperkalemia propagates seizure activity and can have deleterious effects on cardiac electrophysiology.[6] Hypoxemia and increased catecholamine release can lead to cardiac arrest.

After one hour of seizures, glucagon stores are diminished and gluconeogenesis cannot keep pace with ongoing glucose requirements. The end result is life-threatening hypoglycemia. Breakdown of muscle can lead to rhabdomyolysis and kidney failure. Because of the tonic axial muscle contraction, respiration is impaired, and anoxia may result. Patients with SE often aspirate gastric or oral contents during a seizure, producing pneumonia.[6]

Clinical Manifestations

CLASSIFICATION OF SEIZURES

Although far beyond the scope of this chapter, seizures can be classified according to clinical manifestations. The International League Against Epilepsy recommends classifying seizures as either generalized or partial (Table 27-3).[8]

The gold standard for diagnosing seizures is the electroencephalogram (EEG), preferably coupled with a real-time video of the seizure.

Table 27-3
Classification of Seizures

Generalized seizures (consciousness impaired)

- Tonic-clonic (previously known as grand mal)
- Absence (previously known as petit mal)
- Myoclonic
- Tonic
- Clonic
- Atonic (nonconvulsive seizures)

Partial (focal) seizures

- Simple partial (consciousness intact)
- Complex partial (consciousness impaired)
- Partial (simple or complex) with secondary generalization

DEFINITION OF STATUS EPILEPTICUS

The classic definition of SE for both adults and children is seizure activity continuously for 30 minutes or more or a series of seizures followed by a failure to regain full consciousness between ictal episodes.[1,2,5,9] This definition is vague and imprecise, and reflects a lack of understanding the pathophysiology of SE in most instances. As of this writing a consensus still has not been reached, although **most neurologists agree than any seizure lasting 5 minutes or more should be treated aggressively rather than waiting for a seizure to last 30 minutes to meet the classical definition of SE.**[1,5,6]

TONIC-CLONIC SEIZURES

In SE, seizures are ordinarily of the generalized type, and are tonic-clonic in nature. Tonic extension of the trunk and extremities, coupled with loss of consciousness, typically precedes vibration and rhythmic (clonic) extension of the extremities. The cycle of tonicity followed by clonic movements may be repeated several times in SE or the patient may lapse into unconsciousness. These types of seizures were previously described as **grand mal** seizures; this terminology is no longer preferred.

OTHER TYPES OF SEIZURES

Myoclonic seizures are characterized by a series of extremity jerks, increasing in intensity, and eventually leading to generalized tonic-clonic seizure activity. These types of seizures are common in patients with anoxic encephalopathy or metabolic disturbances.[6] Since inborn errors of metabolism can cause these types of seizures, infants with such conditions are also predisposed to developing myoclonic SE.

Nonconvulsive SE

Nonconvulsive SE is a condition that has recently been recognized as a cause of unresponsiveness in up to 8% of hospitalized patients with coma.[8] There is controversy surrounding this term because nonconvulsive SE was initially recognized as EEG evidence of seizures in a patient without the characteristic motor activity. Since infants and children may have SE with minimal motor activity, the term should be reserved for patients with absence SE and partial complex SE.[5] Patients who demonstrate epileptiform activity on the EEG without tonic-clonic activity are more appropriately described as having **subtle status epilepticus.** It is important for the emergency physician or intensivist to recognize this condition because investigators have shown that if abnormal cerebral electrical activity is not suppressed, neuronal damage may occur, even if a patient is not actively seizing.[1]

Management

INITIAL PREHOSPITAL CARE

As with all emergencies, attention should be directed to maintaining the ABCs. SE is a challenging disorder for clinicians because patient access is limited due to the tonic-clonic seizure activity. **Providers should resist the temptation to protect the airway by inserting padded tongue blades or similar devices since these items are more likely to obstruct the airway than maintain it.** Oxygen can be administered either by nonrebreather face mask or blow-by methods. While actively seizing, efforts to protect the patient from further harm should be implemented. **At no time should an actively seizing patient be restrained, especially patients with SE, since these patients are predisposed to severe muscle breakdown** (rhabdomyolysis). Cardiac monitoring, rapid glucose testing, and large-bore intravenous access should be achieved before arrival in the ED. Glucose-containing solutions should be avoided because the drug of choice for SE, phenytoin, is incompatible with glucose.[1,5]

SEQUENCE OF PHARMACOTHERAPY

Benzodiazepines

The initial class of medications used to treat SE are the benzodiazepines. The initial drug of choice is lorazepam (Ativan®). Lorazepam binds to the benzodiazepine receptor sites and increases GABAergic inhibitory neuronal activity. At a dosage of 0.1 mg/kg for both adults and children, lorazepam is the preferred benzodiazepine because of its longer duration of action (4-14 hours) and higher initial response rate.[1,5,6]

If lorazepam is not available, diazepam (Valium®) can be used. Diazepam has weaker binding to the benzodiazepine binding sites and is more lipid soluble, and more likely to redistribute in the bulk of fatty tissues outside the brain after initial administration.[1] The half-life of diazepam is approximately 20 minutes in SE and requires frequent dosing. Rectal diazepam is a viable treatment option when intravenous access is not available, especially in children.[6]

Midazolam (Versed®) is emerging as a drug-of-choice in many systems because of its rapid onset of action and usefulness in refractory SE.[1,6] Many European physicians recommend midazolam as the first agent of choice in SE. Midazolam is a water soluble benzodiazepine with a rapid onset (1-2 minutes) and short half life (20-30 minutes). An infusion is usually required after the initial bolus. Intranasal preparations are available for use in children.

All benzodiazepines have the potential to depress consciousness and respiration. Since gauging the return to consciousness after treatment is a primary goal for physicians evaluating patients with SE, benzodiazepines have a limited role.

The role of early treatment for SE cannot be overemphasized. A study by Alldredge *et al.* **showed significant improvement in children treated with diazepam outside the hospital versus children treated after arrival in the emergency department.**[10]

Phenytoin and Fosphenytoin
After administration of benzodiazepines, phenytoin (Dilantin®) should be administered. For SE, rapid intravenous dosing of phenytoin is not without potential serious complications. Hypotension and severe cardiac disturbances (phenytoin is a class IB antidysrhythmic) may occur due to the 40% propylene glycol (antifreeze), high pH, and sodium hydroxide (drain cleaner) contained in parenteral preparations.[1]

An alternative to phenytoin for rapid anticonvulsant dosing is fosphenytoin (Cerebyx®). Fosphenytoin can be administered rapidly in a wide variety of intravenous solutions and is not associated with the side effects of parenteral phenytoin. Fosphenytoin is the prodrug of phenytoin and can be administered intramuscularly. The main disadvantages to fosphenytoin dosing is higher cost; fosphenytoin is over twenty times more expensive than phenytoin.

Loading of phenytoin and fosphenytoin must be done in the emergency department or intensive care unit with close hemodynamic monitoring.

SECOND- AND THIRD-LINE ANTIEPILEPTIC MEDICATIONS
When seizures cannot be controlled with benzodiazepines and phenytoin, barbiturates are used. Pentobarbital is the choice of many intensivists although phenobarbital is the traditional barbiturate of choice. Propofol (Diprivan®), a powerful short-lived intravenous barbiturate, is becoming another drug of choice for refractory SE. This agent has been shown to control seizures faster than other barbiturate compounds.[1]

SPECIAL PATIENT POPULATIONS

Alcoholics and Malnourished Patients

The alcohol withdrawal syndrome typically begins 24 hours after cessation of alcohol use and can be followed by the symptom complex known as **delirium tremens.** Autonomic hyperactivity is manifested by visual hallucinations, anxiety, tachycardia, hypertension, and tremors of the extremities. Seizures may accompany this syndrome and can occur as early as 6 hours after cessation or up to one week later. Generalized seizures can accompany the signs and symptoms of autonomic hyperactivity and are usually self-limiting but may progress to SE if not treated promptly. Benzodiazepines are the drugs of choice for both prevention and treatment. The EEG is normal in these patients and phenytoin is not indicated.

Eclampsia

A pregnant woman with hypertension, edema, and the development of seizures after 20 weeks gestation has eclampsia. The management of SE in patients with eclampsia is complicated by the potentially serious side effects of antiepileptic drugs on the developing fetus. Although not an anticonvulsant per se, magnesium sulfate has been shown to have superior results over diazepam and phenytoin for pregnant patients with this disorder.[11] The ultimate treatment for eclampsia is delivery of the fetus.

DEFINITIVE CARE FOR PATIENTS WITH SE

All patients with SE should be monitored in an intensive care setting. An EEG is obtained as soon as possible and the exact etiology investigated with a battery of laboratory and radiological tests.

References

1. Leppik IE. *Contemporary Diagnosis and Management of the Patient with Epilepsy.* 5th Edition. Newtown, PA: Handbooks in Healthcare, 2000. 164-176.

2. Gastaut H. *Dictionary of epilepsy.* Part I: Definitions. Geneva: World Health Organization, 1973.

3. Shorvon S. *Status Epilepticus.* Cambridge, MA: Cambridge University Press, 1994.

4. DeLorenzo RJ, Hauser WA, Towne AR, *et al.* A prospective population-based epidemiological study of status epilepticus in Richmond, Virginia. *Neurology* 1996; 46: 1029-1035.

5. Huff SJ, Winograd SM. Status epilepticus: A systematic approach to assessment, differential diagnosis, and outcome-effective management. *Emergency Medicine Reports* 1997; 18(14): 138-147.

6. Weise KL, Bleck TP. Status epilepticus in children and adults. *Crit Care Clinics* 1997; 13(3): 629-646.

7. Crawford RE, Leppik IE, Patrick B, *et al.* Intravenous phenytoin in acute treatment of seizures. *Neurology* 1979; 29: 1474-1479.

8. Commission on Classification and Terminology of the International League Against Epilepsy: Proposal for revised clinical and electroencephalographic classification of epileptic seizures. *Epilepsia* 1981; 22: 489.

9. Epilepsy Foundation of America. Treatment of convulsive status epilepticus: Recommendations of America's Working Group on status epilepticus. *JAMA* 1993; 270: 854-859.

10. Alldredge BK, Wall DB, Ferriero DM. Effect of prehospital treatment on the outcome of status epilepticus in children. *Pediatr Neurol* 1995; 12: 213-216.

11. The Eclampsia Trial Collaborative Group. Which anticonvulsant for women with eclampsia? Evidence from the Collaborative Eclampsia Trial. *Lancet* 1995; 345: 1455.

Review Questions

1. You are called to the scene of a patient with a history of epilepsy. The patient is actively seizing and does not have an intervening return to consciousness between seizures. Which of the following is the most common cause of status epilepticus in patients with a known seizure disorder?
   A. Phenytoin toxicity
   B. Fever and upper respiratory tract infection
   C. Poor compliance with antiepileptic medications
   D. Concussion
   E. Stroke

The answer is C.

2. Reasons for early aggressive treatment for status epilepticus include all of the following EXCEPT:
   A. Depletion of energy reserves in the brain with prolonged seizures
   B. Inability of GABAergic neurons to inhibit excess electrical activity in the brain
   C. Depletion of glucagon stores with life-threatening hypoglycemia
   D. Research shows little impact on mortality and morbidity for status epilepticus patients treated aggressively in the field by prehospital providers
   E. Increased NMDA and AMPA ion channel activity leading to increased calcium release

Research has shown better outcomes for patients treated aggressively in the field with antiepileptic medications. The answer is D.

3. Seizures lasting greater than _____ should be treated immediately.
   A. 30 minutes or more
   B. 60 minutes or more
   C. 5 minutes or more
   D. 20 minutes or more
   E. 15 minutes or more

The answer is C.

4. Airway management of hypoxic patients with status epilepticus should include all of the following EXCEPT:
   A. Aggressive use of tongue blades and airway adjuncts during active seizing to protect the tongue
   B. Supplemental oxygen by face mask or blow-by methods
   C. Intubation for postictal patients unable to sustain respirations
   D. Suctioning as needed to remove excess secretions
   E. Jaw-thrust, chin-lift maneuver after seizures to open the airway

Tongue blades are more likely to obstruct the airway than to protect it during active seizures. The answer is A.

5. The initial class of drugs used for the treatment of status epilepticus is:
   A. Barbiturates
   B. Benzodiazepines
   C. Phenytoin
   D. Fosphenytoin
   E. Thiamine

The answer is B.

6. The primary mechanism of action for the answer to Question 5 is:
   A. Binding to GABAergic inhibitory receptors in the brain
   B. Inhibition of sodium-potassium channels in the brain
   C. Blockage of NMDA channels in the brain
   D. Inhibition of glutamate formation
   E. Replacement of essential coenzymes for proper brain function

The answer is A.

Neurological Trauma

This chapter focuses on the pathophysiology of the two most common serious neurologic traumatic diseases: head trauma and spinal cord injury.

Traumatic Brain Injury

EPIDEMIOLOGY

Traumatic brain injury (TBI) is responsible for half of the 150,000 injury-related deaths each year in the United States and is the **number one cause of death in all Americans under the age of 45.**[1] In the past, the majority of survivors were severely disabled, but in recent years, the mortality rate for patients who survive to the hospital has been reduced from 50% to 25% with a higher proportion of patients returning to a functional existence.[2] Thanks to improved out-of-hospital emergency care and an improved understanding of pathophysiology and pharmacology, TBI is now associated with an improved outcome in many cases.

NORMAL BRAIN PHYSIOLOGY

Autoregulation of Cerebral Blood Flow

Although the brain receives approximately 20% of the cardiac output, only 30% to 40% of the delivered oxygen is used.[3,4] Blood flow to the brain is dependent on autoregulation, complex metabolic factors, and responsiveness to carbon dioxide and oxygen. The perfusion of cerebral tissue is measured as the cerebral perfusion pressure (CPP) and is calculated by subtracting the intracranial pressure (ICP) from the mean arterial pressure.

Cerebral perfusion pressure is a rough indicator of cerebral blood flow. Normal CPP ranges from 50 to 150 mm Hg; ranges above or below these values are associated with loss of autoregulation.[5] The CPP becomes dependent on the mean arterial pressure for maintenance of cerebral blood flow when autoregulation is lost. Dependence on mean arterial pressure at critically low or high cerebral perfusion pressures is described as **pressure passive** cerebral blood flow. This phenomenon can lead to cerebral ischemia and death of brain tissue with progressive edema.[5]

Intracranial Pressure

Intracranial pressure (ICP) is a measurement of pressure within the intracranial compartment. The total volume of the cranial contents is constant; therefore, increases in edema, blood volume, or other mass effects can increase the ICP to the point of decompensation (CPP over 150 mm Hg) since the ICP is one of two critical factors in determining the CPP. This concept is the basis for the Monroe-Kellie Doctrine and is discussed below. Any abnormal increase can severely limit blood flow and can result in brain herniation through the tent of dura mater that supports the occipital lobes and covers the cerebellum (*e.g.*, tentorium cerebelli). The ICP is measured by a device placed directly into the cranium in the intensive care unit setting or neurosurgical operating room.

Responsiveness to Carbon Dioxide

Blood vessel diameter and intracranial pressure are directly regulated by the partial pressure of carbon dioxide in arterial blood ($PaCO_2$). When the $PaCO_2$ decreases, as with hyperventilation, the arterioles in the brain constrict, causing a fall in cerebral blood flow. The opposite effect is observed when the $PaCO_2$ is elevated; the arterioles vasodilate. These changes take place rapidly in the brain due to the high permeability of the blood-brain barrier to carbon dioxide, with changes in $PaCO_2$ affecting the negative decadic logarithm of the H^+ ion concentration (pH) and bicarbonate in the cerebral spinal fluid (CSF). In the brain, pH and bicarbonate are regulated by enzymes (carbonic anhydrase), returning levels to normal within hours. For this reason, **hyperventilation is an ineffective therapy for reducing the intracranial pressure because the pH of the CSF is corrected to prehyperventilation levels within a few hours.**[4] Additionally, if hyperventilation is withdrawn during a period of increased ICP, the arterial pH and partial pressure of carbon dioxide (PCO_2) abruptly return to normal values, leaving the CSF PCO_2 elevated, causing a rebound increase in ICP, exceeding the initial prehyperventilation levels.[4]

Oxygen Metabolism

Since the cerebral blood flow is directly proportional to the $PaCO_2$, when the oxygen level in the brain falls below a partial pressure of 50 mm Hg, cerebral vasodilatation ensues with an increase in cerebral blood flow. Brain tissue will show histologic evidence of neural injury and death within minutes of oxygen deprivation.[6] Free radicals, molecules with an orbiting unstable, highly reactive, unpaired electron, are formed during normal aerobic metabolism, and are produced in higher concentrations during hypoperfusion and cellular ischemia.[6]

PATHOGENESIS

Mechanical Factors

Mechanisms for traumatic brain injury can be categorized according to mechanical, ischemic, and biochemical factors. The Monroe-Kellie Doctrine describes the compensation for expansion of blood, mass, or fluid within the cranial vault. Under normal conditions, the ICP is managed by the process of autoregulation and other physiologic responses to limit the expansion of venous or arterial blood volume. Mass effects (*e.g.*, expanding blood clot) or edema stimulate an elevation of ICP when compensatory mechanisms are exhausted (Figure 28-1).

The end result is an exponential increase in ICP, even when the volume of the mass is marginally increased. Examples of mechanical factors that lead to decompensation and compression of brain tissue include extensive edema, epidural or subdural hematomas, or microscopic neuronal hemorrhage[6] (Figure 28-2).

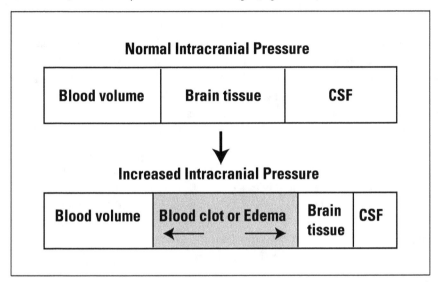

Figure 28-1 The Monroe-Kellie Doctrine: blood clots, masses, or edema compress brain tissue and increase CSF pressure due to the fixed space within the cranial vault.

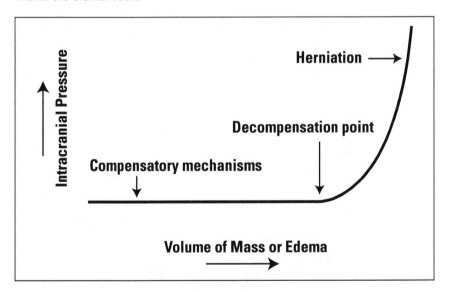

Figure 28-2 The relationship of increasing mass or edema volume to intracranial pressure. Compensatory mechanisms serve to normalize the intracranial pressure up to the point of decompensation. Once this point is reached, intracranial pressure increases exponentially, to the point of brain herniation through the tentorium cerebelli.

Biochemical Factors

Biomolecular cascades run in overdrive after brain injury, producing excessive toxic metabolites and free radicals.[6] Free radicals are highly reactive molecules that have a destructive impact on cells and when produced in high concentrations, may lead to apoptosis (programmed cell death) and DNA mutations. The end result of apoptosis is a shrunken, nonfunctioning cell that eventually dies.[2] Excitotoxins, such as excitatory amino acids, lead to overconsumption of available oxygen, eventually outstripping the limited ability of the brain to sustain a hypermetabolic state in the face of progressive hypoxia and anoxia at the local tissue level. Glutamate has been widely implicated as a toxic excitotoxin in brain injury; this transmitter substance is toxic to cells at high concentrations. Nitric oxide, a normal transmitter substance, is produced in supraphysiologic quantities and leads to destruction of neuronal cell membranes as the result of oxygen free radical reactions.[2]

Brain injury leads to widespread activation of neurons in the brain (depolarization) and promotes excitatory amino acid release with activation of cell receptors. The NMDA receptor is activated in brain injury, allowing the toxic accumulation of intracerebral calcium. Calcium promotes further cell injury by inciting free radical reactions and further release of excitatory amino acids. High intracellular calcium levels cause osmolar shifts leading to edema and necrosis of neurons.

Ischemia

The hypermetabolic state induced by the release of excitatory molecules and other factors lead to a state of increased oxygen demand, often in the face of decreased supply, with ischemia and anoxia as the end result. Since the blood-barrier is frequently compromised as the result of trauma or toxin release, cerebral blood flow is either increased or decreased when the process of autoregulation is disrupted (Figure 28-3).

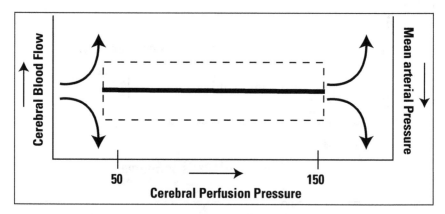

Figure 28-3 The relationship of cerebral blood flow, cerebral perfusion pressure, and mean arterial pressure. When the extremes of cerebral perfusion pressure are breached (under 50- or over 150 mm Hg), autoregulation is lost and cerebral blood flow becomes dependent on mean arterial pressure.

When the cerebral perfusion pressure is below 50 or above 150 mm Hg, autoregulation is lost and cerebral blood flow becomes dependent on the mean arterial pressure.[2,5] If the mean arterial pressure is **low** (hypotension), cerebral blood flow is **decreased**; likewise, if the mean arterial pressure is **elevated** (hypertension), cerebral blood flow may be **abnormally increased**, exacerbating preexisting hemorrhage or edema. The end result in both cases is progressive ischemia and anoxia with eventual cell necrosis or neuronal apoptosis.

Edema

Brain edema is defined as an increase in brain water content with increased brain tissue volume. Two types of edema are described in traumatic brain injury: **interstitial** (vasogenic) and **intracellular** (cytotoxic).[2] Vasogenic edema arises when the blood-brain barrier is disrupted and tissue pressures are increased. Increased tissue pressures impede blood flow in the small vessels of the brain and can cause ischemia.[2] Cytotoxic brain edema is a local form of water accumulation in the brain and results from membrane and ion channel dysfunction. Failure of the sodium-potassium-ATPase pump leads to excessive intracellular sodium concentrations and osmolar shifts. Intracellular calcium increases when the NMDA receptor on neuronal cells is inappropriately activated. Both of these processes cause water to diffuse into cells. Brain edema is maximally demonstrated on a computed tomographic scan of the brain within 24 to 48 hours.[2]

Secondary Injury

Secondary brain injuries are the result of systemic or intracranial pathologic processes. Systemic causes include electrolyte and acid-base disorders, hypotension, hyperthermia, hypoxia, anemia, and hypo- or hypercapnea (decreased or increased PCO_2).[5] Intracranial causes include cerebral edema, intracranial hypertension, infection, and seizures in addition to the complex biochemical and mechanical factors discussed above.[5] Secondary injuries contribute to the pathogenesis of traumatic brain injury by elevating the ICP, decreasing the cerebral blood flow, exacerbating the underlying hemorrhage and complex biochemical cascade.[2] Early treatment of potential causes of secondary brain injuries can lead to vastly improved outcomes (Figure 28-4).

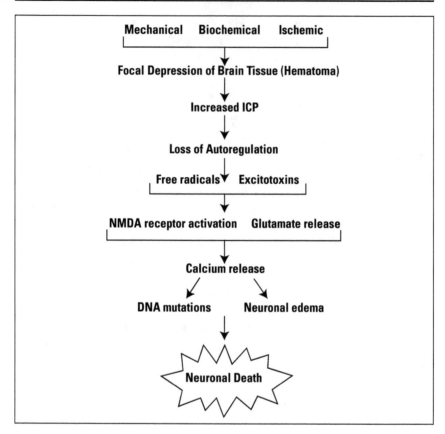

Figure 28-4 Summary of the biochemical cascade in traumatic brain injury.

CLINICAL MANIFESTATIONS

Clinical Classification of Traumatic Brain Injury

Traumatic brain injuries are classified according to the Glasgow Coma Scale (GCS; Table 28-1).

A patient with a severe traumatic brain injury has a GCS score of **less than or equal to 8**, preferably measured after resuscitation, keeping in mind that the GCS is graded according to the best response observed in each of the three categories.[5] A GCS of 8 or less is generally accepted as the definition for coma.[7] A patient with a GCS of 9 to 12 is considered to have a moderate head injury, and a GCS greater than or equal to 13 constitutes a mild head injury.[5]

Unfortunately, there are no easily measured biochemical markers to assess prognosis of traumatic brain injuries; information from magnetic resonance (MR) imaging, computed tomography (CT) scans, and other radiologic studies are not always reliable indicators of the initial underlying pathophysiology.[8] **The GCS remains the most useful clinical too to classify traumatic brain injuries.** Despite the fact that most classification schemes group patients with a GCS of 13 to 15 in the mild category, these patients have been shown in some studies to have a higher degree of neuronal damage with temporary or permanent effects.[9]

Table 28-1
The Glasgow Coma Score for Adults

Variable	Score
Eye	**4** Spontaneous **3** To speech **2** To pain **1** None
Verbal	**5** Oriented **4** Confused **3** Inappropriate words **2** Incomprehensible sounds **1** None
Motor	**6** Obeys commands **5** Localizes pain **4** Normal flexion (withdraws) **3** Abnormal flexion (decorticate) **2** Extension (decerebrate) **1** None (flaccid)
Best Possible Score:	15

Epidural Hematoma

Epidural hematomas exist outside the dura but within the skull, and are most commonly caused by fractures of the cranial bones with associated injury to the anterior branch of the middle meningeal artery. Epidural hematomas are occasionally caused by lacerated venous sinuses in the posterior aspect of the skull or parieto-occipital region. While this injury is relatively uncommon (0.5% of all patients with head injury), patients may present with the characteristic **lucid interval**.[7] This interval is typified by a period of normal level of consciousness followed by rapid progression to coma: the so-called "talk and die" presentation.

Subdural Hematoma

Subdural hematomas are more common than epidural hematomas and may occur in up to 30% of all severe traumatic brain injuries.[7] Subdural hematomas usually are the result of damage to the bridging veins between the cerebral cortex and major venous sinuses but may occasionally be associated with small arterial lacerations. These lesions typically involve far greater brain volume than epidural hematomas and have a worse prognosis overall. Alcoholics and the elderly are especially susceptible to this injury.

Concussion

A concussion is usually the result of acceleration-deceleration forces and ranges from mild to serious in presentation and prognosis. Mild concussions do not result in loss of consciousness although some degree of amnesia may be present. Retrograde (after the injury) and antegrade (before the injury) amnesia suggests a more severe degree of injury. Severe or **classic** concussions are marked by a head injury that results in loss of consciousness. Of all patients with a mild concussion, 30% to 80% report symptoms such as headache, fatigue, memory or learning deficits, and dizziness 3 months after injury; another 15% continue to have symptoms for up to 1 year.[9] While the true rate of complications relating to concussions depends on the area of brain involved and the extent of injury, these clinical post-injury patterns are referred to collectively as the **postconcussive syndrome**.[9]

Diffuse Axonal Injury

Tissue strains applied to the brain cell membranes are usually the result of severe head trauma and are known as diffuse axonal injury. Brain cells are damaged, not killed, and rendered nonfunctional in this disorder. Patients with this diffuse axonal injury have a history of prolonged coma with an initial CT scan that is normal. MR imaging can detect evidence of diffuse axonal injury. Serious neurologic and systemic deficits such as decorticate or decerebrate posturing, hypertension, hyperpyrexia, or other severe disabilities are common.

MANAGEMENT

The following discussion pertains to the initial management of patients with **severe** traumatic brain injury.

Initial Priorities

Airway control, oxygenation, and ventilation are the initial priorities for resuscitation of the patient with a severe head injury. Since patients with a GCS less than 8 are unable to protect the airway, endotracheal intubation, with rapid sequence intubation (RSI) if available, should be accomplished, although there is no GCS score that serves as an absolute threshold for intubation.[6] RSI prevents transient increases in ICP with stimulation of the airway with intubation attempts; pharmacologic agents for use with severe head injuries are discussed separately in the appendix at the end of this book. Studies have shown that endotracheal intubation in the prehospital setting appears to be associated with a decreased incidence of secondary hypoxic brain insults.[5] Indeed, **intubation and ventilation with 100% oxygen is the most crucial step in the early management of severely head injured patients.**[7] When appropriate, full spinal immobilization precautions should be implemented. The percentage of oxygen delivered (FiO₂) may be tapered to keep the peripheral oxygen saturation as measured by a pulse oximeter at 100%.[5]

Hyperventilation

A classic teaching in the past was to use hyperventilation as a means to decrease intracranial pressure by lowering the $PaCO_2$. While hyperventilation does decrease the PaCO$_2$, and may lower the ICP in the short term, cerebral ischemia, the result of cerebral vasoconstriction, will aggravate underlying hypoxia. Cerebral blood flow is reduced with hyperventilation; lower cerebral blood flow is linked with poor outcome.[4] Furthermore, rebound increases in cerebral blood flow and ICP can occur when hyperventilation is withdrawn. It is for the above reasons that the American Association of Neurological Surgeons and Congress of Neurological Surgeons recommend that the **use of prophylactic hyperventilation within the first 24 hour of severe traumatic brain injury be avoided because "it can compromise cerebral perfusion during a time when cerebral blood flow is already reduced."**[4,10] In patients with pupillary dilatation (a sign of brain herniation) or worsening GCS, hyperventilation may be used if end tidal CO$_2$ measurements are available and if the PCO$_2$ can be maintained between 25 and 35 mm Hg.[7]

Fluid Resuscitation

Many practitioners ascribe to the unfounded tenet that head-injured patients should be run dry and kept in a state of relative hypovolemia to avoid increasing the ICP. This teaching, while widely accepted, is not justified with clinical studies. Systolic blood pressures lower than 90 mm Hg are correlated with poor outcomes, but no value has emerged as an adequate resuscitation threshold.[5] Most authors recommend providing isotonic fluids until a target systolic blood pressure of 120 to 140 mm Hg is achieved.[5] Avoid dextrose-containing solutions because even though glucose is an essential substrate for cerebral metabolism, it is abnormally converted to lactate, a neurotoxin, in seriously injured patients.[6] Dextrose-containing solutions such as 5% dextrose in water (D5W) are undesirable because the blood brain barrier is leaky for a short period after brain trauma, and hypotonic fluids exacerbate cerebral edema.[5] In truly hypotensive, hypovolemic patients, whole blood is theoretically the ideal resuscitation fluid because it is neutral with respect to osmotic gradients in and around areas of neuronal tissue injury.[6]

Mannitol

The role of mannitol and diuretics in the immediate management of severe traumatic brain injury remains unclear.[5,6] The diuretic most commonly used is 20% mannitol, a hypertonic preparation given initially as a 1 g/kg bolus.[7] Mannitol works through multiple mechanisms. As a hypertonic solution, mannitol creates a gradient that favors the movement of water out of the brain cells. In the acute setting, this enhances preload, increasing cardiac output, and enhancing oxygen delivery.[1] Blood viscosity (resistance to flow) is reduced by a decreased hematocrit (percentage of circulating red blood cells) through hemodilution. Mannitol may also confer a neuroprotective effect, especially in ischemic tissues, as a free radical scavenger.[1] Furosemide (Lasix®) is a potent diuretic that works at the level of the ascending loop of Henle in the kidney; this agent is sometimes used in conjunction with mannitol to enhance diuresis.

Disadvantages to mannitol include the potential for dehydration, dysrhythmias due to electrolyte abnormalities, renal failure, and hypotension from acute diuresis.[1] Prehospital diuresis is dangerous when used outside of a physiologically-monitored setting because of hypotension, alkalosis, and renal complications.[1] Mannitol can accumulate in the brain over time, causing a paradoxical reversal of the osmotic gradient, worsening intracerebral edema. In general, the use of mannitol is reserved for the intensive care unit when ICP and arterial blood pressure monitoring are available.

Neuroprotective Agents

The 20th century was a time of great progress in the area of neuroprotection. Barbiturates, hypothermia, and novel pharmacologic agents continue to show promise in several major clinical trials. Large-scale outcome studies and laboratory research will likely yield additional data to support the use of neuroprotective agents in the immediate resuscitative phase.

DEFINITIVE CARE

Patients with severe traumatic brain injury are best managed in the neurosurgical intensive care unit. Arterial lines, ICP and central venous pressure monitoring, and other standard intensive care measures are implemented. Prompt neurosurgical intervention is necessary when indicated.

Spinal Cord Injuries

EPIDEMIOLOGY

Spinal cord trauma is a significant cause of morbidity and mortality in the United States with nearly 11,000 individuals sustaining spinal cord injuries annually.[12] The mortality rate ranges from 17% to 50%; many patients who survive suffer permanent disability.[1,13] These injuries are more common in young adults; men are more commonly affected (4:1 ratio) and the average age at the time of injury is 29.[12] The number one cause of spinal cord trauma is injury following motor vehicle accidents, followed by gunshot wounds, falls, and recreational sports.[14]

PATHOGENESIS

Anatomy

The spinal cord is continuous with the base of the brain (medulla oblongata) and extends through the bony canal of the spinal cord, terminating at the level of the first or second lumbar vertebrae. The 33 units that comprise the spinal cord are grouped according to 5 regions: cervical, thoracic, lumbar, sacral, and coccygeal vertebrae. Vertebrae are supported by flexible vertebral disks and supporting ligaments. The spinal cord is a cylinder-shaped bundle of neurons ensheathed by the same three layers of the brain: dura, arachnoid, and pia mater. Each spinal nerve is named for its adjacent vertebral body (*e.g.*, C4, T12).

Two main arteries, the anterior spinal and paired posterior spinal arteries provide the blood supply to the spinal cord. The anterior spinal artery arises from the vertebral and radicular arteries, as well as the artery of Adamkiewicz, and supplies 75% of the spinal cord. The posterior spinal arteries are paired vessels arising from posterior branches of the vertebral arteries and supply the remaining 25%. The spinal cord is bathed by cerebrospinal fluid (CSF) and the perfusion pressure is autoregulated in the same manner as in the brain.[13]. Cord autoregulation is intact between perfusion pressures of 50 and 130 mm Hg.[12]

A cross-sectional view of the spinal cord reveals the location of several important tracts of ascending and descending fibers. These tracts have specific functions and are described in Figure 28-5. The three most clinically significant descending and ascending tracts are the corticospinal, spinothalamic, and posterior columns.

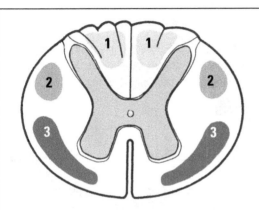

1. **Posterior Columns: Proprioception, Vibration, Light, Touch**
2. **Corticospinal Tracts: Motor Control**
3. **Spinothalamic Tracts: Pain and Temperature Sensation**

Figure 28-5 A cross section of spinal cord, illustrating the anatomical location of the corticospinal, spinothalamic, and posterior columns.

Mechanical Factors

Initial traumatic forces involve compression and contusion of the spinal cord tissue with secondary hemorrhage, swelling, and inflammation. Fractured segments of vertebrae lead to compression of nerve cells with permanent dysfunction frequently the end result.

Although the cord itself is rarely completely transected, trauma often causes immediate and complete disruption of spinal cord function.[13] The cervical and thoracolumbar divisions of the spinal cord are most susceptible to injury because of the greater range of mobility in these segments. Forces of excessive flexion, extension, rotation, lateral flexion, and vertical compression (*i.e.*, axial unloading) are responsible for most cervical spinal injuries.[13]

Biochemical Factors

The biochemical cascade described previously for traumatic brain injury applies to spinal cord trauma as well. Spinal cord contusions cause local disturbances in sodium, potassium, and calcium metabolism, leading to further injury progression.

Ischemia

Any interruption of blood flow to the spinal cord results in permanent neuronal death in a matter of minutes. The biochemical cascade involves the release of potent vasoconstrictors that decrease spinal cord blood flow, leading to ischemia and neuronal demise. Hemorrhage into the gray and white matter results from contusions to the cord. Neuronal cell degeneration and extensive endotheilial injury can be demonstrated as early as 4 hours after injury.[12]

Secondary Effects

As with traumatic brain injury, the concept of secondary injury also applies as the mechanisms are thought to be similar. Abnormal calcium metabolism, inflammation, and free radical formation are thought to be important mechanisms of secondary injury.

CLINICAL MANIFESTATIONS

Neurologic Examination

A complete neurologic examination is too time-consuming to be properly performed in the prehospital arena; however, once in the emergency department, mental status, motor, sensory, proprioceptive (sense of position and vibration), and deep tendon reflex function are assessed. The essentials of a brief neurologic examination are summarized in Table 28-2.

Systemic Effects

Spinal cord trauma is associated with a number of systemic effects. The initial compensatory sympathetic stimulation after injury can be followed by **neurogenic shock**. Neurogenic shock is the result of a loss of sympathetic tone and is characterized by a fall in systemic vascular resistance with an increase in venous capacitance and pooling.[13] The clinical manifestations of neurogenic shock include profound hypotension with bradycardia and warm, rather than cool, skin; **this can help distinguish the syndrome from hypovolemic shock**. Neurogenic shock is often confused with **spinal shock**. The later term describes the flaccidity and loss of reflexes after a spinal cord injury rather than damage to the sympathetic pathways.[7] Spinal shock is the result of direct trauma or shock to the spinal cord.

In lesions above C 3, 4, or 5, the diaphragm can become paralyzed (spinal segments C 3,4 and 5 comprise the phrenic nerve; the innervation of the diaphragm) with associated losses in functional residual capacity, forced vital capacity, and maximum inspiratory and expiratory pressures. Hypoventilation is common and neurogenic pulmonary edema may follow. Patients with spinal cord trauma involving cervical segments are often predisposed to developing pneumonia due to collapsed segments of lung (atelectasis) and impaired cough reflex. In the initial stages, deep tendon reflexes are absent, but over time, spasticity develops with hyperactive reflexes.

Table 28-2
Essentials of a Brief, Focused, Neurologic Exam

Mental Status

- GCS score
- Spell world backwards
- Recall 3 objects after 3 minutes
- AVPU: **A-A**lert **V-V**erbal **P-**Response to **P**ain **U-U**nresponsive

Cranial Nerves

CN1- Smell soap or tobacco leaves	**CN7-** Smile
CN2- Visual acuity; gross visual fields	**CN8-** Hear fingertips moving
CN3- Pupillary light reflex & gaze	**CN9-** Gag reflex
CN4- Pupillary light reflex & gaze	**CN10-** Gag reflex
CN5- Corneal blink reflex; facial sensation	**CN11-** Shrug shoulders
CN6- Pupillary light reflex & gaze	**CN12-** Stick out tongue

Motor

- Pronator drift
- Hand grasp
- Toe dorsi- and plantarflexion

Sensory

- Double simultaneous stimulation with pin or paperclip on hands and feet
- Light touch with cotton swab or brush
- Check vibration with tuning fork

Coordination

- Finger-to-nose
- Heel-to-shin
- Tandem gait (walk with one foot directly in front of other)
- Romberg test (stand with eyes closed, feet together; check for imbalance)

Reflexes

- **C5-6** Biceps
- **C7** Triceps
- **L4** Patellar
- **S1** Achilles

Spinal Cord Syndromes

The diagnosis of spinal cord syndromes is beyond the scope of prehospital care; however, the ability to recognize a limited number of distinctive syndromes is possible if a focused neurologic examination can be performed. Five anatomic spinal cord syndromes are presented here for the sake of completeness.

Anterior Cord Syndrome

Hyperflexion injuries with herniated disks can cause damage to the anterior portion of the spinal cord, resulting in loss of motor function, pinprick, and light touch below the level of the lesion. These clinical manifestations are the result of damage to the corticospinal and spinothalamic tracts. Proprioception is preserved because the posterior columns are spared.

Central Cord Syndrome

The most common partial cord syndrome, this syndrome is usually caused by hyperextension injuries in elderly patients with preexisting cervical vertebral disease. Patients present with bilateral motor impairment with the upper extremities affected more than the lower. Sensory impairment and bladder dysfunction are possible sequelae. The centrally located portions of the posterior columns, corticospinal, and spinothalamic tract are affected, explaining the clinical findings.

Brown-Sequard Syndrome

This syndrome is the rare result of penetrating trauma and is associated with loss of motor and proprioception on the same side of the lesion with contralateral loss of pain and temperature sensation. Brown-Sequard syndrome is the result of cord hemisection (damage to half of the spinal cord). This lesion is reported to have the best prognosis for recovery.

Complete Cord Syndrome

Complete transection of the spinal cord can be caused by trauma (i.e., disk herniation, fracture fragments) or delayed injury (*i.e.*, hemorrhage, ischemia). Neurogenic shock is the usual result and is caused by complete interruption of sympathetic fibers as well as all ascending and descending tracts.

Cauda Equina Syndrome

The terminal end of the spinal cord is known as the conus medullaris and when rarely injured, causes a peripheral rather than central nerve deficit. The bladder can become denervated, resulting in disturbances of urination and loss of sexual function. The characteristic "saddle" distribution of anesthesia occurs when the lower sacral or coccygeal nerve segments are affected. Since this syndrome is ordinarily the result of a peripheral nerve injury in the lower lumbar, sacral, or coccygeal segments, prognosis is very good.

MANAGEMENT

Initial Priorities

Stabilization of a patient with a spinal cord injury begins at the scene. **Full spinal immobilization is the most important initial intervention, and if performed properly, can prevent lifelong disability.** Since the spinal cord is especially sensitive to secondary insults caused by ischemia, an airway should be established with the modified jaw-thrust maneuver, and ventilation provided as needed to maintain the SpO$_2$ at 100%. **Since up to 5% to 6% of trauma patients requiring endotracheal intubation have an unstable cervical fracture, intubation is reserved for experienced personnel only and in most cases can be averted with proper bag-valve ventilation techniques.**[1] Rapid sequence intubation with in-line cervical stabilization is safe and effective when performed by properly trained providers.[14] Shock may be difficult to assess in patients with spinal cord injuries since neurogenic shock is marked by bradycardia rather than tachycardia, and patients often have warm skin due to abnormal vasodilation. If hypovolemia is suspected, isotonic fluids should be administered judiciously. Time permitting, a brief, focused, neurologic exam should be performed.

Steroids
Although significant controversy remains regarding the overall benefit, intravenous steroids are currently the standard of care for patients with acute nonpenetrating spinal cord trauma.[1,7,12,14] The protocol includes an initial bolus of methylprednisolone (Solu Medrol™) at a 30 mg/kg dose, followed by a loading dose administered at 5.4 mg/kg/hour for 24 hours.[7,14] This regimen is most effective when initiated within 8 hours of injury.[14]

DEFINITIVE CARE
Patients with spinal cord trauma should be referred to a center where neurosurgical expertise is readily available. While in the neurosurgical intensive care unit, patients may require inotropes and chronotropes such as dopamine and dobutamine for cardiac support. These agents help maintain perfusion to the spinal cord and may prevent secondary injury. New pharmacologic therapies such as free radical scavengers, N-methyl D-aspartate (NMDA) antagonists, and GM-1 gangliosides hold promise as potential beneficial treatments. Induced hypothermia is also being investigated as a potential neuroprotective modality for spinal cord trauma. After the acute phase, aggressive rehabilitation remains the cornerstone of care.

Regeneration
Transplantation and axonal regeneration techniques represent an exciting and promising facet of neurobiological research. Current techniques in animals have shown that peripheral nerve grafts can be placed, but growth is limited by scar tissue.[12] Schwann cells, the major growth-promoting cells in the spinal cord tissue, improve cell survival and reduce scar tissue formation by forming a living bridge over the site of damaged neurons when given immediately after injury.[12] Trophic factors and antibodies for growth inhibitory factors are potential therapies, and improvements in tissue engineering and gene therapy may pave the way for great progress in the future treatment of spinal cord injury.

References

1. King BS, Gupta R, Narayan RK. The early assessment and intensive care unit management of patients with severe traumatic brain and spinal cord injuries. *Surg Clin North America* 2000; 80(3); 855-870, viii-ix.

2. Zink BJ. Traumatic brain injury outcome: Concepts for emergency care. *Ann Emerg Med* 2001; 37(3): 318-332.

3. Dangor A, Lam AM. Perioperative management of patients with head and spinal cord trauma. *Anesthesiology Clin North America* 1999; 17(1): 155-170.

4. Yundt KD, Diringer MN. The use of hyperventilation and its impact on cerebral ischemia in the treatment of traumatic brain injury. *Crit Care Clin* 1997; 13(1): 163-184.

5. Chesnut RM. The management of severe traumatic brain injury. *Emerg Med Clin North America* 1997; 15(3): 581-604.

6. Gruen P, Liu C. Current trends in the management of head injury. *Emer Med Clin North America* 1998; 16(1): 63-78.

7. The Committee on Trauma of the American College of Surgeons. *Advanced Trauma Life Support for Doctors.* Chicago: The American College of Surgeons, 1997. 186-206.

8. Borczuk P. Mild head trauma. *Emerg Med Clin North America* 1997; 15(3): 563-579.

9. Jaoda A, Riggio S. Mild traumatic brain injury and the postconcussive syndrome. *Emerg Med Clin North America* 2000; 18(2): 355-363.

10. Bullock R, Chesnut RM, Clifton G, *et al.* The use of hyperventilation in the acute management of severe traumatic brain injury. In: Bullock R, Chesnut RM, Clifton G, *et al* (eds.). *Guidelines for the Management of Severe Head Injury.* New York: Brain Trauma Foundation, 1995.

11. Cheng MA, Theard MA, Tempelhoff R. Intravenous agents and intraoperative neuroprotection: Beyond barbiturates. *Crit Care Clinics* 1997; 13(1): 185-198.

12. Girardi FP, Kahn SN, Cammisa FP, Blanck TJJ. Advances and strategies for spinal cord regeneration. *Ortho Clin North America* 2000; 31(3): 465-472.

13. Dangor A, Lam A. Perioperative management of patients with head and spinal cord trauma. *Anesthesiology Clin North Amer* 1999; 17(1): 155-170.

14. Wagner R, Jagoda A. Spinal cord syndromes. *Emerg Med Clin North America* 1997; 15(3): 699-711.

Review Questions

1. You are transporting a patient with a serious head injury. Glasgow coma scale is 8. Hyperventilation for this patient is likely to be ineffective for all of the following reasons EXCEPT:

A. A rebound increase in intracranial pressure is possible due to PCO_2 elevation in the cerebrospinal fluid.

B. A rebound increase in cerebral blood flow can occur after hyperventilation is withdrawn.

C. Hyperventilation is contraindicated in patients with transtentorial herniation when the PCO_2 can be maintained between 25 to 35 mm Hg.

D. Vasoconstriction of cerebral arterioles exacerbates preexisting brain hypoxia.

E. The pH of cerebrospinal fluid returns to pre-hyperventilation levels within hours.

Transtentorial herniation is the only known circumstance where prehospital hyperventilation may be beneficial. The answer is C.

2. Which of the following pathogenic mechanisms explains the progressive clinical deterioration of severely brain-injured patients?

A. Loss of cerebral autoregulation secondary to expansion of blood volume in the cranial vault

B. Progressive edema

C. Ischemia due to a hypermetabolic state

D. Excitotoxin release with widespread neuronal activation

E. All of the above

The answer is E.

3. A male patient sustains a blow to the right temple and loses consciousness. When you assess him, he is conscious, alert, and oriented to person, place, time, and event. He complains of pain at the site of impact. During transport, the patient rapidly progresses to coma. Which of the following would be the most likely etiology for this patient's neurologic deterioration?

A. Meningitis

B. Orbital blowout fracture

C. Concussion

D. Stroke

E. Epidural hematoma

The answer is E.

4. The condition in Question 3 is usually caused by:
   A. Bleeding from the anterior branch of the middle meningeal artery
   B. Ischemia in the distribution of the middle cerebral artery due
      to thrombosis
   C. Inflammation of the meninges secondary to infection
   D. Tripod fracture of orbit and facial bones
   E. Diffuse axonal injury secondary to coup-contra-coup mechanisms

The answer is A.

5. An elderly alcoholic male sustains a head injury and is transported to the
emergency department. Bystanders report that the patient was struck by a car.
The patient is unconscious. What would be a disorder that must be considered
in this patient?
   A. Meningitis
   B. Subdural hematoma
   C. Uncomplicated depressed skull fracture
   D. Orbital blowout fracture
   E. Concussion

The answer is B.

6. The most common cause of the condition described in Question 5 is:
   A Diffuse axonal injury
   B. Laceration of the middle meningeal artery
   C. Tear of the bridging veins between the cortex and venous sinuses
      in the brain
   D. Thrombosis of the anterior cerebral artery
   E. Inflammation of the meninges secondary to infection

The answer is C.

7. Routine prophylactic hyperventilation is not recommended in head-injured
patients for all of the following reasons EXCEPT:
   A. Reduces cerebral blood flow and exacerbates ischemia
   B. Causes rebound increase in intracranial pressure when withdrawn
   C. Aggravates cerebral hypoxia by inducing vasoconstriction
   D. Cerebrospinal fluid pH changes to pre-hyperventilation levels within
      hours, obviating any advantage
   E. Induces cerebral vasodilation and increases blood flow

The answer is E.

8. Which of the following is the most crucial step in managing severely head-injured patients?
   A. Intravenous mannitol with furosemide
   B. Intubation and ventilation with 100% oxygen
   C. Prophylactic hyperventilation with 100% oxygen
   D. Administration of calcium channel blockers
   E. Administration of intravenous corticosteroids

The answer is B.

9. All of the following are advantages of mannitol in head-injured patients EXCEPT:
   A. Prevents dysrhythmias and metabolic alkalosis
   B. Creates favorable osmotic gradient, decreasing cerebral edema
   C. Increases cardiac output, enhancing oxygen delivery to the brain, by reducing preload
   D. Reduces blood viscosity
   E. Acts as a neuroprotective free radical scavenger

Dysrhythmias and metabolic alkalosis, both due to electrolyte losses through diuresis, are known complications of mannitol use. The answer is A.

10. A 43-year-old male falls down a flight of stairs. He states, "I can't feel my legs." Which of the following are signs of neurologic shock?
   A. Hypotension, tachycardia, cool skin
   B. Hypotension, tachycardia, warm skin
   C. Hypertension, tachycardia, cool skin
   D. Hypotension, bradycardia, warm skin
   E. Hypertension, bradycardia, cool skin

The answer is D.

11. The most important initial intervention for the patient in Question 10 is:
   A. Lumbar puncture to decrease cerebrospinal fluid pressure
   B. Intravenous steroids
   C. Full spinal immobilization
   D. Intravenous mannitol
   E. Hyperventilation with 100% oxygen

The answer is C.

12. All of the following are potentially beneficial treatments for spinal cord injuries EXCEPT:
   A. Mandatory endotracheal intubation for patients with respiratory failure, even if done by inexperienced personnel
   B. Judicious use of intravenous fluids for hypotension
   C. Free radical scavengers, NMDA antagonists, GM-1 gangliosides
   D. Full spinal immobilization
   E. Intravenous methylprednisolone within 8 hours of injury

Intubation can be dangerous for patients with spinal cord injuries. The airway can be effectively maintained for short transports with bag-valve ventilation, in-line manual stabilization, and cricoid pressure. The answer is A.

Section IX

Environmental Emergencies

29

Hypothermia

Nearly 700 patients die each year from accidental hypothermia, although this number probably underestimates the total number of deaths since the condition is often unrecognized.[1,2] The death rate for accidental hypothermia is highest for persons 65 years of age or older and is approximately three times higher in men than women.[3]

Pathogenesis

CAUSES OF HYPOTHERMIA

There are many causes of hypothermia; this chapter deals specifically with **accidental** or **primary** hypothermia. Hypothermia can develop in temperate regions and even indoors during the summer, and is not a disorder seen only after exposure to excessively cold environments.

Environmental hypothermia is caused by transfer of heat away from the body through the four processes of conduction, convection, radiation, or evaporation. Since water conducts heat away from the body 20 to 30 times more readily than air, wet clothing or prolonged immersion in water represents a common preventable cause of hypothermia. Immersion in water as warm as 26.6°C (80°F) can lead to hypothermia.[4] **Convection** is the process of heat transfer by the movement of heated material. An example of this mechanism is heat loss in windy conditions. **Radiation** of heat from the body to the environment and evaporation of water can occur over a wide range of temperatures, causing hypothermia in dry, cold environments.

Disorders associated with decreased heat production or increased heat loss can be responsible for hypothermia. Endocrinologic diseases such as hypoadrenalism or hypothyroidism are associated with a decreased metabolic rate, preventing the **nonshivering** compensatory response to cold. Insufficient fuel, as occurs in malnutrition, hypoglycemia, and alcoholism, complicates the normal response to cold due to lack of useable substrates (*i.e.*, glucose) required for normal metabolism.

Hypothermia can be caused by pathologic processes that impair thermoregulation. Peripheral neuropathies, spinal cord disease, and diabetes are important comorbidities for hypothermia because peripheral nerves are necessary for shivering and cutaneous vasoconstriction. Sepsis, pancreatitis, cancers, and progressive neurologic disorders such as Parkinson's disease and multiple sclerosis are risk factors for hypothermia as these diseases are associated with impaired thermoregulation. Nearly half of all trauma patients are found to be hypothermic during and after resuscitation attempts.[4]

Up to 90% of deceased hypothermic patients have detectable blood alcohol levels.[4,5] Alcohol is a vasodilator and inhibitor of antidiuretic hormone (ADH). As a central nervous system depressant, alcohol alters or inhibits the perception of thermal adversity.

NORMAL TEMPERATURE REGULATION

Body temperature is regulated by the preoptic nucleus in the anterior hypothalamus. In conscious individuals, the sensation of cold induces either **shivering** or **nonshivering** mechanisms to maintain body temperature. The hypothalamus conserves heat by producing peripheral vasoconstriction and stimulating muscular activity in the form of shivering. The skin accounts for nearly 50% of the body surface area; one of the most important regulators of heat is blood flow to the skin and extremities.[6] Shivering increases heat production by two to four times and is a vital mechanism for rewarming in hypothermic patients.[2] Inhibition of this mechanism by drugs (*e.g.*, meperidine) or advanced age results in an inability to respond to cold stimuli. Temperatures below 32°C (89.6°F) inhibit this mechanism.[3] Nonshivering mechanisms compensate for heat loss by increasing the output of the thyroid and adrenal gland, increasing circulating levels of epinephrine, norepinephrine, and thyroxine (thyroid hormone) with a subsequent rise in the basal metabolic rate.[6]

Systemic Manifestations of Hypothermia

CLASSIFICATION OF HYPOTHERMIA

The degree of hypothermia depends on the core body temperature. Core temperatures can be approximated by rectal thermometers, although even this technique lags behind the true core body temperature. **Ear lobe devices and oral determinations are not accurate and should not be used in hypothermic patients.** Hypothermia is classified as mild, moderate, or severe according to temperature (Table 29-1).

SYSTEMIC MANIFESTATIONS

Pulmonary

With mild hypothermia, the respiratory rate initially increases, but as the core body temperature drops, depression of the respiratory center occurs with a decreased respiratory rate and tidal volume, and decreased oxygen consumption and CO_2 production. Pulmonary edema is common during rewarming of severely hypothermic patients.

Cardiovascular

The initial cardiovascular response to mild hypothermia is an increase in the heart rate, cardiac output, peripheral vascular resistance, and degree of vasoconstriction. These mechanisms serve to route oxygenated blood to vital organs. At lower temperatures, the myocardium becomes irritable and cardiac output may drop precipitously due to progressive bradycardia. The sequence of dysrhythmias as the core body temperature falls includes bradycardia, atrial fibrillation, ventricular

Table 29-1
Classification Scheme for Hypothermia

Degree of Hypothermia	Core Temperature	Clinical Findings
Mild	32-35°C (89.6-95°F)	Shivering Complaint of cold Mild confusion
Moderate	30-32°C (86-89°F)	No shivering Altered mental status Muscle rigidity Ventricular fibrillation (if patient handled aggressively) Dilated pupils Hypotension Decreased respirations
Severe	<30°C (<86°F)	Comatose Flaccid (no rigidity) Apnea Ventricular fibrillation

fibrillation, and asystole. **Rough handling of the patient, such as moving the patient from the stretcher to the hospital bed, has induced ventricular fibrillation in severely hypothermic patients.**[7,8] Ventricular fibrillation is common at temperatures less than 28°C (82.4°F); asystole occurs at temperatures below 20°C (68°F). The characteristic Osborn or J waves are seen on the ECG in 25% to 30% of patients with moderate to severe hypothermia (Figure 29-1).[3]

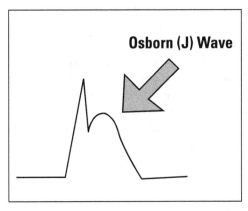

Osborn (J) Wave

Figure 29-1 The Osborn (J) wave associated with hypothermia. The presence of this ECG finding is characteristic of moderate to severe hypothermia, but cannot be used to confirm the diagnosis.

Central Nervous System

As cardiac output decreases in moderate to severe hypothermia, cerebral blood flow decreases, leading to changes in mental status. Patients with mild hypothermia present with confusion, slurred speech, impaired judgment, or amnesia, while lethargy, hallucinations, and coma are associated with moderate to severe hypothermia.[3] Pupillary reflexes are lost in severe hypothermia; hence, **fixed and dilated pupils are not indicative of brain death.**[4] Moreover, cerebral ischemia during cardiopulmonary arrest is tolerated by some patients in contrast with the normothermic state; thus, the axiom that death cannot be pronounced until the patient is "warm and dead" holds true for patients with hypothermia.[3,4]

Renal

Renal-concentrating abilities are impaired in patients with mild hypothermia, triggering a cold diuresis that leads to volume depletion and profound dehydration.[3] Rhabdomyolysis, a condition characterized by muscle breakdown, may be associated with hypothermia and can cause acute tubular necrosis.

Hematologic

Hypothermic patients are prone to bleeding because cold inhibits the enzymes needed for reactions in the coagulation cascade. Increased blood viscosity and hemoconcentration impair the delivery of oxygen to the vital organs and produce ischemia. The oxygen-hemoglobin dissociation curve shifts to the left in hypothermia, increasing the affinity of hemoglobin for oxygen and decreasing the amount of available oxygen for systemic delivery.

Management

INITIAL PRIORITIES

Cardiopulmonary Resuscitation (CPR)

As discussed above, a **rectal** temperature should be taken to confirm hypothermia. Oxygen administration and aggressive airway support should be initiated and CPR started if necessary. Some investigators argue that CPR may be harmful insofar as chest compressions may precipitate ventricular fibrillation in severely hypothermic patients. Nevertheless, severe hypothermia is associated with decreased or absent cardiac output and withholding CPR may subject the patient to further ischemia. Since hypothermic patients are often bradycardic, **the pulse should be taken for at least 30 seconds to 1 minute before starting CPR.** Intubation in hypothermic patients can be difficult owing to the rigidity of the jaw; blind nasotracheal intubation can be considered as an alternative.

Fluid Resuscitation

Patients with moderate to severe hypothermia are volume depleted and require aggressive fluid resuscitation. Vasoactive medications such as dopamine and norepinephrine seldom correct hypotension since peripheral vascular resistance is already maximized in hypothermic patients. Avoid lactated Ringer's because of the decreased ability of the liver to metabolize lactate during hypothermia.[3] Fluids should be heated to about 40°C (104°F) but usually do not provide added heat unless infused in large quantities.[3] Normal saline is the recommended fluid, although since hypothermic patients are often hypoglycemic, a 5% dextrose in normal saline solution may be considered to provide added glucose.[3]

Drug Therapy

The ACLS algorithm for hypothermia should be followed, keeping in mind that medications for cardiac arrest should be given at longer intervals since these drugs may accumulate to toxic levels.[4] As many patients with hypothermia are alcoholics, thiamine and dextrose should be given to prevent Wernicke's encephalopathy and hypoglycemia. **Defibrillation is seldom successful at temperatures below 29°C (84°F) and most hypothermia-induced dysrhythmias improve with rewarming and do not require specific treatment.**[6] Bretylium tosylate is the only antidysrhythmic shown to be effective in animal studies, but lidocaine and procainamide may also be effective.[3] Bretylium is no longer widely available in the United States.

REWARMING TECHNIQUES

Despite the lack of controlled studies to validate optimal method, duration, and rate of administration, **rewarming methods remain the cornerstone of care for hypothermic patients**. All hypothermic patients should be removed from the cold environment, dried, and covered with an insulating material to prevent further heat loss.

Active Rewarming

Active rewarming involves the transfer of heat to the patient by external or internal techniques and can be accomplished through several modalities.[3] In general, **active core rewarming techniques are recommended for any severely hypothermic patient.**[4] Heated humidified oxygen is a simple technique that should be considered, as well as the administration of warmed intravenous fluids. Concerns have been raised relating to the use of heating units such as forced-air rewarming techniques, heating pads, and radiant heat because these methods may stimulate peripheral vasodilation, making the victim more hypothermic.[3,9] **If the skin is warmed without providing heat to the core, the drive to shiver is extinguished and vasodilation may exacerbate hypotension.**[9] Therefore, if external rewarming devices are used, they should be applied around the thorax to provide **core** rewarming.

Invasive Techniques

Once in the emergency department or critical care unit, a variety of invasive core rewarming techniques can be implemented. These techniques include gastric, pleural, or bladder irrigation and peritoneal lavage. Hemodialysis, cardiopulmonary bypass, arteriovenous rewarming, and venovenous rewarming, are the four methods available for extracorporeal blood rewarming. Long-term outcome of patients treated with these techniques has been favorable, but these methods are often fraught with complications.[3,4]

Future Techniques

Two potentially promising modalities for rewarming include the use of very high temperature intravenous fluids and diathermy. Preliminary data from animal models show administration of fluids warmed to 65°C (149°F) to be effective for moderate to severe hypothermia without significant vascular injuries.[10,11] Further studies in humans are pending. Diathermy involves the use of ultrasound or low-frequency microwave radiation to deliver large amounts of heat to deep tissues.[3] Animal studies have provided encouraging preliminary results.[12]

References

1. Hypothermia-related deaths. *MMWR* 1994; 43: 849, 855-856.

2. Josephs JD. Hypothermia and extracorporeal rewarming: The journey toward a less invasive, more accessible methodology. *Crit Care Med* 1998; 26(12): 1944-1945.

3. Hanania NA, Zimmerman JL. Accidental hypothermia. *Crit Care Clin* 1999; 15(2): 235-249.

4. Braun R, Krishel S. Pearls, pitfalls, and updates: Environmental emergencies. *Emerg Med Clin North Am* 1997; 15(2): 451-476.

5. Freedland ES, McMicken DB, D'Onofrio G. Alcohol and trauma. *Emerg Med Clin North Am* 1993; 11: 225-239.

6. Britt DL, Dascombe WH, Rodriguez A. New horizons in management of hypothermia and frostbite injury. *Surg Clin North Am* 1991; 71(2): 345-349.

7. Weinberg AD. Hypothermia. *Ann Emerg Med* 1993; 22 (part 2): 370.

8. Lloyd EL. Accidental hypothermia. *Resuscitation* 1996; 32: 111.

9. Weiss E. Medical considerations for wilderness and adventure travelers. *Med Clin North Am* 1999; 83(4): 893.

10. Sheaff CM, Fildes JJ, Keogh P, *et al.* Safety of 65 degrees C intravenous fluid for the treatment of hypothermia. *Am J Surg* 1996; 172: 52-55.

11. Fildes J, Sheaff C, Barrett J. Very hot intravenous fluid in the treatment of hypothermia. *J Trauma* 1993; 35: 683.

12. Giesbrecht GG, Bristow GK. Recent advances in hypothermia research. *Ann NY Acad Sci* 1997; 813: 663.

Review Questions

1. Aeromedical evacuation is requested for a patient lost for 2 days in an arctic environment. The patient has an altered mental status, cold skin, and fixed, dilated pupils. Core body temperature is 36°C (86°F). The finding of dilated pupils in this patient is:
   - A. Sign of permanent brain injury
   - B. Due to parasympathetic stimulation
   - C. Not indicative of death in hypothermic patients
   - D. A sign of ventricular fibrillation
   - E. A sign of irreversible, impending brain death

The answer is C.

2. All of the following are true regarding ventricular fibrillation in hypothermic patients EXCEPT:
   - A. Common at temperatures less than 28°C (83°F)
   - B. Due to myocardial irritability
   - C. May be precipitated by CPR techniques
   - D. Should be treated immediately with intravenous atropine
   - E. May be caused by rough handling of the patient

The answer is D.

3. All of the following are processes responsible for the development of hypothermia EXCEPT:
   - A. Radiation
   - B. Evaporation
   - C. Sublimation
   - D. Conduction
   - E. Convection

The answer is C.

4. Which of the following is an ECG finding in moderate to severe hypothermia?
   - A. Osborn waves
   - B. U-waves
   - C. Q-waves
   - D. Flutter waves
   - E. Delta waves

The answer is A.

5. All of the following are expected physiologic changes in patients with moderate to severe hypothermia EXCEPT:

A. Bleeding disorders
B. Cold diuresis leading to volume loss
C. Increased myocardial irritability leading to ventricular fibrillation
D. Pulmonary edema in rewarmed patients
E. All of the above are expected physiologic changes in moderate to severe hypothermia

The answer is E.

Heat Stroke and Heat Exhaustion

Despite various structural and functional adaptations for survival in warm environments, human beings have been plagued by heat-related illnesses throughout history. Heat stroke has claimed casualties since as early as King Edward's war against the Arabs for the Holy Land to the U.S. Army's loss of 125 soldiers during basic training for World War II.[1-3] Heat stroke is the most serious manifestation of heat-related illness, and is a true medical emergency that results from an overload or impairment of heat-dissipating mechanisms. Left untreated, this disorder is universally fatal if body temperature is not rapidly lowered.[4] Older adults, obese patients, infants, patients with hyperthyroidism, and those taking certain medications are at the greatest risk, although the true risk for any patient is difficult to quantify since many patients with heat stroke are misidentified because of other disorders associated with an excessively high body temperature.[4,5]

Pathogenesis

HEAT PRODUCTION

Metabolic processes throughout the body normally produce body heat; most body heat production is increased by the metabolic activity of skeletal muscle. In an average adult male, 1700 kilocalories (kcal) are produced each day, increasing to 2500 to 3000 kcal per day with moderate physical activity.[1] Heat production can be increased by up to ten times above normal with excess shivering, tremor, or exertion.[6] In addition to endogenous heat production, heat can be gained by radiation from the sun, ground, or reflected radiation from the sky.

NORMAL RESPONSE TO HEAT

Without mechanisms of heat loss, body temperature would rise by approximately one degree Celsius per hour.[1,7] The four essential methods of heat loss, include conduction, convection, radiation, and evaporation, but these methods are responsible for only 20% to 30% of heat lost from the body.[1] Millions of eccrine and apocrine sweat glands are distributed over the body surface and serve to promote cooling by evaporation. **Eccrine** glands are innervated by cholinergic neurons and are found mostly in the scalp, palms, and soles. **Apocrine** glands are stimulated by epinephrine and the sympathetic nervous system. Apocrine glands are located around nipples and in areas of body creases such as the axilla and groin, secreting sweat rich in protein and carbohydrates. One liter of evaporated sweat on the surface of the human body can lead to the loss of over 500 kcal.[1] In order for heat loss to be accomplished, evaporation must take place; therefore, **when sweat is wiped from the skin, no heat loss occurs.** In areas of high humidity, evaporation takes place more slowly; **it is for this reason that hot, humid environments rather than hot, dry environments are more dangerous for developing heat stroke.**

ACCLIMATIZATION

Humans can physiologically adapt to hot environments within a period of 7 to 10 days.[1] Adaptive responses include onset of sweating at lower core temperatures and increased sweat volume. During acclimatization, skin blood flow increases, stroke volume increases, and heart rate decreases, enabling individuals exposed to heat stress to improve oxygen utilization while initiating mechanisms to assist with evaporative heat loss. **Hydration status is the most important independent factor influencing the development of heat stroke;** aerobic fitness does not influence the tolerance for high temperatures.[6]

PREDISPOSING FACTORS

There are several factors known to increase the risk of heat stroke. These factors are listed in Table 30-1.

Table 30-1

Predisposing Factors for Heat Stroke
Alcoholism
Poverty
Drugs
Nonacclimatization
Obesity
Extremes of age
Dehydration
Lack of sleep
Infections
Chronic illness

HYPERTHERMIA VERSUS FEVER

Although often used interchangeably, the distinction between **fever** and **hyperthermia** is important to appreciate because the pathophysiology and treatment for the two conditions differs. Fever is caused by circulating substances such as microbial products, toxins, microbes, interleukins, or other molecules (*i.e.*, pyrogens). Infections are the most common cause of fever.[8] During fever, the thermostat setting in the hypothalamus shifts upward, much like the way a thermostat for a room is reset to a higher temperature to raise the ambient temperature.[8] Inhibitors of cyclo-oxygenase such as aspirin and nonsteroidal anti-inflammatory drugs (NSAIDs) prevent the release of fever-inducing prostaglandins such as PGE_2.[8]

Hyperthermia differs from fever insofar as the hypothalamic thermoregulatory center remains unchanged as body temperature increases. Eventually the body temperature overrides the body's ability to lose heat, with the end result being perilously high temperature levels.

Clinical Manifestations

DIFFERENTIAL DIAGNOSIS

The differential diagnosis of the patient with increased body temperature is extensive. Sepsis should always be considered in addition to any obvious infectious etiology. Other possible diagnoses include malignant hyperthermia and neuroleptic malignant syndrome.

Malignant Hyperthermia

Malignant hyperthermia is a potentially lethal hyperthermic syndrome afflicting patients with a genetically inherited predisposition. Administration of certain medications to susceptible individuals may increase the permeability of calcium channels on the sarcolemmal membrane, leading to an unpredictable rapid release of calcium into the muscle cells.[6] Medications known to cause malignant hyperthermia are listed in Table 30-2.

The earliest sign of malignant hyperthermia is usually trismus, or spasm of the masticatory muscles, with difficulty opening the mouth. This may occur during the administration of the drug or thereafter, and often proceeds rapidly to cyanosis, tachycardia, tachypnea, and unstable blood pressure.[6] The antidote for malignant hyperthermia is sodium dantrolene. This agent inhibits calcium release from the sarcoplasmic reticulum, decreasing the amount of available calcium for muscle contraction.

Table 30-2
Drugs Known to Cause Malignant Hyperthermia

Drug Class	Agents
Depolarizing agents	Succinylcholine
Volatile anesthetics	Halothane, enflurane, isoflurane, etc.
Other drugs	Lidocaine

Neuroleptic Malignant Syndrome

Neuroleptic malignant syndrome (NMS) is a rare idiosyncratic disorder, developing in approximately 0.2 % of all patients taking certain antipsychotic agents or with abrupt withdrawal of dopamine agonists[6] (Table 30-3).

NMS is believed to be the result of dopaminergic blockade or depletion in the central nervous system.[9] Dopamine depletion in the hypothalamus, corpus striatum, basal ganglia, and spinal cord, has been shown to produce the symptoms of NMS in animal models, and is the most favored hypothesis for the pathogenesis of NMS.[9] This syndrome has a more insidious onset than heat stroke or malignant hyperthermia, developing over days rather than minutes or hours, and is initially marked by an altered level of consciousness, followed by autonomic hyperactivity (tachycardia, tachypnea, and blood pressure irregularities). The treatment of NMS is similar to that for heat stroke, with the addition of nondepolarizing agents as an added measure to terminate increased muscle tone, fever, and lactic acidosis.[6] Supportive care measures are the mainstay of treatment and include aggressive airway management, fluid therapy, cooling, and antipyretics.[9] The offending agent should be promptly discontinued (*e.g.*, patients with Parkinson's disease); in instances where dopaminergic therapy has been abruptly discontinued, therapy should be reinstituted.

Table 30-3
Drugs Known to Cause Neuroleptic Malignant Syndrome

Drug Class	Examples
Neuroleptics (butyrophenones, phenothiazines)	Haloperidol (Haldol) Fluphenazine (Prolixin)
Tricyclic antidepressants	Amitriptyline (Elavil) Amoxapine (Asendin) Desipramine (Norpramin)
Benzodiazepines	Diazepam (Valium) Lorazepam (Ativan)
Anticonvulsants	Carbamazepine (Tegretol) Phenytoin (Dilantin)
Parkinson's Disease medications	Amantadine (Symmetrel) Bromocriptine (Parlodel) Levodopa (Larodopa)
MAO inhibitors	Phenelzine (Nardil) Tranylcypromine (Parnate)
Other dopamine antagonists	Metoclopramide (Reglan) Lithium (Eskalith) Reserpine (Serpasil) Hydroxyzine (Atarax)

Other Heat-Related Illnesses
Heat stroke can be preceded by a variety of heat-related illnesses. The clinical manifestations of heat cramps, heat tetany, heat syncope, heat edema, and heat exhaustion are reviewed in Table 30-4.

TEMPERATURE MEASUREMENT
Heat stoke is usually defined in the literature as an elevation of the body temperature to greater than 41°C (106°F).[1] Temperatures as high as 46°C (114.8°F) were measured in some patients who achieved full recovery, but severe elevation of body temperature has been shown to denature enzymes, damage mitochondria, liquefy membrane lipids, and impair a variety of physiologic processes.[1]

Table 30-4
Clinical Manifestations Of Heat-Related Illnesses

Heat-Related Condition	Clinical Manifestations	Pathophysiology
Heat exhaustion	Weakness, dizziness, headache, tachycardia, syncope, sweating	Volume depletion, hyperthermia
Heat cramps	Cramps in large muscle groups	Disorder of cellular levels of sodium, potassium, calcium, magnesium
Heat tetany	Carpopedal spasm, perioral numbness (often confused with heat cramps)	Electrolyte imbalance (same as heat cramps)
Heat edema	Peripheral edema	Orthostatic pooling of blood; vasodilation with interstitial fluid accumulation
Prickly heat	Rash; lesions with red base; at first itchy	Blockage of sweat pores by macerated stratum corneum; occasional staphylococcal infection

Exertional Heat Stroke
Two types of heat stroke are encountered: **exertional** and **nonexertional**. Exertional heat stroke is common in environments where heat stress is maximal. Military recruits, athletes, or other individuals engaged in strenuous activity while exposed to heat stress are mostly affected. Mental status changes such as loss of consciousness or delirium are frequent early findings. Other signs and symptoms include constricted pupils, tachycardia, tachypnea, nausea, vomiting, diarrhea, or seizures.

Nonexertional Heat Stroke
Victims of nonexertional heat stroke are by and large the elderly, infants, or others lacking the ability to counteract heat exposure through normal thermoregulatory mechanisms. Access to water, especially in infants, is an important consideration. The elderly may succumb to heat stroke as the result of poorly ventilated housing or lack of air conditioning. The signs and symptoms of nonexertional heat stroke are the same as exertional heat stroke, but early signs such as irritability, aggressiveness, or nausea may be subtle or attributed to other factors.

SYSTEMIC EFFECTS

Neurologic impairments are nearly universal findings in heat stroke and are the result of cerebral edema, hemorrhages, and neuronal degeneration. Heart rates as high as 150 beats per minute may be observed, but as heat exposure persists, myocardial damage can occur, progressing to total circulatory collapse. Pericardial effusion, edema, degeneration, and necrosis are common findings on autopsy.[1] Disorders in the coagulation system manifest as bruising, bleeding, or other systemic signs of internal hemorrhage. Acute renal failure, severe hepatic injury, and pulmonary edema are other findings in heat stroke. Absence of sweating, although classically taught as the *sine non qua* of heat stroke, is not a reliable sign; patients with heat stroke may still produce sweat.[1,3,6]

Management

INITIAL SUPPORT

Supportive care for heat stroke, as for any emergency situation, requires following the appropriate algorithms for the primary assessment, including the ABCs. Endotracheal intubation should be performed if the airway is not secured and supplemental oxygen administered for patients with evidence of hypoxemia. Large bore intravenous lines should be established and isotonic fluids such as 0.9% saline or lactated Ringer's solutions should be used for volume replacement. **Since patients with heat stroke are prone to develop pulmonary edema and acute renal failure, fluids should always be administered judiciously.**[1] During the process of cooling, peripheral vasoconstriction occurs, requiring mild to moderate fluid replacement to increase blood pressure.

COOLING METHODS

Rapid reduction of body temperature is the first priority in heat stroke and should begin in the field.[1] Although the optimal cooling method remains controversial, all patients should be removed from the hot environment, with clothing removed and skin kept wet. Ice packs may be placed over the groin, axilla, and neck, to help decrease the core body temperature. Ice water immersion, a controversial technique, is not practical outside the hospital, but can be accomplished in the emergency room. Hazards associated with this technique include peripheral vasoconstriction with shunting of blood away from the skin, induced shivering, patient discomfort, and difficulties with patient monitoring.[1]

Antipyretics such as aspirin or acetaminophen are contraindicated in heat stroke and may be harmful. Acetaminophen can aggravate liver damage and aspirin may worsen heat-induced bleeding disorders.[1] Alcohol sponge baths should not be used because a large amount of alcohol can be absorbed through the skin, leading to alcohol toxicity.

DEFINITIVE CARE

Once stabilized in the emergency room, cooling should be discontinued in order to avoid hypothermia. If other methods fail, evaporative cooling can be done by spraying the patient's body with atomized water while blowing warm air across the skin surface.[10] Since shivering is a common complication of cooling, intravenous chlorpromazine may be used to prevent this complication.[6] The systemic complications of heat stroke can be severe and are best managed in the intensive care unit.

References

1. Khosla R, Guntupalli KK. Heat-related illness. *Crit Care Clin* 1999; 15(2): 251-263.

2. Malamud N, Haymaker W, Custer RP. Heat stroke: A clinicopathologic study of 125 fatal cases. *Mil Surg* 1946; 99: 397.

3. Shibolet S, Lancaster MC, Danon Y. Heat stroke: A review. *Aviat Space Environ Med* 1976; 47: 280.

4. Worfolk JB. Heat waves: Their impact on the health of elders. *Geriatr Nurs* 2000; 21(2): 70-77.

5. Waters TA. Heat illness: Tips for recognition and treatment. *Cleve Clin J Med* 2001; 68(8): 685-687.

6. Caramori-Kriger AC. Chapter 1—Case studies in hyperthermia. *In:* Gluck EH, Franklin CM (eds.). *Critical Care Medicine Board Review Manual: Environmental Hazards.* Crit Care Med 1998; 3(2): 1-9.

7. Keel CA, Neil E, Joels N. Regulation of body temperature in man. *In:* Wright, S. *Applied Physiology.* 13th Edition. New York: Oxford University Press, 1982. 346.

8. Dinarello CA. Infectious complications of cancer therapy: Thermoregulation and the pathogenesis of fever. *Infect Dis Clin North Am* 1996; 10(2): 433-439.

9. Bottoni TN. Neuroleptic malignant syndrome: A brief review. *Hospital Physician* 2002; 58-63.

10. Weiner JS, Kogali M. A physiological body cooling unit for treatment of heat stroke. *Lancet* 1980; 1: 507.

Review Questions

1. A 73-year-old is found in her apartment with a rectal temperature of 42°C (107°F). The patient is diagnosed with nonexertional heat stroke. All of the following statements about this condition are true EXCEPT:
   A. Hydration status is the most important independent risk factor for developing heat stroke
   B. Heat stroke is generally defined as a temperature above 41°C (106°F)
   C. The hypothalamic thermoregulatory center remains unchanged with hyperpyrexia
   D. Dry, hot environments place patients at greater risk for heat stroke than hot, humid environments
   E. Untreated heat stroke can cause myocardial damage that leads to full cardiopulmonary arrest

Hot, humid environments place a patient at the greatest risk for developing heat stroke. The thermoregulatory center changes with fever, not hyperpyrexia. The answer is D.

2. Field management of the patient in Question 1 includes which of the following:
   A. Judicious administration of intravenous fluids
   B. Sodium dantrolene intravenously
   C. Acetaminophen
   D. Alcohol sponge baths
   E. Gradual reduction of body temperature with cooling techniques

The answer is A.

3. Risk factors for heat stroke include all of the following EXCEPT:
   A. Alcoholism
   B. Infections
   C. Obesity
   D. Poverty
   E. All of the above

The answer is E.

Match the following patients with heat-related conditions to the correct patho-physiologic processes. Answers may be used once, more than once, or not at all.

    A. Volume depletion, hyperthermia
    B. Electrolyte imbalances
    C. Orthostatic pooling of blood
    D. Vasodilation with interstitial fluid accumulation
    E. Blockage of sweat pores by macerated stratum corneum; occasional infection

4. A 55-year-old patient with weakness, dizziness, headache, sweating, and elevated body temperature
5. A 26-year-old military recruit with bilateral carpopedal spasm and perioral numbness
6. Cramps in both calves of an 18-year-old soccer player
7. 6-month-old female with an itchy, red rash

4. The answer is A. (Heat exhaustion)

5. The answer is B. (Heat tetany)

6. The answer is B. (Heat cramps)

7. The answer is E. (Prickly heat)

Appendices

I. Pharmocology of Rapid Sequence Intubation

II. Essentials of 12-Lead Electrocardiograph Interpretation

III. Essentials of Acid-Base Interpretation

Pharmacology of Rapid Sequence Intubation

Introduction

Rapid sequence **induction** is the term used by anesthesiologists to describe the initiation of anesthesia. Rapid sequence **intubation** (RSI) pertains to emergency intubation facilitated by the use of sedative and paralytic agents. The use of RSI is predicated on several principles. RSI is indicated when less invasive means to maintain an airway and ventilation are unsuccessful in a patient with a suspected full stomach or when intubation without RSI is unlikely to be successful. RSI optimizes the safety of emergency intubation by allowing combative patients to be sedated, by decreasing upper airway muscle tone to simplify atraumatic intubation, and by preventing adverse sympathetic responses (*e.g.*, increased intracranial pressure) to direct laryngoscopy and intubation. The only contraindication for RSI includes any condition preventing bag-valve mask (BVM) ventilation because this is the alternative means of ventilating a patient after a failed RSI attempt. **RSI is not indicated for cardiac arrest patients or in patients with an anticipated difficult airway.** The RSI provider must be skilled at performing back-up airway techniques such as BVM ventilation and needle cricothryoidotomy.

Sequence of RSI

The 7 Ps describe the order of events when preparing a patient for RSI (Table A-1). The first step in RSI is pre-oxygenation with 100% oxygen by nonrebreather mask. **BVM ventilation is not part of the normal RSI protocol, but gentle ventilatory assistance can be provided in near-apneic patients.** Premedication with agents such as fentanyl, lidocaine, atropine, or defasiculating paralytics is accomplished next to help prevent the side effects of RSI. After 3 minutes, a sedative agent is administered to induce anesthesia. Paralytics such as succinylcholine or rocuronium are then administered to provide upper airway relaxation and suppression of gag reflexes. Once these agents are given, cricoid pressure (Sellick's maneuver) is applied for 30 seconds. During this time, the patient should be assessed for jaw relaxation, decreased resistance to BVM ventilation if used, and apnea. Intubation is performed next and should be accomplished **within 20 seconds.** Once the endotracheal tube is in place, placement should be assessed by 5-point lung auscultation, bilateral chest rise and fall with ventilations, pulse oximetry, and end-tidal CO_2. Bulb aspiration devices such as the esophageal detector device (EDD) are another means of secondary confirmation of successful tube placement. The tube should be secured appropriately and additional sedative and paralytic infusions are given to maintain anesthesia.

Table A-1
The 7 Ps of Rapid Sequence Intubation

RSI Step	Time Interval	Pharmacologic Agents
Preoxygenation	0-3 minutes	Oxygen
Premedication	3 minutes	Fentanyl, lidocaine, atropine, defasciculating agents (*e.g.*, vecuronium)
Paralysis after sedation	3.5-5.5 minutes*	Thiopental, midazolam, ketamine, etomidate; **then**: succinylcholine, rocuronium (see text)
Placement/performance	6-6.5 minutes	Oxygen, BVM
Placement/primary confirmation	6.5-7 minutes	Oxygen, BVM
Placement/secondary confirmation	7-7.5 minutes	Oxygen, BVM
Post-intubation management	7.5 + minutes	Nondepolarizing agents, midazolam infusion, etc.

*Wait 30 seconds after paralytic administered

Pharmacology of Premedication Agents

LIDOCAINE AND ATROPINE

Lidocaine can be given either topically or parenterally to help suppress coughing and other adverse airway reflexes such as laryngospasm and bronchospasm during instrumentation of the pharynx. Lidocaine is reported to help prevent a rise in intracranial pressure during intubation, conferring a possible cerebroprotective effect in head injured patients. Atropine, a parasympathetic blocker, is useful for preventing secretions and bradycardia when RSI is used in children. It is also reported to help reduce nausea and is recommended for any pediatric patient receiving succinylcholine. Glycopyrrolate (Robinul®) is similar to atropine, although due to its quaternary ammonium structure, is ionized at physiologic pH and does not cross the blood brain barrier, producing less sedation and central nervous system side effects than atropine.

FENTANYL

Fentanyl citrate (Sublimaze®) is an injectable opioid analgesic with an onset of action of 7 to 8 minutes and duration of 1 to 2 hours. 100meg of fentanyl is equivalent to approximately 10 mg of morphine sulfate. All opiates act at the $\mu1$, $\mu2$, sigma, and kappa opioid receptors. Activation of the mu1 receptor provides analgesia and activation of $\mu2$ receptors are responsible for the sedative and respiratory depressive properties of opiates. Hemodynamic responses to intubation, such as elevation of the ICP, can be blunted when fentanyl is administered because of an attenuation in sympathetic output; however, if fentanyl is abruptly discontinued in a patient hemodynamically dependent on increased sympathetic stimulation, catastrophic cardiovascular collapse can occur. Fentanyl provides analgesia and sedation but not amnesia. The effect of respiratory depression is synergistic with benzodiazepines such as midazolam and can be antagonized by naloxone (Narcan®) or nalmefene (Revex®).

Fentanyl can be used for the preanesthetic medication, induction, and maintenance of anesthesia for short duration and is often used to supplement general anesthetics. It is a useful agent for RSI in patients with head injury or hypertensive patients with pulmonary edema. It should not be used in hypotensive patients even though unlike morphine, fentanyl does not release histamine and is usually only associated with hypotension in a severely compromised patient dependent on excessive sympathetic outflow for hemodynamic support. Fentanyl is contraindicated in pediatric patients or patients with status epilepitcus. High doses of fentanyl prolong clinical effects because of the high lipid solubility and widespread distribution in adipose tissue. Respiratory depression is a known complication of all parenteral opioids, and may be significantly increased when fentanyl is co-administered with benzodiazepines, alcohol, or any central nervous system depressant. Chest wall rigidity is a rare, dose-dependent complication and cannot be reliably reversed with naloxone.

NONDEPOLARIZING PARALYTICS
Nondepolarizing paralytics reversibly block the acetylcholine receptor at the neuromuscular junction, but do not activate it. As such, they do not cause effects such as elevated potassium and fasciculations that are associated with depolarization at the neuromuscular junction. Unlike succinylcholine, ICP is not increased with nondepolarizing agents, although ICP is nearly always elevated during direct larngoscopy. Representative agents include vecuronium (Norcuron®), rocuronium bromide (Zemuron®), and rapacuronium (Rapalon®). Vecuronium has a dramatically slower onset of action than succinylcholine (5 minutes) and is therefore not an agent of choice for paralysis since BVM ventilation may be required if intubation attempts are prolonged. This drug is used primarily as a defasciculant and can also be given as an infusion to maintain paralysis after intubation. Rocuronium bromide has a faster onset of action than vecuronium (90-120 seconds) and is therefore an acceptable paralytic agent for use in RSI. As with vecuronium, this agent has a long duration of action (45 minutes - 1 hour) and can also be used to maintain paralysis after intubation. Rapacuronium has nearly the same onset of action as succinylcholine (30-60 seconds) but has a shorter duration of action than the other nondepolarizing agents (20 minutes). It should be used with caution in patients with hypotension, asthma, or COPD because it causes moderate histamine release as the result of mast cell degranulation, leading to hypotension in susceptible patients. Benadryl is the appropriate antidote if hypotension develops in a patient treated with rapacuronium.

Pharmacology of Sedative Agents

ETOMIDATE

Etomidate (Amidate®) is an imidazole compound, unrelated to benzodiazepines or barbiturates, that has a rapid onset of action (30 seconds) and short duration of action (3-5 minutes). It decreases ICP and intraocular pressure while maintaining cerebral perfusion, and reliably produces adequate sedation for RSI, although without analgesia or amnesia. Etomidate has a favorable hemodynamic profile when compared to other sedatives used in RSI. **For these reasons, etomidate is widely regarded as the current sedative of choice for use with RSI.** Side effects associated with use include nausea, local pain at the injection site, and occasional reemergence reactions. Reemergence phenomenon are attributed to etomidate's moderate dissociative effects. Other side effects include persistent muscle movement (myoclonus) and an occasional increase in seizure activity. In critically ill patients, etomidate may cause adrenal insufficiency. Etomidate should be used with caution in asthmatics.

MIDAZOLAM

Midazolam (Versed®) is a rapid-acting water-soluble benzodiazepine used to provide sedation and amnesia in RSI. Midazolam, like all benzodiazepines, activates gamma-aminobutyric acid (GABA) receptors, inducing muscle relaxation and sedation, and is also an anticonvulsant. This agent does not have analgesic properties, so if pain control is a priority, premedication with fentanyl or other analgesics is suggested. **Of all the sedative agents available, midazolam is the most likely to cause respiratory depression, especially when used with fentanyl.** Since all benzodiazepines have myocardial depressant properties, hypotension due to decreased cardiac output is an important potential adverse effect; for this reason, midazolam is not recommended for hypotensive patients. The antidote for benzodiazepines, Flumazenil (Romazicon®), can reverse sedation and respiratory depression, but can not reverse hypotension since this is a direct effect not mediated by GABA receptors. For hypotension, fluid boluses are the treatment of choice. Midazolam is rapid acting (3-5 minutes) and lasts about 30 minutes, but may have a delayed onset and inconsistent effect in some patients.

PROPOFOL

Propofol (Diprivan®) is an emulsified sedative with a very rapid onset of action (5-10 minutes) and short duration of action. It is widely used for maintenance sedation rather than RSI, and has potent antiemetic and anticonvulsant properties, without an analgesic effect. Since propofol lowers ICP to the point of decreasing intracranial blood flow, it is not recommended for patients with head injury and hypotension. Propofol is not recommended for patients with heart failure or asthma, as it has the potential for myocardial and respiratory depression as well as bronchospasm and laryngospasm.

KETAMINE

Ketamine (Ketalar®) is a dissociative agent with a rapid onset (3-5 minutes) with analgesic, amnestic, and sedative properties that last only 5 to 10 minutes. As a dissociative agent, ketamine works to remove the sense of the physical from the conscious. It is also a potent bronchodilator and does not affect airway control or ventilation at low doses, making it an ideal choice for use in asthmatic patients. Since blood pressure is usually preserved with ketamine, it may be used in patients with hypotension. Side effects associated with ketamine include excessive salivation, increased intraocular pressure, occasional laryngospasm, increased heart rate, nausea, and vomiting. Use of ketamine should be avoided in patients with glaucoma, uncontrolled hypertension, or eye injuries; atropine can be used to diminish secretions. Emergence reactions are common after the effects of ketamine wear off and are described by patients as severe nightmares upon reawakening. Benzodiazepines are the drugs of choice for this side effect. Ketamine is a sedative of choice for RSI in children; the risk of re emergence phenomenon is reported to be low for patients under the age of 10.

METHOHEXITAL

This rapidly acting (30-60 seconds) barbiturate sedative decreases ICP but has no analgesic properties. Barbiturates are highly lipid-soluble compounds and readily cross the blood-brain barrier. The action of the inhibitory neurotransmitter gamma-aminobutyric acid (GABA) is enhanced by barbiturates at the postsynaptic membranes, depressing neural activity in both nerve and muscle tissue. Methohexital (Brevital®) has a short duration of action (5-10 minutes) and should not be used in hypotensive patients or in patients with seizure disorders. Respiratory depression, laryngospasm, blood abnormalities (porphyria) and hiccupping are other potential side effects.

THIOPENTAL

Thiopental (Pentothal®) is another ultra short acting (10-20 minutes) barbiturate used in RSI. This agent is an anticonvulsant and decreases ICP, therefore making it another agent of choice in head-injured patients. Disadvantages include hypotension, myocardial and respiratory depression, and histamine release. Use should be avoided in asthmatics, hypotensive patients, and patients with porphyria.

SCOPOLAMINE

As a minimally sedative inductive agent, scopolamine does not have any analgesic properties, but it is a potent amnestic. This agent can be considered for patients in extremies, when other induction agents are contraindicated for fear of exacerbating preexisting hypotension. Onset of action occurs in 10 to 20 seconds and lasts up to an hour. Like atropine, this medication is an anticholinergic parasympathetic blocker, so atropine should never be co-administered. Tachycardia, mental status changes, and other anticholinergic side effects are common. The toxicity of anticholinergic compounds such as scopolamine and atropine can be remembered with the mnemonic provided in Table A-2.

Table A-2

Mnemonic for Remembering the Signs of Anticholinergic Toxicity
Hot as Hades
Blind as a bat
Dry as a bone
Red as a beet
Mad as a hatter

Pharmacology of Paralytic Agents

SUCCINYLCHOLINE

For most RSI situations, succinylcholine (Anectine®) is the paralytic of choice because of its rapid onset, short duration, and reliable pharmacodynamic profile. Succinylcholine provides neuromuscular blockade by irreversibly binding to nicotinic muscle receptors. It remains bound to these receptors, maintaining the motor end plate in a state of constant depolarization. By keeping the end-plate from repolarizing, the drug causes muscle relaxation leading to flaccid paralysis until plasma levels decline and the drug dissociates from the receptors (Figure A-1).

Paralysis produced by succinylcholine is preceded by transient contractions (fasciculations); for this reason, low doses of nondepolarizing paralytics should be given beforehand to attenuate this side effect. Muscle pain, fasciculations, muscle breakdown, hyperkalemia, and hypertension are adverse effects associated with succinylcholine. For these reasons, this agent is contraindicated in burns, preexisting hyperkalemia, renal failure, or neuromuscular disorders. Succinylcholine increases intraocular, intragastric, and intracranial pressures and should not be used in patients with eye injury, glaucoma, or increased ICP. In some instances, malignant hyperthermia, discussed briefly in Chapter 30, is a potentially fatal drug reaction; sodium dantrolene is the antidote. Rarely, succinylcholine can lead to bradycardia or asystole. Succinylcholine should only be used in pediatric patients older than 5 years of age when a nondepolarizing agent can be administered in conjunction to prevent fasciculations. Succinylcholine should be avoided if a difficult airway is anticipated or if doubt exists regarding the potential success of providing BVM ventilations in the event of a failed RSI attempt. The agent should not be used in patients with a known family or personal history of malignant hyperthermia.

NONDEPOLARIZING PARALYTICS

Due to an improved side effect profile, rocuronium and rapacuronium are becoming alternative agents of choice to succinylcholine. These agents have been discussed in detail previously in this appendix.

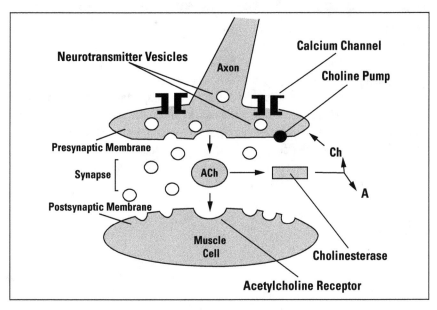

Figure A-1 The neuromuscular junction.

Maintenance of Paralysis and Sedation

Once RSI is successful and endotracheal placement is confirmed, sedative and paralytic infusions should be started to maintain induction and to prevent extubation. Infusions of nondepolarizing paralytics such as rocuronium, vecuronium, pancuronium, and atracuronium have a duration of action that varies according to agent, but usually last longer than 20 minutes and less than 1 hour. **It is important to remember that whenever a paralytic is administered, an appropriate sedative must be co-administered.** Paralysis in an otherwise awake patient is a frightening condition for the patient and leads to adverse effects related to agitation such as tachycardia and hypertension. Midazolam and propofol are the two most commonly used sedative agents administered by parenteral infusion (Tables A-3 and A-4).

Table A-3
The Onset and Duration of Action for Pharmacologic Agents Used in RSI

Class	Agent	Onset	Duration (Minutes)
Sedatives	Etomidate	30-45 seconds	10-20
	Midazolam	2-3 minutes	20-30
	Propofol	10-30 seconds	8-10
	Ketamine	30-60 seconds	5-20
	Methohexital	30-60 seconds	5-10
	Thiopental	10-40 seconds	10-20
	Scopolamine	10-20 seconds	60
Paralytics	Succinylcholine	45-60 seconds	6-12
	Rapacuronium	45-75 seconds	20-30
	Rocuronium	45-75 seconds	30-60
	Vecuronium	2-5 minutes	25-40
	Atracuronium	3-5 minutes	20-35
	Pancuronium	3-5 minutes	45-60

Table A-4
RSI Agents for Different Clinical Scenarios

Condition	Premedication	Sedation	Paralytic
Isolated mild hypotension	Defasciculating paralytic	Etomidate, midazolam*, ketamine	Succinylcholine, rocuronium
Isolated head injury	Lidocaine, fentanyl	Etomidate, thiopental, propofol	Rapacuronium, rocuronium
Hypotension and head injury	Lidocaine, fentanyl	Etomidate, thiopental, propofol, midazolam	Rapacuronium, rocuronium
Severe hypotension	Lidocaine, defasciculating paralytic	Ketamine, etomidate*, midazolam*, scopolamine	Succinylcholine, rapacuronium, rocuronium
Status asthmaticus	Defasciculating paralytic	Ketamine, etomidate, propofol	Succinylcholine, Rapacuronium, Rocuronium
Status epilepticus	Lidocaine	Thiopental, propofol, midazolam	Rapacuronium, rocuronium
Pulmonary edema	Fentanyl, defasciculating paralytic	Etomidate, midazolam *	Succinylcholine, rapacuronium, rocuronium
Burns	Fentanyl, lidocaine	Etomidate, midazolam	Rapacuronium, rocuronium
Pediatric patients	Atropine, defasciculating paralytic	Ketamine, etomidate, midazolam	Succinylcholine, rapacuronium, rocuronium

* Lower dosages

References

American Society of Anesthesiologists Task Force on management of the Difficult Airway: Practice Guidelines for Management of the Difficult Airway. *Anesthesiology* 1993; 78:597.

Blackburn P, Vissers R. Pharmacology of emergency department pain management and conscious sedation. Emerg Med Clin North Am 2000; 18(4): 803-827.

Gerardi MJ, Sacchetti AD, Cantor RM *et al.* (Pediatric Emergency Medicine Committee of the American College of Emergency Physicians). Rapid-sequence intubation of the pediatric patient. Ann Emerg Med 1996; 28(1): 263-267.

Hazinski MF, Cummins RO, Field JM (Eds.). *2000 Handbook of Emergency Cardiovascular Care for Healthcare Providers.* Dallas, TX: American Heart Association, 2000.

Horak J, Weiss S. Emergent management of the airway: New pharmacology and the control of comorbidities in cardiac disease, ischemia, and valvular heart disease. *Crit Care Clin* 2000; 16(3): 411-427.

Ho IK, Harris RA. Mechanisms of action of barbiturates. *Annu Rev Pharmacol Toxicol* 1981; 21:83.

Medical Economics: Thompson Healthcare (Editorial Staff). *Physician's Desk Reference: 2001.* 55th Edition. Montvale, NJ: Medical Economics Co., 2001.

Orebaugh SL. Succinylcholine: Adverse effects and alternatives in emergency medicine. *Amer J Emerg Med* 1999; 17(7): 715-721.

Rodricks M, Deutschman CS. Emergent airway management: Indications and methods in the face of confounding conditions. *Crit Care Clin* 2000; 16(3): 389-409.

Sivilotti MLA, Ducharme J. Randomized, double-blind study on sedative and hemodynamics during rapid-sequence intubation in the emergency department: The SHRED study. *Ann Emerg Med* 1998; 31: 313.

Tintinalli JE, Kelen GD, Stapczynski JS. *Emergency Medicine: A Comprehensive Study Guide.* 5th Edition. New York: McGraw-Hill, 2000.

Wadbrook PS. Advances in airway pharmacology: Emerging trends and evolving controversy. *Emerg Med Clin North Am* 2000; 18(4): 767-788.

Essentials of 12-Lead Electrocardiograph Interpretation

The key to successfully interpreting the electrocardiograph (ECG) is to employ a structured, systematic approach.

Lead Placement

PRECORDIAL LEADS

The precordial leads evaluate electrical impulses from the heart in the horizontal or transverse plane (Figure AA-1).

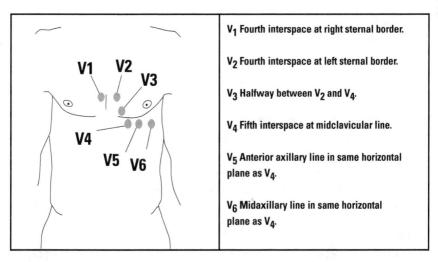

Figure AA-1 Precordial Leads.

Posterior Precordial Leads

Three posterior precordial leads can be placed along the fifth intercostal space starting laterally (V_7) at the posterior axillary line, medially next to the vertebral column (V_9), and between V_7 and V_9 (V_8). To use these leads, simply place the precordial leads at these locations and label the ECG appropriately according to the changed V leads.

STANDARD LIMB LEADS

The standard limb leads evaluate electrical impulses generated from the edges of the frontal plane as if it were flat or uni-dimensional (Figure AA-2).

Bipolar limb leads are placed at the right anterior shoulder (white), the left lateral aspect of the rib cage (red), and the left anterior shoulder (black). A memory device for remembering limb lead placement is, **"white for right, smoke (black) over fire (red)."** The unipolar limb leads consist of aVR, aVL, and aVF. Lead aVR is placed on the right arm, usually at the right wrist, and aVL is placed on the left arm. Lead aVF is placed near either foot, typically at the ankle.

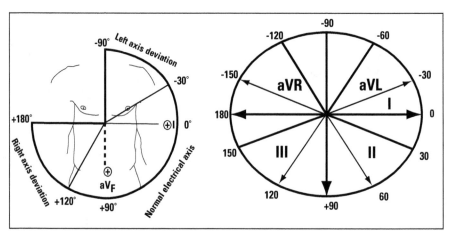

Figure AA-2 Hexaxial Reference System.

Systematic Approach to Interpretation

SYSTEMATIC ANALYSIS

A systematic analysis should be used when interpreting an ECG. A six-step sequence is recommended, with a stepwise analysis of **rate, rhythm, axis, intervals, infarct, and chambers.**

Rate

There are two methods for measuring rate. The large squares between R-waves can be counted for a rough estimation (Table AA-1).

For a more precise determination, 300 is divided by the number of large boxes in any given R-R interval. For example, if 5 large boxes are within one R-R interval, 300 divided by 5 equals 60 beats per minute. This method should only be used for regular rhythms.

Rhythm

Axis deviation can be determined by finding the most isoelectric QRS complex in leads I, II, II, aVR, aVL, or aVF. The isoelectric QRS complex is that with the lowest voltage and approximately 50% deflection above and below the isoelectric line (*i.e.,* ECG baseline).

Table AA-1

1 Square = **300** bpm
2 Squares = **150** bpm
3 Squares = **100** bpm
4 Squares =   **75** bpm
5 Squares =   **60** bpm
6 Squares =   **50** bpm

The perpendicular arrow to the isoelectric lead is identified on the hexaxial reference chart, and the indicated degree of axis deviation is found by following the arrow (Figure AA-3).

Another quick and easy method for determining axis deviation involves checking the QRS complexes in leads I and aVF (Table AA-2). If both QRS complexes in leads I and aVF are positive, the axis is normal.

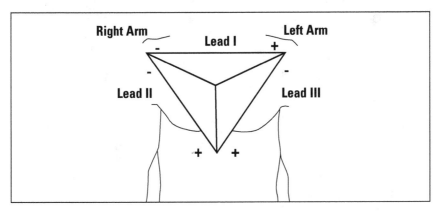

Figure AA-3 Limb Leads.

Table AA-2

Axis Deviation			
Normal Axis	**Right Axis** (90 to180°)	**Left Axis** (0 to -90°)	**Pathological Left Axis** (greater than -30°)
Lead I positive	Lead aVF positive	Lead I negative	Lead aVF positive
Lead I positive	Lead aVF negative	Lead I positive	Lead aVF negative

Intervals

The P-R interval, QRS complex, and QT interval should be checked for normalcy. A normal P-R interval is 0.12 to 0.21 seconds long; a normal QRS complex is 0.04-0.10 seconds. A widened QRS complex should raise the suspicion for a bundle branch block (BBB; Table AA-3).

The QT interval should be less than half the R-R interval and can be calculated by dividing the measured QT interval (QTc) by the square root of the R-R interval. A reference should be consulted for normal male and female values since the QTc varies according to age, sex, and heart rate. In general, if the QTc is greater than 0.40 seconds with a heart rate of 70, it is considered abnormal. The QTc is abnormally shortened in conditions such as hypercalcemia and abnormally prolonged with certain medications. An abnormally prolonged QTc interval is a risk factor for developing the dysrhythmia **torsades des pointes.**

Table AA-3

Bundle Branch Blocks (BBB)			
Right BBB	**Left BBB**	**Left Anterior Hemiblock**	**Left Posterior Hemiblock**
1. Wide QRS (>0.11)	1. Wide QRS (>0.12)	1. Normal QRS; no ST-segment changes	1. Normal QRS; no ST-segment changes
2. Wide S in I and V_6	2. Upright QRS in lead I and V_6	2. Abnormal left axis	2. Right axis deviation
3. RSR' in V_1	3. Negative QRS in lead V_1	3. Small Q in lead I	3. Small Q in lead III
4. Positive QRS in left leads	4. No Q waves	4. Small R in lead III	4. Small R in lead I

Infarct

Electrocardiographic evidence of myocardial infarction manifests as ST-segment changes, Q waves, T wave abnormalities, and poor R wave progression. **ST-segment elevation is significant if greater than 1 mm in two or more contiguous leads** (Table AA-4).

Q waves can be a normal variant in leads I, aVL, and V 4-6, but if greater than one-third the height of the QRS complex, they are clinically significant. T waves may be inverted as a normal variant in leads III, aVF, aVL, and V1. Biphasic T waves are discussed in the chapter on myocardial infarction; these abnormal T waves are common in non-Q wave myocardial infarction. Large, tented T waves are a common finding with hyperkalemia.

Chambers

Signs of atrial or ventricular enlargement may be evident on the ECG (Table AA-5).

Two sets of criteria used to determine left ventricular hypertrophy (LVH) are the Sokolow-Lyon indices and Cornell voltage criteria.

Table AA-4

Myocardial Infarction

Location	Inferior Wall	Anterior Wall	Lateral Wall	Right Ventricle	Posterior Wall
Leads	II, III, aVF	V_1-V_4	I, aVL, V_5, V_6	V_4R	V_1-V_3*, V_7-V_9
Anatomy	Right coronary (90%) left circumflex (10%)	Left anterior descending (LAD)	Left circumflex, LAD, right coronary	Right coronary	Left circumflex, dominant right coronary
Caveats	Associated with high degree of AV block	RBBB, left anterior hemiblock, type II AV blocks possible since ventricular septum involved	Isolated lateral wall MI usually involves the left circumflex	Associated with reduced cardiac output	*ST depression in these leads, not elevation
	Associated with higher mortality and lower ejection fraction when reciprocal changes are present			Commonly associated with inferior wall MI	Common with either inferior or lateral MI
				Associated with high degree AV block	

Table AA-5

Chamber Enlargements			
Left Ventricular Hypertrophy	**Right Ventricular Hypertrophy**	**Left Axis Deviation**	**Right Axis Deviation**
Sum of S in V_1 and R in V_5 or V_6 greater than 35 mm	Right axis deviation	M shape of P wave in lead II	Increased initial deflection of P wave in lead II and/or V_1
R in aVL greater than or equal to 11 mm	QRS slightly negative in lead I	Biphasic P wave in V_1	P wave duration not prolonged
(men): S in V_3 plus R in aVL greater than 28 mm	R > S in V_1	P wave duration > 0.12	P wave amplitude increased > .25 mV
	S > R in V_6	No increased P wave amplitude	
	Right atrial enlargement		
(women): S in V_3 plus R in aVL greater than 20 mm	Strain pattern in leads II, III, aVF, $V_{1\text{-}3}$		

References

Stein E. *Rapid Analysis of Electrocardiograms-A Self Study Program.* Second Edition. Lea and Febiger, 1992.

Wagner G. *Marriot's Practical Electrocardiograph.* 9th Edition. New York: Lippincott Williams & Wilkins, 1994.

Hurst JW. *Ventricular Electrocardiography.* Georgia: JW Hurst, 1998.

Essentials of Acid-Base Interpretation

Prehospital providers are not required to interpret acid-base problems, but an elementary understanding is strongly encouraged. As many providers progress to teach advanced level courses such as ACLS and PALS—courses that use acid-base data in testing scenarios, the ability to solve these problems is essential for effective instruction. Other readers, including medical students and allied health professionals involved in emergency medicine, will benefit from the simplified approach to solving acid-base problems presented here.

Physiologic Basis

A buffer is any substance that reversibly binds hydrogen ions. Bicarbonate is the foremost extracellular buffer in the human body; that is, bicarbonate helps regulate the hydrogen-ion concentration in the fluids outside of cells.

$$CO_2 + H_2O \underset{\text{Carbonic anhydrase}}{\rightleftharpoons} H_2CO_3 \rightleftharpoons H+ + HCO_3^-$$

Carbonic acid   Bicarbonate

$$H^+ \text{ Buffer} \longleftarrow H^+ + \text{ Buffer}$$

The bicarbonate extracellular buffer system. Bicarbonate reversibly binds to hydrogen to neutralize free hydrogen ions.

The physiology of the bicarbonate-buffer system is discussed in Chapters 3 and 17.

Acid-base data is obtained from an arterial blood gas analysis. This analysis provides information on levels of arterial oxygen, carbon dioxide, bicarbonate, pH, and base excess.

Normal Values

A prerequisite for interpreting acid-base problems is an understanding of normal values for pH, PCO_2, and bicarbonate (HCO_3), the rules of interpretation, and the formulas for expected changes in certain instances. The first step is understanding the normal values (Table AAA-1).

Table AAA-1

Normal Values for pH, Carbon Dioxide, and Bicarbonate

$$pH = 7.35\text{-}7.45$$
$$PCO_2 = 35\text{-}45 \text{ mm Hg}$$
$$HCO_3 = 22\text{-}26 \text{ mEq/L}$$

Rules of Interpretation

Rules 1 and 2 apply to metabolic disorders; rules 3 and 4 apply to respiratory disorders.

1. For metabolic disorders, the pH is abnormal and the pH and PCO_2 change in the same direction.

2. A superimposed (secondary) respiratory acid-base disorder is present if any of the following is/are present:

- The PCO_2 is normal
- The PCO_2 is higher than the expected PCO_2 (see formula below)
- The PCO_2 is less than the expected PCO_2 (see formula below)

3. For respiratory disorders, the PCO_2 is abnormal and the PCO_2 and pH change in opposite directions.

4. The expected change in pH (see formulas below) is used to determine whether the respiratory condition is acute or chronic and whether a superimposed (secondary) metabolic acid-base disorder is present.

5. A mixed disorder (acidosis and alkalosis) is present if the PCO_2 is abnormal and the pH is unchanged or normal, or if the pH is abnormal and the PCO_2 unchanged or abnormal. The pH never returns to normal in an acid-base problem. Also, if a true mixed acid-base disorder is present, you cannot determine the primary or secondary disorder; the disorder is simply referred to as a mixed disorder.

These rules are summarized in the following table (Table AAA-2).

Table AAA-2
A Summary of the Rules for Acid-Base Interpretation

Disorder	pH	PCO₂	HCO₃
Metabolic acidosis	↓	↓	↓
Metabolic alkalosis	↑	↑	↑
Respiratory acidosis	↓	↑	↑
Respiratory alkalosis	↑	↓	↓

Compensation Formulas

Formulas are used to determine the expected changes in PCO_2 and pH. The formulas presented here have been taken from *The ICU Book* by Dr. Paul Marino, and are in the author's opinion, the easiest to use for solving acid-base problems (Table AAA-3).

Table AAA-3

Compensation Formulas		
Metabolic acidosis[*]	$PCO_2=$	1.5 x HCO_3 + (8+/-2)
Metabolic alkalosis	$PCO_2=$	0.7 x HCO_3 + (21+/-2)
Acute respiratory acidosis	pH change=	0.008 x (PCO_2-40)
Chronic respiratory acidosis	pH change=	0.003 x (PCO_2-40)
Acute respiratory alkalosis	pH change=	0.008 x (40-PCO_2)
Chronic respiratory alkalosis	pH change=	0.017 x (40-PCO_2)

*For metabolic acidosis, the Winter's formula is used. The other formulas do not have formal names.

The **anion gap** should be calculated if a triple or hidden (mixed) disorder is suspected (*e.g.*, metabolic acidosis, metabolic alkalosis, and respiratory acidosis). The conditions most commonly associated with mixed disorders are lactic acidosis, salicylate intoxication, and diabetic ketoacidosis. The anion gap is a simple formula that can be calculated from the results of a standard serum chemistry laboratory report. The physiology of the anion gap is beyond the scope of this text, but is explained in detail in the references listed at the end of this chapter. In some instances, calculation of the **osmolar** gap may reveal an acid-base problem related to methanol or ethylene glycol intoxication.

Anion Gap (normal 4-11)	serum sodium- [bicarbonate + chloride]
Osmolar Gap (normal 280-295)	2x sodium + glucose/18 + BUN /2.8

Applying the Three-Step Process

The above information can be used to solve any acid-base problem. Simply apply the following three-step process:

1. Identify the most apparent disorder by comparing with normal values

2. Apply the appropriate compensation formula

3. Calculate the anion gap

A potential fourth step would be to diagnose and correct the underlying disorder, but this can only be accomplished once the problem is solved to begin with. The following diagrams detail the extensive differential diagnosis for metabolic acid-base problems. Respiratory acid-base problems strongly correlate with a patient's clinical condition (*e.g.*, respiratory alkalosis in a hyperventilating patient) and usually have an uncomplicated differential diagnosis (Figures AAA-1 and AAA-2).

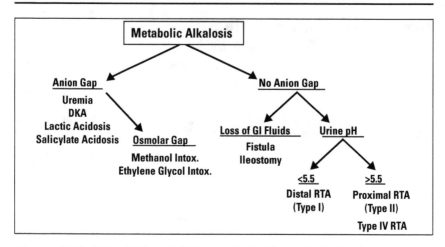

Figure AAA-1 The Differential Diagnosis For Metabolic Acidosis.

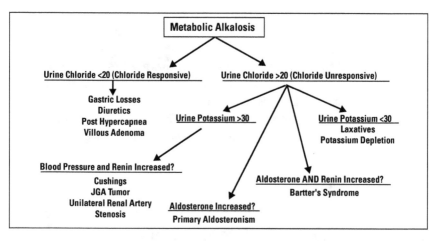

Figure AAA-2 The Differential Diagnosis for Metabolic Alkalosis.

Acid Base Notation

The results of arterial blood gases are usually abbreviated as shown in Table AAA-4.

Table AAA-4

An Example of Acid-Base Notation
pH / PCO$_2$ / HCO$_3$ / pO$_2$ / base excess
for example:
7.45/35/24/99/-1

References

Marino PL. *The ICU Book.* 2nd Edition. Philadelphia: Williams & Wilkins, 1998.

Preston RA. *Acid-Base, Fluids, and Electrolytes Made Ridiculously Simple.* Miami: MedMaster Inc., 1997.

Vander AJ, Sherman JH, Luciano DS. *Human Physiology: The Mechanisms of Body Function.* 6th Edition. New York: McGraw-Hill, 1994.

Index

Page numbers followed by an *f* indicate a figure; page numbers folowed by a *t* indicate a table.

A

Abciximab, 140*t*

ABCs

for gastrointestinal bleeding, 267
for heat stroke, 366
for hypovolemic shock, 190
for status epilepticus, 323-324
for subarachnoid hemorrhage, 313, 318

Abdomen
pain in
acute, 249, 254*t*, 256*t*
intra-abdominal, 251-252
periumbilical, 258
topography of, 251

Abdominal aortic aneurysm, 251, 252
diagnostic test for, 256*t*
ruptured, misdiagnosis of, 255*t*

Abdominal wall
lesions of, 259
pain of, 253

Absorption, 37

Acclimatization, 362

Acebutolol, 106*t*

Acetaminophen (Tylenol)
for acute ischemic stroke, 309-310
in heat stroke, 366

Acetoacetate, 221

Acetone, 221

Acetylcholine, 29, 31

Acidic drugs, protein binding of, 39 Acidosis. *See also* Ketoacidosis, diabetic; Metabolic acidosis
hemoglobin-oxygen dissociation curve in, 22

ACLS algorithm, 355

Action potentials, 89-92
altered automaticity on, 102*f*
biochemical activation of, 92
in cardiac contractility, 94-95
correlation of in S-A node and ventricles, 91*f*
electrophysiologic events in, 92
pacemaker, 90
phases of, 90
for ventricular muscle cells, 91*f*

Active transport, 7

Acute abdomen, 249, 258-259
dangerous mimics of, 255*t*

definitive care of, 256
extra-abdominal pain in, 252-255
intra-abdominal pain in, 251-252
physiology of, 250-251

Acute abdominal pain, 249
diagnostic tests for, 256*t*
eponyms or signs of, 254*t*

Acute coronary syndromes, 126-127
clinical classifications of, 119-120
management of, 123-124
myocardial infarction, 129-148
pathogenic mechanisms of, 120-122
pathologic processes in, 116*f*
pathophysiology of, 113-118
Venn diagram of, 113*f*

Acute surgical abdomen, 249

Acyclovir (Zovirax, Avirax), 287

Adamkiewicz artery, 338

Addison's disease
clinical diagnosis and management of, 236-237
pathogenesis of, 235-236

Adenosine, 107, 110

Adenosine triphosphate (ATP)
in active transport, 7
release of, 30*f*

Adenovirus, 288

Adenylate cyclase, 30
activation of, 51, 52*f*
at beta receptors, 31

Adrenal emergencies, 233-245

Adrenal glands
anatomical vulnerability of, 235-236
anatomy and physiology of, 235
cortex of, 235
histological layers of, 53*f*
medulla of, 235

Adrenal insufficiency, acute
clinical diagnosis and management of, 236-237
definitive care for, 237
factors increasing susceptibility for, 243
hallmark of, 243
pathogenesis of, 235-236
signs of, 244

Adrenergic agonists, 49-50

Adrenergic receptors, 30-31

Adrenocorticotrophic hormone (ACTH), 235
in adrenal insufficiency, 236

Adrenocorticotrophic hormone (ACTH) stimulation test, 237

Afterload, 92-93
  in myocardial ischemia, 120

Air embolus, 83

Air pollution, 71

Airway management
  for croup, 289
  for status epilepticus, 328

Airway zones, 45-46
  arborization of, 45*f*

Airways
  diameters of in adults versus children, 289*f*
  obstruction of
    in asthma, 63
    chronic, 71
  physiology of, 45
  upper, infections of, 287-289

Albumin, drug binding to, 39

Albuterol (Ventolin, Proventil)
  activating adenylate cyclase, 52*f*
  for asthma, 64
  for chronic obstructive pulmonary disease, 73-74
  mechanism of action of, 70
  pharmacology of, 51-52

Alcohol
  in gastrointestinal bleeding with, 267
  in hypoglycemia, 232
  in hypothermia, 352

Alcohol sponge baths, 366

Alcoholics, status epilepticus in, 325

Aldosterone, 150
  release of, 235

Aldosterone antagonists, 162

Allergens
  in anaphylactic reaction, 199
  in asthma, 60, 62

Allergic asthma, 59

Allergic reaction, 197-198

Alpha-1 receptors, 30

Alpha-2 receptors, 30

Alpha$_1$-antitrypsin deficiency, 71

Alpha receptors, 30

Alveolus, 46
  physiology of, 48-49

Amaurosis fugax, 306

Aminophylline, 52
  for asthma, 65

Aminosalicylic acid, 239

Amiodarone (Cordarone, Cordarone X)
  for dysrhythmia, 108
  in hypothyroidism, 239
  mechanism of action of, 106*t*, 112

Amniotic fluid embolus, 83

Amrinone, 163

Anaerobic metabolism, 186

Anaphylactic reactions, 197-199

Anaphylactic shock, 202-203
  agents for, 203
  anaphylactic reactions in, 197-199
  clinical manifestations of, 199
  definition of, 197
  Gell and Coombs classification of, 197, 198*t*
  management of, 199-200
  pathogenesis of, 197

Anaphylactoid reactions, 198

Anaphylaxis, late-phase, 203

Androgens, 235

Anemia, 27

Angina, 126-127
  clinical classifications of, 119-120
  ECG changes in, 122
  management of, 123-124
  pathogenic mechanisms of, 120-122
  stable or typical, 119
  unstable or pre-infarction, 119, 126
    definition of, 119
    diagnostic criteria for, 120*t*
  variant or vasospastic, 119

Angiodysplasia, 263

Angiography, 82

Angiotensin-converting enzyme (ACE), 150

Angiotensin-converting enzyme (ACE) inhibitors
  for angina, 127
  for chronic heart failure, 161-162, 163*t*
  for myocardial infarction, 140*t*, 141

Angiotensin I, 150

Angiotensin II, 150
  in hypertension, 171

Angiotensin receptor blockers, 162

Anoxia
  progressive cerebral ischemia and, 332, 333
  in status epilepticus, 320

Anterior cord syndrome, 342

Antianginal agents, 123, 127

Antibiotics
  for acute infective endocarditis, 292

hypersensitivity reaction to, 198
for meningitis, 285
for mucormycosis, 293
for pneumonia, 278

Anticholinergic agents
for asthma, 65
for chronic obstructive pulmonary disease, 74
pharmacology of, 53-54

Anticoagulants
in adrenal insufficiency, 236
for angina, 123, 127

Anticoagulation, 85

Anticonvulsants, 364*t*

Antidiuretic hormone, 186

Antidysrhythmics
Class I, 105, 106*t*
Class II, 106*t*, 107
Class III, 106*t*, 107
Class IV, 106*t*, 107
for dysrhythmias, 105-108
miscellaneous, 107-108
Vaughan-Williams classification of, 105-108

Antiepileptic drugs
poor compliance with, 327
for status epilepticus, 325

Antihistamine, 200

Antihypertensives, 178

Anti-inflammatory agents, 64, 68

Antioxidants, 131

Antiplatelet therapy, 123

Anti-shock positioning, 192-193

Antitussive agents, 273

Anxiety-related hypertension, 172

Aorta, coarctation of, 172

Aortic stenosis, 153

Apical impulse, 157

Apocrine glands, 361

Appendicitis, 250-251
diagnostic test for, 256*t*
early symptoms of, 258
misdiagnosis of, 255*t*

Arachidonic acid metabolites, 128

Arachidonic acid pathway, 199

Arterial blood gas analysis, 278

Arterial blood pressure, 330

Arterial occlusion

in acute ischemic stroke, 303-304
in stroke, 317

Arterioles, autonomic nervous system of, 32*t*

Arteriovenous malformations
in lower gastrointestinal bleeding, 263
in subarachnoid hemorrhage, 312

Arteriovenous rewarming, 355

Arthropod-borne encephalitis, 285-286
treatment of, 287

Aspirin
for acute myocardial infarction, 147
for angina, 123, 127
first-pass hepatic effect of, 40
in heat stroke, 366
for myocardial infarction, 138, 140*t*
with thrombolytics, 310

Asthma, 59, 68-70
beta-2 agonists in, 51-52
bronchial hyperresponsiveness in, 60
bronchodilators for, 54
cardiac, 158
clinical assessment of, 62-63
cough with, 275
diagnosis of, 56
early response in, 60*f*
emergency treatment of, 68
episodic, 62
extrinsic, 59, 69
incidence of, 59
intrinsic, 59
late response to, 62
lung capacity in, 48
management of, 64-65
chronic, 65-66
mediators of, 128
monitoring clinical response in, 65
pathogenesis of, 60-61
secondary phase of, 69
severity classification of, 63
silent chest in, 70
treatment of, 57
triggers of, 60-61

Asystole, with hypothermia, 353

Atenolol (Tenormin)
for angina, 123
for chronic heart failure, 163*t*
for myocardial infarction, 140*t*, 141

Atherosclerosis
in acute ischemic stroke, 303-304
with chronic or poorly controlled hypertension, 178*t*
hypertension and, 304
pain in, 252
risk factors for, 129-131

ATPase pumps, active transport, 9

Atrial fibrillation
with hypothermia, 352-353
intracardiac thrombi in, 304
thrombosis in, 316

Atrial natriuretic peptide, 152

Atrioventricular (A-V) bundle, 101

Atrioventricular (A-V) node, 101
action potentials of, 90
in cardiac contractility, 94-95

Auscultatory findings, in pneumonia, 276, 281

Autoimmune disease, 235-236

Automaticity, altered, 102

Autonomic nervous system
adrenergic receptors in, 30-31
in cardiac contractility, 94-95
cholinergic receptors in, 31
division of, 29, 32t
drug action sites in, 33f
hyperactivity of in neuroleptic malignant
syndrome, 363
neurotransmitters in, 31
organization of, 29
receptors of, 35
synapses in, 29-30

Axonal regeneration techniques, 343

B

B-complex vitamins, 239

Bacteremia
in septic shock, 205-206
sources for, 127

Bacterial pathogens
in meningitis, 283
in necrotizing skin and soft tissue infections, 293
in peritonitis, 252
in pneumonia, 272-273
in septic shock, 127-128
toxins of, 128

Bacteroides infections, 127

Barbiturates
for status epilepticus, 325
for traumatic brain injury, 338

Basophils
activation of, 199
in asthma, 62

Beck's triad, 291

Beclomethasone (Vanceril, Beclovent), 54

Benzodiazepines

mechanism of action of, 328
in neuroleptic malignant syndrome, 364t
for status epilepticus, 324, 328

Bernoulli's law, 98

Beta-2 agonists, 51-52
for asthma, 65
bronchodilatory effect of, 57
for chronic obstructive pulmonary disease, 73-74

Beta-1 receptors, 31

Beta-2 receptors, 31
bronchioles, 49-50
pharmacology of activation of, 51-52

Beta-adrenergic agonists, 64

Beta-blockers, 147
for angina, 123, 127
for chronic heart failure, 162, 163t
clinical trials for, 142t
contraindication to, 111
for dysrhythmia, 106t, 107
for myocardial infarction, 140t, 141
for thyroid storm, 239

Beta-carotene, 131

Beta-lactam antibiotics, 278

Beta receptors, 31

Bicarbonate
for diabetic ketoacidosis and hyperosmolar
hyperglycemic syndrome, 225
formation of, 24f
for hypovolemic shock, 192

Bicarbonate buffer system, 24
biochemistry of, 189f

Bi-level positive airway pressure (BiPAP), 159-160, 167

Biliary tract disease, 256t

Bioavailability, 38

Bioavailability curve, 39f

Biochemical cascade
in spinal cord trauma, 340
in traumatic brain injury, 332, 334f

Bisoprolol fumarate (Zebeta), 162, 163t

Bitolterol (Tornalate), 51-52

Bleeding, hypothermia-related, 354

Blindness, 306

Blood-brain barrier, 284f
bacteria passing, 285
compromise of in brain injury, 332-333

Blood coagulation cascade, 129

Blood cultures
for acute infective endocarditis, 292

for pneumonia, 278

Blood flow
catheter selection and, 190, 195
to myocardial layers, 121f
physics of, 190
pressure gradient driving, 94
to spinal cord, 340
through catheter, 98

Blood groups, 191t

Blood pressure
changes in with hypovolemic shock, 187-188
complications of indirect measurements of, 181
decreased in septic shock, 214
differences in, 94
measurement of in hypertension, 172-173
patient positioning and cuff placement for
measuring, 173
rate of rise of, 169
sympathetic nervous system effect on, 170f

Blood substitutes, 191-192

Blood transfusion
for gastrointestinal bleeding, 265
for hypovolemic shock, 191-192
Ringer's lactate solution and, 14, 18

Blood vessels
fluid flow into, 13
fluid out of, 12, 13f
permeability of, 12

Blood volume changes, 188

Bloody diarrhea, 263
causes of, 264t

Blue bloaters, 73

Blunt trauma, abdominal wall, 253

Body fluids, 11-19
distribution of, 12
forces affecting movement of, 12-13

Body temperature
regulation of, 352
response to heat in, 361-362

Bohr effect, 22

Bowel obstruction
diagnostic test for, 256t
misdiagnosis of, 255t

Boyle's law, 46, 98

Bradycardia
with hypothermia, 352-353
with myocardial infarction, 131

Brain
biopsy of for encephalitis, 286
edema of, 333

in cerebral stroke, 306
limited blood flow in, 303
normal physiology of, 329-330
oxygen metabolism in, 330
secondary injury of, 333
traumatic injury of
biochemical cascade in, 332, 334f
clinical classification of, 334-335
clinical manifestations of, 334-336
effects of hyperventilation for, 345
epidemiology of, 329
management of, 336-338, 347
pathogenesis of, 330-333

Brain cell, diffuse axonal injury of, 336

Brain death, 354

Brain imaging, 310

Bretylium, 106t

Bretylium tosylate, 355

Bronchial hyperresponsiveness, 60

Bronchial musculature, drug-induced relaxation of, 51

Bronchioles, 46
receptors of, 49-50

Bronchitis, 71
in chronic obstructive pulmonary disease, 72, 73
pathogenesis of, 73

Bronchoconstriction, 70

Bronchodilators
for asthma, 64
in asthma management, 66t
pharmacology of, 52

Bronchus, 46

Brown-Sequard syndrome, 342

Brudzinski's sign, 285

Budesonide (Pulmicort), 54

Bumetanide (Bumex)
for acute pulmonary edema, 160t
for chronic heart failure, 161, 163t

Bundle branches, 101

Burns
in hypovolemic shock, 185
in septic shock, 127

C

Calcium
in brain cell injury, 332
in cardiac action potentials, 92
in cell membrane action potential, 90
in depolarization, 89

intracellular, 31
metabolism abnormalities of in hypertension, 172

Calcium channel blockers
in angina, 123
for asthma, 65
contraindication to, 111
for dysrhythmia, 106*t*, 107

Candesartan, 162

Candida albicans, 287

Capillary, Starling's law of, 12-13, 18, 153, 154*f*, 167

Captopril (Capoten)
for chronic heart failure, 163*t*
clinical trials for, 142*t*
for myocardial infarction, 141

Carbon dioxide
bicarbonate formation from, 24*f*
brain responsiveness to, 330
end-tidal, 25
in metabolic acidosis, 192
transport of, 24

Carbon monoxide poisoning, 23
pulse oximetry in, 27

Cardiac action potentials, 89-92
pacemaker, 90
phases of, 90

Cardiac arrest, 25

Cardiac asthma, 158

Cardiac catheterization, 137

Cardiac contractility
control of, 94-95
Frank-Starling mechanism in, 97

Cardiac cycle, 95

Cardiac glycoside, 107-108

Cardiac injury, serum markers of, 136-137

Cardiac monitoring, 324

Cardiac output, 93
in heart failure, 99
with hypothermia, 352
with sympathetic hyperactivity, 170

Cardiac physiology, basic, 89-99

Cardiac risk factors, 129-131, 147

Cardiogenic shock
with heart failure, 163
mechanisms and causes of, 185*t*

Cardiomyopathy, 153

Cardioprotective pharmacologic therapy, 139-141

Cardiopulmonary bypass, 355

Cardiopulmonary resuscitation, 354

Cardiopulmonary stabilization, 292

Cardioselective beta-blockers, 141

Cardiothoracic surgery, 292

Cardiovascular disease, 172

Cardioversion, 104-105

Carnett's sign, 253, 254*t*

Carotid arteries, internal, 304*f*
in ischemic stroke, 306
three main branches of, 307*t*

Carvedilol (Coreg), 162, 163*t*

Catabolism, 221

Catecholamines, 221

Catheter fluid administration, 98

Cauda equina syndrome, 342

Cell-mediated delayed hypersensitivity, 198*t*

Cell membrane channels, 90

Cell membranes
diffusion across, 4
phospholipids in, 3
potential of, 89
proteins in, 4
structure of, 4*f*

Cell-signaling pathways, 152

Cells
active transport in, 7
damage to in status epilepticus, 321
diffusion in, 4
osmosis in, 5
physiology of, 3-9
response of in hypovolemic shock, 187
tonicity of, 6-7

Cellular organelles, 3

Cellulitis, 292

Central cord syndrome, 342

Central nervous system, 29
changes in with hypovolemic shock, 188

Cephalosporins, hypersensitivity to, 198

Cerebral arteries, 307*t*

Cerebral blood flow
autoregulation of, 329
cerebral perfusion pressure and, 332*f*
decreased with hypothermia, 354
mean arterial pressure and, 333
pressure passive, 329
reduction of, 316

Cerebral infarction
  acute, 316-317
    clinical manifestations of, 306-309
    diagnosis of, 310
    incidence and mortality of, 303
    initial management of, 309-310
    management of, 310-312
    pathogenesis of, 303-306
  evolution of, 305

Cerebral ischemia
  events of, 309
  with hypothermia, 354
  pressure passive cerebral blood flow in, 329

Cerebral perfusion pressure, 177, 329
  cerebral blood flow and, 332f
  factors in determining, 330
  in hypovolemic shock, 188

Cerebrospinal fluid, 339
  analysis of for meningitis, 285

Cerebrovascular accident, 303

Cerebrovascular occlusion, 309

Chemoreceptors
  central, 50, 57
  peripheral, 50, 58
  in respiratory system, 49

CHESS mnemonic, 264t

Chest pain
  in angina, 119
  pathophysiology of, 131
  pleuritic, 291
  substernal, 146
  in unstable angina, 126

Chest x-ray
  for heart failure, 158-159
  for pneumonia, 277-278

Children
  hypoglycemia in, 227
  pneumonia in, 276-277

Chlamydia pneumoniae, 272, 273

Chlorpromazine, 367

Cholesterol
  in fibrolipid plaque, 114
  in hypertension, 171-172
  LDL, 130

Cholinergic receptors, 30, 31

Chronic obstructive lung disease, 71

Chronic obstructive pulmonary disease, 56, 71, 76-77
  beta-2 agonists in, 51-52
  clinical characteristics of, 77
  clinical manifestations of, 72-73
  management of, 73-74
  medications for, 76
  risk factors for, 71, 76

Chronotropic effects, 94, 95

Cimetidine (Tagamet), 200

Cincinnati Prehospital Stroke Scale, 306, 308t

Cirrhosis, 263

CK-MB, 136

Clopidogrel, 140t

Clot formation
  in acute ischemic stroke, 303-304
  progression of, 118

Coagulation cascade, 354

Coagulation disorders, 312

Coagulopathy, 236

Cocaine abuse, ECG patterns in, 135

Cold diuresis, 354

Collagen
  reduced synthesis of, 115
  thrombogenic, 115

Colloid fluid preparations, 16
  for hypovolemic shock, 191
  in resuscitation, 18
  for septic shock, 130
  tonicity of, 9

Colonic bleeding, 262

Coma
  definition of, 334-335
  progression to, 335, 345

Complement cascade, 188

Complete cord syndrome, 342

Compression stockings, 83

Computed tomography (CT)
  in acute ischemic stroke, 310
  for encephalitis, 286
  for subarachnoid hemorrhage, 313
  for traumatic brain injury, 334

Concussion, 336

Conducting zone, 46

Conduction
  heat transfer, 351
  pathways of, 101

Congestive heart failure, 97

Consciousness, loss of, 345

Continuous positive airway pressure, 159-160

Convection, 351

Cooling methods, 366

Core body temperature, 358

Coronary arteries
anatomy of, 133
calcification of, 113
to myocardium, 121

Coronary artery disease
in heart failure, 149, 168
incidence and mortality rate of, 113
pathophysiology of, 113-118
plaque formation in, 113-115, 116*f*

Corticosteroids
for anaphylactic shock, 200
in asthma management, 66*t*
for chronic obstructive pulmonary disease, 74
for croup, 289
pharmacology of, 53-54

Corticotropin releasing hormone, 236

Cortisol, 235

Co-transmitters, 29-30

Cough, 275

Cough test, 254*t*

Coumadin. *See* Warfarin (Coumadin)

Crackles, 276

Craniosacral division, 29

Creatine kinase, 136

Cricothyrotomy, 288

Crohn's disease, 263

Cromolyn sodium (Intal), 54
for asthma, 65
mechanism of action of, 70

Croup
spasmodic, 288, 289
viral, 288
clinical manifestations of, 288-289, 299
definitive diagnosis and treatment of, 289
pathogenesis of, 288, 299

Crystalloids
for hypotension in anaphylactic shock, 200
hypotonic, 16
for hypovolemic shock, 190
isotonic, 14
for septic shock, 130

Culprit plaque, 113-114

Cyclic adenosine monophosphate (cAMP)
in adenylate cyclase activation, 52*f*
at beta receptors, 31
in cardiac action potentials, 92
elevation of, 51

Cytokine antibodies, 131

Cytokines
in asthma, 62
release of, 199
in septic shock, 128

Cytomegalovirus pneumonia, 273*t*

Cytotoxic edema
of brain, 333
in cerebral stroke, 306

Cytotoxic hypersensitivity reaction, 198*t*

D

Daltaparin, 140*t*

Debridement, surgical
for host response to injury, 131
for mucormycosis, 293
for toxic shock syndrome, 294

Deep vein thrombosis, 79
pain in, 252

Defibrillation
for dysrhythmias, 104-105
for hypothermia, 355

Dehydration, 354

Depolarization, 89
of atrial muscles, 92
electrolyte exchange during, 90*f*
spontaneous, 102

Depolarizing agents, 363*t*

Depression-related hypertension, 172

Dexamethasone (Decadron)
for Addison's disease, 237
for croup, 289

Dextrose solutions
5%, 16
for acute ischemic stroke, 309
for hypoglycemia, 228, 231, 232
hypotonicity of, 18
for myxedema coma, 240
reasons to avoid, 19
tonicity of, 6*t*
for traumatic brain injury, 337

Diabetes
emergencies of, 219-232
mellitus
incidence of, 219
in myocardial infarction, 130
in necrotizing skin and soft tissue infections, 293
pathogenesis of, 219
silent myocardial infarction with, 131
types I and II, 219, 230

Diaphragm, respiratory, 46

Diarrhea, bloody, 263-264

Diastolic failure, 152, 153

Diastolic pressure, 92

Diathermy, 356

Diazepam (Valium)
  drug binding of, 39
  for status epilepticus, 324

Diffuse axonal injury, 336

Diffusion, 4

Digitalis
  for chronic heart failure, 162, 163*t*
  contraindication to, 112
  for dysrhythmia, 107-108
  increased automaticity with, 102

Digoxin, 162, 163t

Diltiazem
  for dysrhythmia, 107
  mechanisms of action of, 106*t*

Diphenhydramine (Benadryl), 200

Distribution, 38

Distributive shock, 185*t*

Diuretics
  for acute pulmonary edema, 160*t*
  for chronic heart failure, 161, 162, 163*t*
  effect of, 168
  for heart failure, 167
  sites of action for, 161*f*

Diverticulitis
  diagnostic test for, 256*t*
  misdiagnosis of, 255*t*

Diverticulosis, 263

Dobutamine
  contraindications to, 163
  for heart failure, 168
  for septic shock, 130

Dopamine
  adrenal secretion of, 235
  antagonists of, 364*t*
  depletion of in neuroleptic malignant syndrome, 363
  for hypotension in anaphylactic shock, 200
  for hypothermia, 354-355
  release of, 30*f*
  for septic shock, 130

Doppler flow studies
  for heart failure, 159
  for myocardial infarction, 137

^{23}-DPG synthesis, 22-23

Dromotropic effects, 94, 95

Drug-related seizures, 320

Drugs
  absorption of, 37
  bioavailability of, 39
  distribution of, 38
  elimination of, 38
  first pass hepatic effect of, 40
  free versus bound, 39
  metabolism of, 38
  organ impairment by, 39-40
  protein binding by, 39
  sites of action of, 33*f*
  toxic effects of, 42

Duodenal ulcers, 262

Duplex Doppler exams, 82

Dyspnea, 56
  in heart failure, 155
  in pulmonary embolism, 81, 85

Dysrhythmia, 101-112
  in heart failure, 159
  with hypothermia, 352-353
  mechanism of action of, 110
  mechanisms of formation of, 102-104
  treatment of, 104-108
  triggered, 104
  Vaughn-Williams classification of, 110

E

Eastern equine encephalitis, 285-286

Eccrine glands, 361

Echocardiography
  for acute infective endocarditis, 292
  for heart failure, 158-159
  for myocardial infarction, 137

Eclampsia, 178
  status epilepticus with, 325

Ectopic pregnancy, 253
  diagnosis of, 259
  diagnostic test for, 256*t*
  misdiagnosis of, 255*t*

Edema, 12. *See also* Pulmonary edema
  of brain tissue, 329
  in croup, 288
  cytotoxic, 306, 333
  heat, 364, 365*t*
  peripheral, 156, 167
  in pneumonia, 274

Ejection fraction, 93

Elderly
heat stroke in, 365
pneumonia in, 277

Electrocardiography
in acute myocardial infarction, 131
changes of in angina, 122
confounding patterns of in myocardial
infarction, 133-135
electrophysiologic events in, 95
for heart failure, 158-159
for myocardial infarction, 146
for pericarditis, 291
recovery phase of, 148

Electroencephalography
for encephalitis, 286
for seizures, 322
for status epilepticus, 325

Electrolytes
distribution of, 3
exchange of
during cardiac depolarization, 90f
during muscle contraction, 89

Elimination, pathways for, 38

Embolectomy, 83

Embolus
air, 83
amniotic fluid, 83
in cerebral arterial occlusion, 304
fat, 83
pulmonary, 79-85

Emesis, coffee grounds, 262, 264, 267

Emphysema, 71
in chronic obstructive pulmonary disease, 72-73
lung capacity in, 48
pathogenesis of, 73
pathology of, 76
treatment of, 58

Enalapril (Vasotec)
for chronic heart failure, 163t
for myocardial infarction, 140t, 141

Enalaprilat, 176t

Encainide, 106t

Encephalitis, 285
clinical manifestations of, 286, 298
definitive diagnosis and treatment of, 286-287
pathogenesis of, 285-286
in status epilepticus, 320

Encephalopathy, hypertensive, 177

End-systolic volume, 93

End-tidal carbon dioxide detectors, 28

End-tidal carbon dioxide measurement, 25

Endocarditis, acute infective, 291
clinical manifestations of, 291-292
definitive diagnosis and treatment of, 292
differential diagnosis of, 300
pathogenesis of, 291

Endocrine system
adrenal anatomy and physiology in, 235
disorders of, 235-245
locations of organs of, 233f
organization of, 233
thyroid physiology in, 234

Endoscopy, 264-265, 268

Endothelin, 152

Endothelin-1, 171

Endotoxins, 128

Endotracheal intubation
for spinal cord trauma, 343
for traumatic brain injury, 336

Energy
ATP as source of, 7
deficiency of in angina, 120

Enflurane, 363t

Enoxaparin
for myocardial infarction, 140t
for pulmonary embolism, 82

Enteric nervous system, 29

Enterobacter infection, 127

Enteroviruses, 285-286

Environmental hypothermia, 351

Eosinophils, 62

Ephedrine, 74

Epidural hematoma, 335, 345

Epiglottitis, 287
clinical manifestations of, 287, 298
definitive diagnosis and treatment of, 288
pathogenesis of, 287
pathophysiology of, 298

Epilepsy, 320, 327

Epinephrine
activating adenylate cyclase, 52f
for anaphylactic shock, 199-200
for asthma, 64
for chronic obstructive pulmonary disease, 74
for croup, 289
in diabetic ketoacidosis, 221
in heart failure, 152
in hypoglycemia, 227-228

release of, 235
in respiration, 49-50

Epstein Barr virus, 253

Eptifibatide, 140*t*

Equilibrium, 4

Escherichia coli, 127

Esmolol
for hypertensive emergencies, 176*t*
mechanisms of action of, 106*t*

Esmotol (Brevibloc), 141

Esophageal intubation, 25, 28

Esophagus
thoracic pain in disease of, 252
varices of in upper GI bleeding, 263

Etomidate, 313

Evaporation, 351, 361-362

Evaporative cooling, 367

Excitotoxins, 332

Expiration, 46
muscles of, 56

Expiratory reserve volume, 48, 56

Extravascular fluid, 11

Eyes, 32*t*

F

Factor VII, 129

Factor X, 129

Fat embolus, 83

Fatty acid tails, 3

Fenoldopam, 176*t*, 177

Fever
in acute infective endocarditis, 291
versus hyperthermia, 362
in immunocompromised patients, 295
in infective endocarditis, 300
in status epilepticus, 320

Fibrinogen, 130

Fibrolipid plaque, 114
in acute ischemic stroke, 303-304
in myocardial infarction, 130
ruptured, 114, 115, 129

Filtration, 12

First-pass hepatic effect, 40, 42

Flecainide, 106*t*

Fluid compartments, 11

Fluid resuscitation. *See also* Intravenous
fluid preparations
for diabetic ketoacidosis and hyperosmolar
hyperglycemic syndrome, 224-225
for gastrointestinal bleeding, 265
for heat stroke, 366
for hyperglycemic hyperosmolar syndrome and
diabetic ketoacidosis, 231-232
for hypothermia, 354-355
for hypothyroidism, 245
for hypovolemic shock, 190
intravenous fluid preparations in, 14-15
for pericarditis, 291
for septic shock, 130, 215
for traumatic brain injury, 337

Fluids. *See also* Water
administration of, 98
body, 11-19
in cellular diffusion, 4
cellular distribution of, 3
distribution of, 12
isotonic, 9, 18, 215, 291
movement through alveolar capillaries, 49
osmolarity of, 5
overload of, 13
reabsorption into intravascular space, 16
tonicities of, 6*t*, 9

Flunisolide (AeroBid), 54

Fluoroquinolone antibiotics, 278

Fluticasone (Flovent), 54

Foam cells, 113-114

Food allergies, 197-198

Forced expiratory volume in 1 second (FEV1), 63

Fosinopril (Monopril), 163*t*

Fosphenytoin (Cerebyx), 325

Fourth heart sound, 158

Frank-Starling curve, 93, 151

Frank-Starling mechanism, 97

Free fatty acids, elevation of, 221

Free radical scavengers, 343

Funduscopy, 169-170

Fungal infections, of skin, 293

Furosemide (Lasix)
for acute pulmonary edema, 160*t*
for chronic heart failure, 161, 163*t*
drug binding of, 39
for heart failure, 168
for traumatic brain injury, 337

G

Gamma aminobutyric acid (GABA), 31

Gangrene, progressive, 293

Gastric erosions, 262

Gastroesophageal reflux disease (GERD), 252

Gastrointestinal anatomy, 261

Gastrointestinal bleeding, 261, 267-268
    definitions of, 261-262
    diagnosis of, 264-265, 268
    indications of, 268
    management of, 265
    pathogenesis of
        lower, 263-264
        upper, 262-263

Gastropathy, hemorrhagic, 262, 267

Genetics, 71

Glasgow Coma Scale, 345
    for traumatic brain injury, 334-335

Glomerular filtration rate, decreased, 223

Glucagon
    for anaphylactic shock, 200
    catabolic effect of, 221
    in hypoglycemia, 227-228
    insulin and, 220f
    release of in diabetic ketoacidosis, 220-221

Glucocorticoids
    pharmacology of, 53-54
    synthesis of, 54

Glucometers, 228

Glucose
    in anaerobic metabolism, 186
    cellular diffusion of, 4
    elimination of, 223
    for hypoglycemia, 227-228
    impaired formation of, 227-228
    loading of for hypoglycemia, 228
    low levels of, 228
    peripheral tissue uptake of, 222
    serial determinations of, 228
    serum levels of in septic shock, 129
    for thyroid storm, 244

Glucose-containing solutions, 19

Glutamate, 332

Glutamic acid, 31

Glycerol backbone, 3

Glycine, 31

Glycoprotein, 39

Glycoprotein IIb/IIIa inhibitors
    clinical trials for, 142t
    for myocardial infarction, 140t

Glycoprotein IIb/IIIa receptor antagonists, 118
    for angina, 123, 124

GM-1 gangliosides, 343

Graded exercise testing, 137

Grand mal seizures, 323

Granulocyte-monocyte colony stimulating factor, 128

Grave's disease, 237-238

Grave's triad, 238

Grunting, 277

Gunshot wound, 195

H

H$_2$ receptor antagonists, 200

H$_1$ receptor blockers, 200

Haemophilus
    influenzae
        in chronic bronchitis, 73
        in epiglottitis, 287
        in meningitis, 283-284
        in pneumonia, 272, 273
        type B vaccine of, 287
        in septic shock, 127

Hagen-Poiseuille equation, 94, 98, 190, 195

Half-life, 38, 42

Halothane, 363t

Head injury
    effects of hyperventilation for, 345
    management of, 347

Headache
    with hypertension, 181
    sentinel, 313
    in stroke, 309
    in subarachnoid hemorrhage, 313, 317

Heart
    anatomy of blood supply to, 133f
    autonomic nervous system of, 32t
    basic physiology of, 89-99
    infections of, 290-292

Heart failure, 166-168
    cardiogenic shock with, 163
    causes of, 168
    with chronic or poorly controlled hypertension, 178t
    clinical manifestations of, 155-158
    diagnosis of, 158-159
    downward spiral of, 155f
    drug distribution in, 40

etiology of, 149, 150*t*
incidence of, 149
increased pressure and volume in, 152*f*
management of, 159-163
mechanisms of, 149-152
New York Heart Association's classification of, 155-156
pathogenesis of, 149-154
pathophysiology of, 166
with pulmonary embolism, 82
signs of, 167
systolic versus diastolic, 152, 153
treatment of, 167

Heart murmur, 300

Heart rate
accelerated, 112
in cardiac output, 99
parasympathetic nervous control of, 95

Heat
normal response to, 361-362
transfer of, 351

Heat cramps, 364, 365*t*
physiologic process of, 370

Heat-dissipating mechanisms, impaired, 361

Heat edema, 364, 365*t*

Heat exhaustion, 361, 364, 365t, 369-370
physiologic process of, 370

Heat loss, 361-362
compensation for, 352
increased, 351

Heat production, 361
decreased, 351
in thermoregulation, 352

Heat stroke, 361, 369-370
clinical manifestations of, 363-366
exertional, 365
management of, 366-367, 369
nonexertional, 365, 369
pathogenesis of, 361-364
predisposing factors for, 362
risk factors for, 369
systemic effects of, 366

Heat syncope, 364, 365*t*

Heat tetany, 364, 365*t*
physiologic process of, 370

Helicobacter pylori, 262

Helium-oxygen mixtures (Heliox), 289

Hematemesis, 262

Hematochezia, 262

Hematoma
epidural, 335, 345
subdural, 335, 346

Hemodialysis, 355

Hemoglobin, 21
affinity of for oxygen, 22
carbon monoxide binding to, 23
reversible reactions of oxygen and, 21*f*

Hemoglobin-oxygen dissociation curve, 21-22
shifting to left, 23
shifting to right, 22-23

Hemorrhage
in hypovolemic shock, 185
oxygen supply-demand imbalance with, 191
with spinal cord injury, 340
subarachnoid, 312-313

Hemorrhagic shock, 14

Hemorrhagic stroke, 306

Hemorrhoids, 263

Heparin
in acute ischemic stroke, 310
for myocardial infarction, 140*t*
for pulmonary embolism, 82

Hepatic impairment, drug-induced, 39-40

Hernia, incarcerated or strangulated, 255*t*

Herpes simplex viral encephalitis, 286
treatment of, 287

His, bundle of, 101

Histamine
in asthma, 60
mast cell release of, 199

Hoarseness, 287

Hollow viscus, obstruction of, 252

Hormones, release of, 233

Host response, 131

Human immunodeficiency virus, 236

Hydralazine
contraindications to, 162
for hypertensive emergencies, 176*t*
for preeclampsia, 178

Hydration status, 362

Hydrochlorothiazide (Microzide), 161, 163*t*

Hydrocortisone, 237t

Hydrostatic pressure, 12, 153

3-Hydroxybutyrate, 221

5-Hydroxytryptamine. *See* Serotonin

Hyperbaric oxygen, 293

Hypercholesterolemia, 130

Hypercoagulable states, 79*t*

Hyperdynamic, hypermetabolic state
 manifestations of, 130*t*, 215
 in septic shock, 129

Hyperglycemia, 309

Hyperglycemic hyperosmolar syndrome, 219
 clinical assessment for, 223-224
 management of, 224-225, 231-232
 manifestations of, 231
 pathogenic mechanisms in, 223
 pathophysiologic mechanism of, 231

Hypermetabolic state, 332-333

Hyperosmolar hyperglycemic syndrome, 223

Hyperosmolar solution, 6

Hyperosmotic solution, 5

Hypersensitivity reaction
 causes of, 202
 Gell and Coombs classification for, 197, 198*t*
 IgE-mediated, 197-198, 202
 mast cell activation in, 198-199
 type I, 199

Hypertension, 118
 in diastolic failure, 153
 essential, 170
 headache with, 181
 in heart failure, 149
 malignant, 169
 in myocardial infarction, 130
 risk group stratification of, 175*t*
 secondary, 172
 sequelae of chronic or poorly controlled, 178*t*
 in stroke, 304

Hypertensive emergencies, 181-182
 definitions of, 169-170
 diagnosis of, 172-175
 epidemiology of, 169
 management of, 175-178
 pathogenesis of, 170-172, 181
 permanent sequelae of, 178
 sublingual nifedipine in, 182

Hypertensive encephalopathy, 177

Hypertensive urgencies, 169

Hyperthermia
 versus fever, 362
 malignant, 363

Hyperthyroidism
 cause of, 237-238
 clinical features of, 238*t*

drug metabolism in, 40
 thyroid storm and, 237-239

Hypertonicity, 6

Hyperventilation, 27, 345
 for elevated intracranial pressure, 330
 in hypovolemic shock, 188
 indications for, 346
 mechanisms of, 57
 for traumatic brain injury, 336-337

Hypoglycemia, 226
 alcohol abuse and insulin in, 232
 causes of, 226*t*
 diagnosis and management of, 227
 differential diagnosis of, 226
 disposition in, 227-228
 management of, 232
 pathogenesis of, 226-227
 pediatric considerations in, 227

Hypo-osmotic solution, 5
 hypotonicity of, 6

Hypotension, 200

Hypothalamic thermoregulatory center, 362

Hypothalamus, 234

Hypothermia, 358-359
 cardiovascular response to, 352-353
 causes of, 351-352, 358
 central nervous system response to, 354
 classification of, 352, 353t
 hematologic response to, 354
 management of, 354-356
 mortality from, 351
 with myxedema coma, 240
 pathogenesis of, 351-352
 physiologic changes in, 359
 pulmonary response to, 352
 renal response to, 354
 for spinal cord trauma, 343
 systemic manifestations of, 352-354
 for traumatic brain injury, 338

Hypothyroidism
 diagnosis of, 239-240
 drug metabolism in, 40
 pathogenesis of, 239
 signs of, 245
 treatment of, 245

Hypotonic crystalloids, 16

Hypotonic solutions, 18

Hypotonicity, 6

Hypoventilation, 27
 in hypoxia, 23

Hypovolemia, 185, 186*t*

Hypovolemic shock, 195-196
   classification of, 185
   clinical manifestations of, 187-189
   compensatory mechanisms in, 186-187
   with diabetic ketoacidosis and hyperosmolar
      hyperglycemic syndrome, 224
   management of, 190-193
   orthostatic vital sign changes in, 196
   pathogenic mechanisms of, 185-187, 195
   resuscitation endpoints in, 193

Hypoxemia, 49
   in asthma, 63
   cellular response to, 187
   in pneumonia, 276, 281
   with pulmonary embolism, 81
   with ventilation-perfusion mismatch, 274

Hypoxia, 23
   causes of, 23, 27
   lactate formation during, 187f
   ventilation and PO_2 in, 51f

Hypoxic drive, 50

I

Ibuprofen, 262

Ibutilide, 106t

Ice water immersion, 366

IgE antibody
   in asthma, 69
   B-cell production of, 199
   in hypersensitivity reaction, 202
   mast cell release of, 197

Immune complex hypersensitivity, 198t

Immune reactions, 127

Immunocompromised states, 295t
   fever in, 295

Immunodeficiency disorders, 273

Infections/infectious diseases
   in adrenal insufficiency, 236
   emergencies of, 283-300
   in sepsis and septic shock, 205-206, 207
   in subarachnoid hemorrhage, 312

Infectious droplets, 273

Inflammation
   in coronary artery disease, 115
   peritoneal, 252

Inflammatory bowel disease, 263

Inflammatory cell mediators, 114

Inflammatory cells, recruitment of, 199

Inflammatory cytokines, 128

Inflammatory factor of anaphylaxis (IF-A), 199

Inflammatory response
   in asthma, 60, 69
   in pneumonia, 274

Influenzae A/B, 288

Inositol triphosphate, 31

Inotropes, 130

Inotropy, 94, 95

Insect stings, 197

Inspiration, 46

Inspiratory regulators, 50

Inspiratory reserve volume, 48

Insulin
   counter regulatory hormones of, 220, 223
   deficiency of, 222f, 223
      absolute or relative, 220
      complete, 219
   for diabetic ketoacidosis and hyperosmolar
      hyperglycemic syndrome, 225
   glucagon and, 220f
   in hypoglycemia, 232
   potassium homeostasis and, 225f

Insulin counter regulatory hormones, 230
   in hypoglycemia, 227-228

Insulin resistance, 222
   in hypertension, 171-172

Interleukins, 128

Interstitial fluid, 11
   in peripheral edema, 167

Intestinal ischemia/infarction, 256t

Intestinal obstruction, 252

Intoxication-related seizures, 320

Intracellular fluid, 11

Intracerebral hemorrhage, 178t

Intracranial pressure, 329-330
   exponential increase in, 330-331
   reduction of, 336-337

Intrathoracic pressures, 46
   negative, 276

Intravascular fluid, 11

Intravenous fluid preparations, 14-15
   compositions of, 15t
   for heat stroke, 369
   for hypothermia, 356
   for hypovolemic shock, 190, 195
   tonicities of, 6t

Ion channels
disturbances of in status epilepticus, 321
opening of, 31

Ion pump dysfunction, 187

Ipratropium, 65

Ischemia
in brain injury, 332-333
in myocardial infarction, 132*f*
pathogenesis of, 120-121
in septic shock, 127
of spinal cord, 340

Ischemic penumbra, 305
thrombolytics for, 316

Isoetharine, 73-74

Isoflurane, 363*t*

Iso-osmotic solution, 5
isotonicity of, 6

Isosorbide dinitrate
contraindications to, 162
for myocardial infarction, 140*t*

Isotonic crystalloids, 14
for septic shock, 130

Isotonic fluids, 9, 18
for pericarditis, 291
for septic shock, 215

Isotonic saline solution, 224-225

Isotonicity, 6

J

J receptors, 49

J waves, 353*f*

Japanese B encephalitis, 285-286

Joint National Commission-VI Classification, 174
hypertension risk group stratification in, 175*t*

Jugular venous distension, 156

Junctional conducting zone, 101

Junctional rhythm, 97

K

Kehr's sign, 254*t*

Kernig's sign, 285

Ketoacidosis, diabetic, 219, 221
clinical assessment for, 223-224
epidemiology of, 220
management of, 224-225, 231, 232
pathogenic mechanisms in, 220-223

pathophysiology of, 230

Ketoacids, 221, 222

Kidney stones, 250

Kidneys
in diabetic ketoacidosis, 222
drug-induced impairment of, 39-40
efferent arteriolar constriction in, 171*f*
in glucose elimination, 223

Kilocalories, 361

Kininase II, 161

Kinins, 161

Klebsiella infection, 127

Korotkoff sounds, 167
five phases of, 173*t*
in hypertension, 172-173

Kussmaul's sign
in heart failure, 156-157
in pericardial tamponade, 290*f*

L

Labetalol
for hypertensive emergencies, 176*t*, 177
for preeclampsia, 178

Lactate
accumulation of in hypovolemic shock, 186
formation of during hypoxia, 187*f*

Lanoxin, 163*t*

LaPlace's law, 48, 98

Laryngoscopy, 288

Laryngotracheitis, 288

Laryngotracheobronchitis, 288

Larynx, 45

Latex allergy, 198

Left bundle branch block
in acute myocardial infarction, 135*t*
ECG patterns of, 133
new onset, 138, 147

Left ventricular function, impaired, 149

Left ventricular hypertrophy, 178*t*

Legionella infection, 273

Leukotriene inhibitors, 54
for asthma, 65, 66*t*

Leukotrienes
in asthma, 60
in septic shock, 128
synthesis pathway of, 53*f*

Levalbuterol (Xopenex), 51-52

Lidocaine
in malignant hyperthermia, 363*t*
mechanisms of action of, 106*t*

Lipase, inhibition of, 221

Lipid bilayer, 3

Lipid soluble drugs, 3, 9

Lipoproteins
drug binding to, 39
phagocytosis of, 113-114

Lisinopril (Prinivil, Zestril)
for chronic heart failure, 163*t*
for heart failure, 168
for myocardial infarction, 140*t*, 141

Lithium, 239

Liver
in diabetic ketoacidosis, 221
fibrosis of with alcohol abuse, 267

Loop diuretics
for acute pulmonary edema, 160*t*
for chronic heart failure, 161, 163*t*

Lorazepam (Ativan), 324

Lorcainide, 106*t*

Los Angeles Prehospital Stroke Screen, 306, 308*t*

Losartan, 162

Lower extremity venous system, 80*f*

Lung stretch receptors, 49

Lung volumes, 48, 56

Lungs
autonomic nervous system of, 32*t*
capacities of, 48, 56
inflation of, 46
physiology of, 45-46

M

Macrolide, 278

Macrophages, 113-114

Magnesium
for asthma, 65
for dysrhythmia, 107
mechanism of action of, 70
for torsades de pointes, 111

Magnetic resonance imaging (MRI)
in acute ischemic stroke, 310
for encephalitis, 286

Malignancy, gastrointestinal, 264

Mallory-Weiss tears
diagnosis of, 264
in upper gastrointestinal bleeding, 262

Malnutrition, 325

Mannitol, 337-338, 347

MAO inhibitors, 364*t*

Mast cell stabilizers, 54
for asthma, 65, 66*t*

Mast cells, 51
activation of, 198-199, 202
mediators released by, 197
stimulation of, 69

McBurney's point, 254*t*

Mean arterial pressure (MAP), 92
cerebral blood flow and, 332*f*, 333l
cerebral perfusion pressure related to, 332*f*
reduction of, 177

Measles, 288

Medical anti-shock trousers (MAST), 192

Medulla oblongata, 338

Melanocyte stimulating hormone, 236

Melena, 262

Membrane potential, 89
resting, 90

Meningeal artery, bleeding from, 346

Meningitis, 283
clinical manifestations of, 285, 297
definitive diagnosis and treatment of, 285
pathogenesis of, 283-285
pathophysiology of, 297
in status epilepticus, 320

Mental status
in diabetic ketoacidosis, 230
in hypovolemic shock, 187-188
in septic shock, 129

Mesenteric ischemia/infarct, 251, 252
misdiagnosis of, 255*t*

Metabolic acidosis
hemoglobin-oxygen dissociation curve in, 22
in hypoglycemia, 227
in hypovolemic shock, 186
ketoacids in, 221
in septic shock, 129
treatment for, 192

Metabolic disorders, 320

Metabolism
of drugs, 38
process of in heat production, 361

Metaproterenol (Alupent, Metaprel, ProMeta)
  for chronic obstructive pulmonary disease, 73-74
  pharmacology of, 51-52

Methimazole (Tapazole), 239

Methyldopa, 178

Methylprednisolone (Solu-Medrol), 54
  for Addison's disease, 237
  for anaphylactic shock, 200
  mechanism of action of, 70
  for spinal cord trauma, 343

Metoprolol (Lopressor/Toprol)
  for angina, 123
  for chronic heart failure, 162, 163t
  clinical trials for, 142t
  mechanisms of action of, 106t
  for myocardial infarction, 140t, 141

Midazolam (Versed), 324

Milrinone, 163

Monroe-Kellie Doctrine, 330, 331f

Montelukast (Singulair), 54

Morphine
  for acute pulmonary edema, 160t
  for angina, 123
  first-pass hepatic effect of, 40, 42
  for heart failure, 167
  for myocardial infarction, 138, 140t

Mucormycosis, 293

Multi-system trauma, 196

Multiple organ dysfunction syndrome
  in hypovolemic shock, 187
  in septic shock, 128, 205

Murphy's sign, 254t

Muscarinic receptors, 31

Muscles, respiratory, 46, 56

Mycoplasma pneumoniae, 272, 273

Myocardial contraction
  biochemical activation of, 92
  Frank-Starling mechanism in, 93, 97
  inadequate, 152-153
  preload and afterload in, 92-93
  pressure differences and blood flow in, 94
  pressures during, 92

Myocardial infarction
  acute, 146-148
    clinical manifestations of, 131
    diagnostic modalities for, 136-137
    ECG findings in, 131-135
    landmark studies of, 141, 142t
    mortality from, 129

pathogenesis of, 129
risk factors for, 129-131
serum markers for, 136-137
silent, 131
treatment of, 137-141
anatomical localization of, 133, 134t
in heart failure, 159
ischemia zones in, 132f
non-Q wave, 119, 122, 135
  pathogenesis of, 129
plaque rupture in, 115
posterior wall, 135, 148
Q waves in, 127
risk factors for, 147
thoracic pain of, 252

Myocardium
  blood flow to, 121f
  cellular oxygen supply and demand in, 120
  hypertrophy of, 151
    concentric and dilational, 152f
  innervation of, 101
  ischemia of
    in angina, 120-121
    in heart failure, 159
    plaque in, 115
    in unstable angina, 126
  oxygen supply and demand in, 120

Myoclonic seizures, 323

Myxedema, 240

Myxedema coma, 245
  clinical diagnosis of, 239-240
  incidence of, 239
  management of, 240
  parameters of, 241t
  pathogenesis of, 239

N

N-methyl D-aspartate (NMDA) antagonists, 343

NADIR mnemonic, 263

Narcotics, 239

National Institute of Neurological Diseases and
  Stroke study, 310-311, 312t

National Institutes of Health Stroke Scale, 309

Necrotizing fasciitis, 293

Necrotizing skin infections, 293

Nedocromil (Tilade), 54
  for asthma, 65

Negri bodies, 286

Neisseria meningitidis
  in adrenal insufficiency, 236

in meningitis, 283-284

Neonatal respiratory distress syndrome, 48-49
diagnosis of, 57

Neoplasms, gastrointestinal, 263

Nervous system infections, 283-287

Neurogenic shock, 340
with spinal cord trauma, 343

Neurohormonal factors, suppression of, 162

Neurohormonal mediator serum assays, 158-159

Neurohormonal substances, 152

Neuroleptic malignant syndrome, 363-364

Neurologic examination
essentials of, 341*t*
for spinal cord injury, 340

Neurologic shock, 347

Neurological trauma, 329-348

Neuromuscular junction, nicitonic receptors at, 31

Neuronal cell degeneration, 340

Neuroprotective agents
for cerebral infarction, 305
for spinal cord trauma, 343
for traumatic brain injury, 338

Neurosurgery, 338

Neurotransmitters, 31
at synapses, 29
synaptic transmission of, 31

Newton's law, 98

Nicotinic receptors, 31

Nifedipine
adverse effects of, 177
in angina, 123
contraindications to, 182

Nitrates
for acute pulmonary edema, 160*t*
for angina, 123
for myocardial infarction, 140*t*

Nitric oxide, 332

Nitroglycerin
for acute pulmonary edema, 160*t*
for heart failure, 168
for hypertensive emergencies, 176*t*
for myocardial infarction, 138, 140*t*

Nitroprusside
for acute pulmonary edema, 160*t*
for hypertensive emergencies, 176*t*, 177

Nondepolarizing agents, 363-364

Nonshivering compensatory response, 351, 352

Nonsteroidal anti-inflammatory drugs, 262

Norepinephrine, 29, 31
in heart failure, 152
for hypothermia, 354-355
release of, 235
in respiration, 49-50
for septic shock, 130

Nose, 45

O

Obesity, 171-172

Obstructive lung disease, 49*f*

Obstructive shock, 185*t*

Obturator sign, 254*t*

Octreotide, 265

Omeprazole (Prevacid), 265

Ophthalmic artery occlusion, 306

Organ impairment, 39-40
drug-induced, 42

Orthostatic vital signs changes, 188

Osborn waves, 353*f*, 358

Osler, Sir William, 271

Osmolarity, 5

Osmosis, 5

Osmotic pressure, 153
in dextrose solution, 16
in fluid reabsorption, 16
in interstitial fluid movement, 12

Ovarian torsion, 256*t*

Oxygen
for acute pulmonary edema, 160*t*
chemical reactions of, 21
for chronic obstructive pulmonary disease, 74
for croup, 289
for heart failure, 168
metabolism of in brain, 330
for myocardial infarction, 137, 140*t*
partial pressure of, 21
reversible reactions of, 21*f*
for septic shock, 130
for status epilepticus, 324
transport of, 21-28

Oxygen-carrying capacity
decreased, 23, 27

Oxygen debt, 195

Oxygen-hemoglobin dissociation curve, 192

right shift, 27
shift in with hypothermia, 354

Oxygen supply-demand balance, 120

Oxygen supply-demand imbalance, 126
in hypovolemic shock, 191

P

P-R interval, 94-95
shortened, 103

P waves, 92

Pacemaker action potentials, 90

Pain
abdominal
acute, 249-252
physiology of, 250-251
extra-abdominal, 252-255
pelvic, 253

Pancreatitis
diagnostic test for, 256t
in septic shock, 127

Paradoxical embolism, 304

Parainfluenza viruses, 288

Paralysis, 340

Parasympathetic ganglia, 29

Parasympathetic nervous system
in cardiac contractility, 95
overstimulation of, 131

Parasympathetic neurons, 29
organization of, 30f

Parasympathetic response, 98

Parietal pain, 250, 258

Parkinson's disease medications, 364t

Partial pressure of oxygen (PO₂), 21
approximate values of, 25f
in bronchitis, 73
decreased, 23, 58
pulse oximetry for, 24
ventilation and, 51f

Passive diffusion, 4

Patient positioning, 173

PCO₂
in bronchitis, 73
in respiratory regulation, 50

Peak expiratory flow
in asthma, 63, 65
measurement of, 68
monitoring of, 65

Pelvic inflammatory disease, 253
diagnosis of, 259
diagnostic test for, 256t

Pelvic pain, 253

Penicillins, hypersensitivity to, 198

Pentobarbital, 325

Peptic ulcers, 262

Percutaneous transluminal coronary angioplasty
clinical trials for, 142t
for myocardial infarction, 139

Pericardial effusions, 290

Pericardial tamponade, 290f

Pericarditis, 290
clinical manifestations of, 291
definitive diagnosis and treatment of, 291
pathogenesis of, 290
ST-segment elevation in, 299

Peripheral edema
cause of, 167
in heart failure, 156

Peritoneal inflammation, 252

Peritonitis, 252

Permeability, 12

Phagocytosis, 113-114

Pharmacokinetics, 9, 37-42
processes of, 37f

Pharmacology, pulmonary, 51-54

Phentolamine, 176t

Phenytoin (Dilantin)
drug binding of, 39
mechanisms of action of, 106t
for status epilepticus, 324

Pheochromocytoma, 172

Phospholipids, 3

Phosphorus, 225

Phosphorylation, 51

Phrenic nerves, 46

Piloerection, 32t

Pink puffers, 72-73

Pirbuterol, 73-74

Plaque
formation of, 113-115, 116f
rupture of, 114f, 115
platelet aggregation with, 121f

Plasma
colloid osmotic pressure of, 49

composition of, 15t
drug binding to proteins of, 39
fluid of, 11

Plasma-lyte, 15t

Plasminogen, 138

Platelet-activating factor
in asthma, 60
in septic shock, 128

Platelet-fibrin complex, 291

Platelets
activation of, 146
aggregation of, 118, 121f
in myocardial infarction, 129
pathway for, 123

Pleural fluid analysis, 278

Pneumatic anti-shock garment, 192

Pneumocystis pneumonia, 273t

Pneumonia, 271, 280-281
aspiration, 272
auscultatory findings in, 281
CDC criteria for hospital-acquired, 277t
clinical manifestations of, 275-277
definition of, 280
diagnosis of, 277-278
factors increasing susceptibility to, 271t
geriatric considerations in, 277
hypoxemia with, 281
pathogenesis of, 272-274
pathophysiology of, 280
pediatric considerations in, 276-277
poor prognostic factors for, 272t
predisposing factors in, 280
risk factors for, 271-272
thoracic pain of, 252
treatment of, 278

Pneumothorax
pathophysiology of, 46, 47f
thoracic pain of, 252

Pons, 50

Postconcussive syndrome, 336

Postganglionic fibers, 29

Postsynaptic membrane, 31

Potassium
in cell membrane action potential, 90
in depolarization, 89
insulin and homeostasis of, 225f

Potassium sparing diuretics, 162

Potential, definition of, 89

Prednisone

for Addison's disease, 237t
for anaphylactic shock, 200

Preeclampsia, 178
causes of, 182
triad associated with, 182

Preload, 92-93
in myocardial ischemia, 120
reduction of, 97

Pressure gradient, 94

Prickly heat, 365t
physiologic process of, 370

Prinzmetal's angina, 119

Procainamide, 106t

Propofol (Diprivan), 325

Proportional pulse pressure, 157

Propranolol
for angina, 123
first-pass hepatic effect of, 40
mechanisms of action of, 106t
for thyroid storm, 239

Propylthiouracil, 239

Prostacyclin, 188

Prostaglandins
in asthma, 60
in diabetic ketoacidosis, 221
in heart failure, 152
synthesis of, 161
synthesis pathway of, 53f

Prosthetic valves, 292

Proteins
binding of, 39
of cell membranes, 4

Proteus infection, 127

Proton pump inhibitors, 265

Pseudomonas
in acute infective endocarditis, 291
aeruginosa
in adrenal insufficiency, 236
in septic shock, 127

Pulmonary capillary pressure, 49

Pulmonary defense mechanisms, 273

Pulmonary edema
cardiogenic, 153
causes of, 49
in heart failure, 153-154, 158
with hypothermia, 352
signs of, 158
stabilization of, 159-160, 167

Pulmonary embolism, 85
 clinical manifestations of, 81-82
 complications of, 82
 diagnosis and treatment of, 82-83
 incidence of, 79
 pain in, 252
 pathogenesis of, 80-81
 risk factors for, 79, 85
 signs and symptoms of, 85

Pulmonary infarction, 82

Pulmonary pharmacology, 51-54, 57-58

Pulmonary physiology, 45-50, 56-57

Pulse, 187

Pulse oximetry, 24, 27, 28
 in asthma, 65

Pulsus paradoxus, 63, 167
 in heart failure, 157

Purkinje fibers, 101

Q

Q wave myocardial infarction, 127, 132

QRX complex, 92

Quinapril (Accupril), 163*t*

Quinidine, 106*t*

R

Rabies virus
 encephalitis and, 286
 vaccine for, 287

Radiation, heat, 351

Radiocontrast media, 198

Radiology, 169-170

Radionuclide scanning, 137

Rales, 276

Ramipril (Altace)
 for chronic heart failure, 163*t*
 for myocardial infarction, 141

Ranitidine (Zantac), 200

Rapid glucose testing, 324

Rapid sequence intubation (RSI)
 for spinal cord trauma, 343
 for traumatic brain injury, 336

Reabsorption, 13

Rectal bleeding, 262

Red blood cells

 oxygen-carrying capacity of, 191
 tonicity effect on, 7*f*

Reentry, 103-104

Referred pain, abdominal, 250-251

Refractory periods, 92

Rehabilitation, 343

Renal impairment, drug-induced, 39-40

Renin, 150
 release of, 171
 suppression of, 162

Renin-angiotensin-aldosterone system
 activation of, 150, 186
 heart failure and, 152
 mechanism of, 151
 overstimulation of in hypertension, 171

Reperfusion, myocardial, 138-139

Repolarization, 90
 impairment of, 131

Residual volume, 48

Respiratory distress, 287

Respiratory dynamics, 46

Respiratory syncytial virus
 in croup, 288
 in pneumonia, 272

Respiratory system
 airway zones of, 45-46
 filtration in, 45-46
 goal of, 45
 neurophysiology of, 49-50
 neuroregulatory mechanisms of, 50
 physiology of, 47-49

Respiratory zone, 46

Resuscitation. *See also* Fluid resuscitation
 colloids in, 18
 endpoints of in hypovolemic shock, 193
 fluids in, 19
 goals of in septic shock, 130

Reteplase, 140*t*

Retractions, 276

Rewarming techniques, 355-356

Rhabdomyolysis, 136
 with hypothermia, 354
 in status epilepticus, 321, 324

Right subscapular referred pain, 254*t*

Right ventricular failure, 149

Ringer's lactate solution, 14
 blood transfusion and, 18

composition of, 15*t*
for diabetic ketoacidosis and hyperosmolar
hyperglycemic syndrome, 224
for heat stroke, 366
for hypovolemic shock, 190
medications incompatible with, 14, 16*t*
for septic shock, 130, 215
tonicity of, 6*t*

Rocky Mountain spotted fever, 286

Rosvig's sign, 254*t*

S

Saccular aneurysms
rupture of, 318
in subarachnoid hemorrhage, 312

St. Louis encephalitis, 285-286

Saline solutions
0.9%, 14
for diabetic ketoacidosis and hyperosmolar
hyperglycemic syndrome, 224-225
for hypothermia, 355
for septic shock, 130, 215
tonicity of, 6*t*

Sarcoplasmic reticulum, 92

Seizures/seizure disorders. *See also* Status epilepticus
with acute ischemic stroke, 309
classification of, 322-323
generalized, 322*t*
partial (focal), 322*t*
physiologic effects of, 321
precipitants of, 319-320
status epilepticus with, 327

Semipermeable membrane, 4
osmosis across, 5*f*

Sepsis, 213
mediators in, 214
in septic shock, 205-206

Septic shock, 213-215
causes of, 213
clinical assessment of, 209-210
definition of, 205-206
etiology of, 207
management of, 210-211
mediators in, 208
pathogenesis of, 207-208
two-hit theory of, 208

Serotonin, 31

Serratia marcescens, 127

Serum markers, 136-137

Serum sickness, 198*t*

Shivering, 352

Shock
anaphylactic, 197-203
cardiogenic, 185*t*
clinical syndromes of, 185*t*
distributive, 185*t*
four stages of, 189*t*
hypovolemic, 185-196
neurogenic, 340
neurologic, 347
obstructive, 185*t*
septic, 205-215
with spinal cord trauma, 343

Shunting, 23

Sigmoidoscopy, 265

Sinoatrial (S-A) node action potentials, 90
altered automaticity on, 102*f*
in cardiac contractility, 94

Skin
autonomic nervous system of, 32*t*
infections of, 292-293

Smooth muscle relaxants, 65

Smooth muscles
muscarinic receptors in, 31
relaxation of, 52

Sodium
in cell membrane action potential, 90
in depolarization, 89

Sodium chloride solution, 15*t*

Sodium-potassium-ATPase pump, 7, 150
in depolarization, 89

Soft tissue
infections of, 292-293
necrotizing infections of, 293

Solubility, 3

Somatostatin, 265

Somogyi phenomenon, 228

Sotalol, 106*t*

Spinal arteries, 338-339

Spinal cord
anatomy of, 338-339
compression and contusion of, 339
cross section of, 339*f*
injuries to
clinical manifestations of, 340-342
epidemiology of, 338
management of, 342-343
pathogenesis of, 338-340
regeneration of, 343

trauma to
  immobilization for, 347
  treatment of, 347-348
Spinal cord syndromes, 341
  anterior, 342
  central, 342
Spinal immobilization, 342-343, 347
Spinal shock, 340
Spirogram, 47
  with obstructive lung disease, 49*f*
Spironolactone (Aldactone), 162
Spleen
  rupture of, 253
  traumatic injury to, 259
SpO₂, 25*f*
Sputum culture, 275, 278
ST-segment
  depression of, 122
  elevation of, 122, 146
    in myocardial infarction, 132
    in pericarditis, 299
Standard Treatment with Alteplase to Reverse
  Stroke study, 310-311, 312*t*
Staphylococcus
  in acute infective endocarditis, 291
  in adrenal insufficiency, 236
  aureus
    in epiglottitis, 287
    in septic shock, 127
Starling curve
  agents causing shift in, 168
  for heart failure, 159
Starling's forces, 154*f*
Starling's law of the capillary, 12-13, 16, 18, 49,
  153, 167
Status epilepticus, 327-328
  clinical manifestations of, 322-323
  definition of, 319, 323
  management of, 323-325, 328
  nonconvulsive, 323
  pathogenesis of, 319-321
  physiologic effects of, 321
  precipitants of, 319-320
  reasons for early aggressive treatment of, 327
  rule of thirds of, 319
Steroids
  for Addison's disease, 237*t*
  for anaphylactic shock, 200
  for asthma, 64, 68
  for chronic obstructive pulmonary disease, 74
  pharmacology of, 53-54

for spinal cord trauma, 343
  withdrawal of in adrenal insufficiency, 236
Streptococcus
  in chronic bronchitis, 73
  in epiglottitis, 287
  group B, in pneumonia, 273*t*
  in necrotizing skin and soft tissue infections, 293
  pneumoniae
    in adrenal insufficiency, 236
    in meningitis, 283-284
    in pneumonia, 272
  in septic shock, 127
  in toxic shock syndrome, 293-294
Streptokinase
  clinical trials for, 142*t*
  for myocardial infarction, 140*t*
Stridor, 287
Stroke. *See also* Cerebral infarction, acute;
  Subarachnoid hemorrhage
  acute ischemic
    clinical manifestations of, 306-309
    diagnosis and management of, 309-312
    pathogenesis of, 303-306
  causes of, 317
  characteristics of, 303
  with chronic or poorly controlled hypertension, 178*t*
  embolic, 303
  hemorrhagic, 303, 306
  National Institutes of Health scale of, 309
  pathophysiology of, 303
  prehospital scales of, 306-308
  risk factors for, 316
  thrombotic, 303
Stroke volume, 93
  in cardiac output, 99
Subarachnoid hemorrhage, 312, 317-318
  clinical manifestations of, 313
  definitive diagnosis and management of, 313
  pathogenesis of, 312
  sentinel headache with, 313, 317
Subdural hematoma, 335, 346
Substance P, 152
Succinylcholine, 363*t*
Superantigen infection, 294
Supraglottitis, 287
Supraventricular pathway, 101
Supraventricular tachycardia, 104, 110
Surface M proteins, 293
Surfactant, 48-49
  lack of, 57

Surgery, 185

Sweat
absence of, 366
in thermoregulation, 361-362

Sympathetic nervous system
in cardiac contractility, 94-95
hyperactivity of, 170
overstimulation of, 131

Sympathetic neurons, 29
organization of, 30*f*

Sympathetic response, 98

Synapses, 29-30
neurotransmitters at, 31

Synaptic transmission, 31, 33*f*

Systemic inflammatory response syndrome
(SIRS), 205-206
criteria for, 206*t*
diagnosis of, 214
events in, 213
in hypovolemic shock, 187
infection and sepsis relationship to, 206*f*
mediators in, 214
in septic shock, 128

Systolic failure, 152-153

Systolic pressure, 92

T

T_3, 234
conversion of T_4 to, 239

T_4, 234, 239

T cells
in asthma, 62
cytokine release by, 199

T wave, 92
inversion of, 122

Tachycardia
in anaphylactic reaction, 199
persistent, 99
supraventricular, 104, 110
ventricular, 102, 104, 111, 159

Tachydysrhythmia, narrow-complex, 104

Tachypnea, 276

"Talk and die" presentation, 335

Temperature, measurement of, 364

Terbutaline (Brethine, Bricanyl, Brethaire)
for asthma, 64
for chronic obstructive pulmonary disease, 73-74
mechanism of action of, 70
pharmacology of, 51-52

Testicular torsion, 256*t*

Theophylline
for asthma, 65
for chronic obstructive pulmonary disease, 74
pharmacology of, 52

Thermoregulation
impaired, 351
normal, 352

Thiamine, 309

Thiazide diuretics, 161, 163*t*

Thienopyridine derivatives, 140*t*

Thiopental, 313

Third heart sound, 157-158

Third space, 11

Third-spacing, 12
pathology in, 13

Thoracolumbar division, 29

Thorax, pain of, 252

Thrombin inhibitors, 124

Thromboembolism, pulmonary, 79-83

Thrombolysis
for acute ischemic stroke, 310-311, 312*t*
for pulmonary embolism, 83, 85

Thrombolytics
in acute ischemic stroke, 310
aspirin with, 310
for cerebral infarction, 305
for ischemic penumbra, 316
mechanisms of action of, 139*f*
for myocardial infarction, 138, 140*t*
safe use of, 317

Thrombosis
in atrial fibrillation, 316
deep vein, 79, 252
in plaque formation, 114
with plaque rupture, 121*f*

Thromboxane, 188

Thrombus
in myocardial infarction, 129
pulmonary, 79-83

Thyroglobulin, 234

Thyroid emergencies, 233-245

Thyroid function tests, 238

Thyroid gland, physiology of, 234

Thyroid hormone, 234
for adrenal insufficiency, 243
homeostasis of, 234*f*
for myxedema coma, 240

reducing circulating levels of, 239

Thyroid stimulating hormone (TSH), 234

Thyroid storm, 237, 244
clinical diagnosis and management of, 238-239
definitive care for, 239
parameters of, 241t
pathogenesis of, 237-238

Thyrotoxic crisis, 237

Thyrotoxicosis, 237
parameters of, 241t

Thyrotropin releasing hormone (TRH), 234

TIA. *See* Transient ischemic attack

Tick-borne ricketsial infection, 286

Ticlopidine, 140t

Tidal volume, 48

Tirobifan, 140t

Tissue growth factors, 114

Tissue plasminogen activator (t-PA)
for acute ischemic stroke, 310-311, 312t
clinical trials for, 142t
for myocardial infarction, 140t
recombinant (rt-PA), 310-311

TNK-TPA, 140t

Tobacco smoking
in chronic obstructive pulmonary disease, 71
in myocardial infarction, 130

Tonic-clonic seizures, 323

Tonicity, 6
effect of on red blood cells, 7f

Torsades de pointes, 104, 111

Torsemide (Demadex)
for acute pulmonary edema, 160t
for chronic heart failure, 163t

Total body water, 11
replacement of for diabetic ketoacidosis and
hyperosmolar hyperglycemic syndrome, 224-225

Total lung capacity, 48

Toxic shock syndromes, 283
clinical manifestations of, 294
definitions of, 293
diagnosis and treatment of, 294
pathogenesis of, 294
streptococcal, 293-294

Trachea, 45

Tracheal intubation, 25, 28

Tracheostomy, 288

Transesophageal echocardiography, 292

Transient ischemic attack, 309

Transmural infarct, 131

Transmural infarcts, 129

Transplantation, spinal cord, 343

Transtentorial herniation, 345

Trauma
host response to, 131
in hypovolemic shock, 185
multi-system, 196
neurological, 329-348
in septic shock, 127
in subarachnoid hemorrhage, 312

Trendelenburg positioning, 192-193

Triacyglycerol, breakdown of, 221

Triamcinolone acetonide (Azmacort), 54

Tricyclic antidepressants, 364t

Trietz, ligament of, 261f

Triggered activation, 104, 111

Triglycerides, 171-172

Troponins, 136-137

Tumor necrosis factor, 128

Tumors
in status epilepticus, 320
in subarachnoid hemorrhage, 312

U

Ulcerative colitis, 263

Ulcers, gastrointestinal, 262, 267

Upper airway infections, 287-289

Urinary stone disease, 256t

V

Valsalva's maneuver, 166
in heart failure, 158

Vascular disorders, 252

Vascular malformations, 312

Vasoactive medications, 354-355

Vasoconstriction
in coronary artery disease, 115
with plaque rupture, 121f
sympathetic hyperactivity and, 170

Vasoconstrictors, 130

Vasodilators, 162-163

Vasogenic edema, 333

Vasopressin, 152

Vena cava filters, 83

Venous system, lower extremity, 80f

Venovenous rewarming, 355

Ventilation
PO$_2$ and, 51f
regulation of, 49-50

Ventilation, infusion, and pump regimen, 190

Ventilation-perfusion inequality, 27
in hypoxia, 23

Ventilation-perfusion mismatch
in asthma, 63
with lung occlusion, 80-81
in pneumonia, 274, 277
in pulmonary embolism, 82

Ventilator-associated pneumonia, 272

Ventilatory rate, regulation of, 50

Ventricular fibrillation, 352-353, 358-359

Ventricular hypertrophy
ECG patterns of, 133
in heart failure, 159

Ventricular muscle cell action potentials, 91f

Ventricular-paced rhythm, 135t

Ventricular pathway, 101

Ventricular tachycardia, 102
in heart failure, 159
polymorphic, 104, 111
reentry in, 104

Verapamil
contraindication to, 111
for dysrhythmia, 107
mechanisms of action of, 106t

Vertebrae, 338

Vertebral arteries, 339

Viral pneumonia, 272-273

Virchow's triad, 79

Visceral pain, 258
abdominal, 250

Viscus perforation, 255t

Vital capacity, 48, 56
in emphysema, 73

Vital sign abnormalities, 275

Volatile anesthetics, 363t

Volume expansion, 130, 215

Volume replacement, 366

W

Warfarin (Coumadin)
for acute ischemic stroke, 311
contraindications to, 162
drug binding of, 39
for pulmonary embolism, 82-83

Water
in cellular diffusion, 4
osmosis of, 5
as percentage of total body weight, 11
tonicity in movement of, 6

Waterhouse-Friderichsen syndrome, 236

Wernicke-Korsakoff syndrome, 309

Wheezing
in anaphylactic reaction, 199
in asthma, 62
heterophonous, 276
homophonous, 276

Whipple's triad, 226

Wigger's diagram, 95

Wolff-Parkinson-White syndrome, 103-104
treatment of, 107, 108, 111

X

Xanthines, methylated
for asthma, 65
for chronic obstructive pulmonary disease, 74
pharmacology of, 52

Xanthochromia, 313

Z

Zafirlukast (Accolate), 54
for asthma, 65
mechanism of action of, 70

Zileuton (Zyflo), 54
for asthma, 65

Printed in the USA
CPSIA information can be obtained
at www.ICGtesting.com
LVHW020558170924
791293LV00001B/27